Documents on Health and Social Services 1834 to the present day

Brian Watkin

Methuen & Co Ltd

First published 1975
by Methuen & Co Ltd
11 New Fetter Lane, London EC4P 4EE

© 1975 Brian Watkin

Printed in Great Britain by
Butler & Tanner Ltd Frome and London

ISBN hardbound 0 416 15170 1
ISBN paperback 0 416 18080 9

Documents on Health and Social Services

1834 to the present day

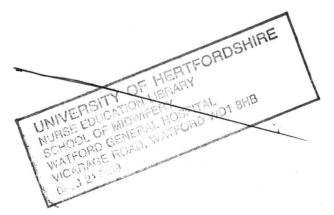

Contents

Preface

I hope this book will be useful to students of social administration, and to trainee and practising administrators in the health and social services. Many of the documents I have cited are now difficult to get hold of outside the major centres, but in any case the task of locating and reading through some eighty reports and Acts of Parliament would be a formidable one.

It would have been nice to have produced a book which included a detailed introduction to and representative extracts from every significant report or Act on health and welfare subjects in the last 140 years, but it quickly became apparent that this was not possible. Such a book would have been too bulky and too expensive to be useful to any but the most earnest of students. I have therefore had to be highly selective and I have at times been arbitrary in my selection.

The idea for this book came from J. Stuart Maclure's *Educational Documents: England and Wales 1816 to the present day*, but I have not followed the pattern he set at all closely. It seemed to me that my field demanded a rather different treatment. Hence this book is divided into Parts, with a brief introduction to each which attempts to do no more than pick out some of the issues and points for discussion which are raised by the material which follows. Within each part, a separate section is devoted to each document. Each section opens with such details as the title and date of publication, and where applicable, the membership and terms of reference of the working party or committee, followed by an often brief essay setting the document in its context and tracing some of the consequences that flowed from its publication or enactment. In many, but not all, cases this essay is followed by extracts from the document itself which for one reason or another I feel to be of particular interest, and which give the flavour of the original in the way which a mere summary cannot do. Some reports are more quotable than others, so the length of the extracts does not always reflect the importance of the documents.

A degree of prejudice and bias will colour any commentator's choice of material, and this is true both of my selection of documents and what I have said about them. To understand the present I believe we need to know something of the Victorian Poor Law and of the sanitary revolution that took place in Victorian times, but the majority of the documents I have cited were published during the last fifty years. My particular interest in the health service, and in the professions working in the health and social services, will be obvious.

One of the problems of the health and social services is the extreme touchiness of many of the groups who work in them where their professional status is concerned. However, one cannot please everyone all the time and the pharmacists will probably not be pleased that they are included in a part bearing the title 'The Paramedical Professions'. It was not practicable to give them a part to themselves and so this was the best I could do.

Similarly I must apologize to those hospital administrators who may be offended by it for the use in certain sections of the terms 'lay administration' and 'lay administrator'. 'Lay' is not a good term to describe a task that no 'layman'—in the strict sense of one without special training or experience—could do at all satisfactorily, but on the other hand it has as a term the overriding advantage, as I see it, that it will be universally understood.

Another apology is perhaps due for the retention of the typographic conventions derived from the various documents which are, in part, reproduced here. I have never been able to understand why so many government publications, even in modern times, give capital initials to almost every second word, but I could not justify making any changes in the passages that are reproduced. I have, however, tried to give the reader's eye a rest in the passages for which I am responsible.

As far as the lists of members of working parties and committees are concerned, I have not always adhered to the style of the original. I have dropped such titles as 'Mr' and 'Esq' that add no useful information, and I have dropped 'Dr' where it is rendered unnecessary by the qualifications appearing after a person's name. I have retained 'Miss' and 'Mrs' where I have known the marital status of lady members.

I have printed eponymous titles where these are generally used, but not otherwise. I have never, for example, heard the Majority Report of the Royal Commission on the Poor Laws and Relief of Distress referred to as the Hamilton Report. Generally I have confined myself to England and Wales, but the Farquharson-Lang Report from Scotland is included because it was subsequently in large measure 'adopted' by the English Ministry of Health, who commended certain of its recommendations to English hospital authorities in a circular.

I hope that some of those who use this book will be stimulated (perhaps particularly by reading the extracts I have reproduced from the documents themselves) to go back to the originals. For any student, these documents contain a wealth of factual information and statistics, sometimes tucked away in appendices, as well as detailed discussion of issues and ideas. They are often well written and readable, which is not what most people expect when they open a blue book.

My last words must be words of thanks to those who have helped me. But for Annette Watkin's sticky fingers this book would never have been completed, for the extracts from the documents themselves had to be carefully pasted up and she has done most of this for me. But beyond that I owe her much for her constant encouragement and the occasional stern reminder, when I felt like doing something else, that I had a book to complete.

I am grateful to the editor of the *Lancet* for his kind permission to reproduce extracts from the Report of the Lancet Commission on Nursing, and to the Secretary of the British Medical Association for allowing me to use extracts from *A General Medical Service for the Nation*. Extracts from Crown copyright documents are reproduced by permission of the Controller, HM Stationery Office.

1 The New Poor Law

Introduction

Edwin Chadwick described the Poor Law Amendment Act of 1834 as 'the first great piece of legislation based upon scientific or economical principles'. It is possible to quarrel with that statement on a number of grounds, but there is no doubt that the Victorian Poor Law must have a fascination for anyone interested in the translation of abstract principles into legislative action. It was far more than a measure to set up certain administrative arrangements that seemed right in their day, but which might well be discarded when circumstances changed. To an unusual degree it embodied a coherent set of beliefs about the nature of society and the nature of man, about the mainsprings of human behaviour and about how human beings may be controlled and influenced. It was thus possible, seventy years later, to refer to 'the principles of 1834' and to refer to them as having a continued relevance. The 'principles of 1834' were of course spelt out in the Report of the Royal Commission on the Administration and Practical Operation of the Poor Laws and when another Royal Commission was set up in the early years of the twentieth century it was with the hope, on the part of the Poor Law administrators, that the commissioners would echo the sentiments of their predecessors.

Most of our existing arrangements in the field of health and welfare have their roots either in the Victorian Poor Law, or in reaction against it. The voluntary hospitals represent a separate tradition going back to the eighteenth century, but the Poor Law infirmaries provided services for those in whom the voluntary hospitals, by and large, were not interested—the chronic sick, the aged and infirm, the incurable. Edwardian social legislation was largely an attempt to save the deserving poor from needing to turn to the Poor Law, while public assistance, national assistance and supplementary benefit in turn took the place of poor relief for those who in spite of all other provisions lacked the ability to command the necessities of life. It would seem that, whatever we choose to call it, the Poor Law, like the poor, will always be with us.

The two great Poor Law reports are well worth reading. Both contain memorable passages and the prose of the earlier report is a real pleasure to read. But they should be read with an open mind, and a consciousness that the thinking of yesterday is not to be despised because we have formed a different view of the matter. In some instances we may yet find there is more wisdom buried in these reports than their authors have ever been given credit for. Perhaps a case in point is the passage from the 1909 report which I quote on page 20. Only relatively recently have we realized that the demand for health care is potentially infinite, and it may be that the majority commissioners in 1909 had a more sophisticated view of what is involved than Beveridge's rather naive belief that spending on health care was a form of investment which would be realized in greater productive efficiency.

1.1 Report of the Royal Commission on the Administration and Practical Operation of the Poor Laws

Published: 1834

Members: *C. J. Blomfield, Bishop of London; J. B. Sumner, Bishop of Chester; W. Sturges Bourne; Nassau W. Senior; Henry Bishop; Henry Gawler; W. Coulson; James Traill; Edwin Chadwick*

Terms of Reference (1832): *To make a diligent and full inquiry into the practical operation of the Laws for the Relief of the Poor in England and Wales, and into the manner in which those laws are administered, and to report ... whether any and what alterations, amendments, or improvements may be beneficially made in the said laws, or in the manner of administering them, and how the same may best be carried into effect.*

The Royal Commission on the Poor Laws, 1832-4, was an early example of the use of a Royal Commission to sift opinion and evidence and to prepare the way for legislation; and it was so successful, at least in the eyes of contemporaries, that the setting up of a Royal Commission became in Victorian times a customary way of dealing with contentious issues and both sounding and moulding opinion. The Royal Commission, as distinct from the Parliamentary Commission, had the advantage that members could include experts and others who did not happen to be members of Parliament, and in the 1832-4 Commission this category included, for example, the economist Nassau Senior and (co-opted at a late stage) the lawyer disciple of Jeremy Bentham, Edwin Chadwick.

The Poor Laws which the Royal Commission was set up to examine had been inherited by nineteenth-century England, with its much increased population and its burgeoning industrial towns in the north and midlands, from the age of Elizabeth. The operation of the Elizabethan Poor Laws had been modified in the Napoleonic Wars and after by what became known as the Speenhamland system of allowances, paid from the

rates, to supplement wages on a scale which varied with the price of
bread and the size of the labourer's family. The Speenhamland system—
named after the place of its inauguration by the Berkshire magistrates in
1795—proved expensive in its direct effect on the rates, and disastrous
in its effect on those it was intended to help. Farmers had little incentive
to pay a living wage when wages would in any case be made up to subsistence level by the rates, and labourers sometimes found themselves
better off if they relied on the parish in which they were born, and on
which they had a legal claim, than if they travelled further afield in search
of work. By the 1830's the ratepayers were alarmed and the rural poor
were discontented with a system of relief which in spite of its expense
failed to meet the problem of rural poverty.

In 1776, before the long war, the poor rates had amounted to £1
million; in 1802 to £4,250,000; but by 1832, despite several post-war
years of falling prices, the cost was £7 million. In 1830 there were hang-
ings and transportations after the labourers of southern England marked
their protests against the system with rick-burning, riots and the breaking of machines.

The remedies suggested for these social and economic ills by the
Royal Commission had a logical coherence that gave them immediate
appeal. The fact that they were based on inadequate analysis did not
immediately appear, although it was not many years before it became
evident to the discerning that remedies devised with an eye mainly to
the agricultural counties of southern England could not be successfully
applied in the industrial north.

The report recommended that new legislation and a new pattern of
administration should be based on the principles of 'less eligibility' and
the 'workhouse test'. 'Less eligibility' meant that incentives for able-
bodied men to rely on the parish for support should be removed by ensuring that the lot of the pauper in receipt of relief from public funds
would always be 'less eligible'—less favourable—than that of the least
well-off labourer in independent employment. The 'workhouse test'
derived from the recommended abolition of 'out-relief'—assistance,
whether financial or in kind, given to men and women who continued to
live in their own homes. It was argued that if the principle of the administration of poor relief was to confine assistance to those who were truly
destitute and had no other means of support open to them, then this
purpose would be served by offering to all who applied for help the opportunity to enter the workhouse where, according to the principle of less
eligibility, the regime and diet would be more spartan than would be
experienced by any but the utterly destitute outside.

Such arguments were clearly directed at the able-bodied poor, but it
was recognized that some of those who applied for relief were sick, or
aged and infirm, and that if parents were admitted to the workhouse then

children would have to be provided for too. The Royal Commission condemned the old type of mixed workhouse in which the able-bodied and the infirm, the young and old, were all accommodated together, and recommended instead that parishes should combine into 'unions', large enough to make it feasible to provide separate workhouses for the able-bodied and the infirm, and to accommodate separately men, women and children. There was a mixture of motives here. The separation of husbands and wives and their children was an aspect of the policy of deterrence designed to ensure that the prospect of entering the workhouse was not unduly attractive. The separation of the able-bodied and the infirm was intended both to make it possible to impose on the able-bodied a regime of salutary harshness, and to provide a more appropriate and humane regime for the elderly and the sick. Some at least of the subsequent criticisms of the Victorian workhouse regime would have been avoided or softened if this policy of classification had been fully implemented. As it was, the old and—in contemporary terms—deserving often had to suffer the rigours of a regime designed to daunt the young and shiftless.

The administrative recommendations of the report were designed to achieve the implementation of a national policy while at the same time avoiding the creation of a centralized bureaucracy. The solution of making the poor a national charge was rejected as likely to lead to lax administration at local level and further increases in cost. The relief of the poor would continue to be charged to the rates and administered by locally elected guardians, assisted by paid full-time officials. But the guardians and their officials would be watched over by a central Poor Law Commission, with power to make regulations, and would be visited and their workhouses inspected by assistant commissioners. The guardians' discretion was to be strictly limited in the belief that if it were not, then either direct intimidation or a preference for being popular in their own districts would make them unsuitably generous with the ratepayers' money.

The report dealt in advance with many of the criticisms likely to be advanced against the policies suggested. The abolition of out-relief would not lead to the flooding of the workhouses, or to great expense in the building of new workhouses, because the number of applicants for relief would fall dramatically once the workhouse test was applied. Statistics and experiences from parishes where relief had been stringently administered were quoted in support of this view. Undue hardship might be caused to deserving individuals from time to time, but this was a price that had to be paid for the sake of benefit to the many, and the report waxed earnest on the danger of legislating for extreme cases.

Some nineteen pages of the report were devoted to review of the bastardy laws and to pointing out the injustices and abuses which arose from the eighteenth-century statutes. A single woman who found herself pregnant could charge any man she chose with being the father and he might be hard put to clear himself of the charge and avoid being forced to reimburse the parish for the cost of maintaining the child. The Royal Commission recommended that all laws purporting to punish the putative father of children born out of wedlock should be repealed. It was argued that if it was clear that an illegitimate child would be a burden on its mother, or on her parents, and not a possible means of blackmailing a man into marrying her, then illegitimacy would become 'as rare as it is among those classes in this country who are above parish relief, or as it is among all classes in Ireland'.

The final paragraph of the report declared that its recommendations were intended to have a negative rather than a positive effect, 'rather to remove the debasing influences to which a large portion of the Labouring Population is now subject, than to afford new means of prosperity and virtue'. But it was at the same time hoped that the removal of these 'debasing influences' would allow the education of the working classes to be improved and would allow them to profit more freely from education based on moral and religious principles, the promotion of which was seen as 'the most important duty of the Legislature'.

Report of the Royal Commission on the Poor Laws, 1834

DEFECTS OF THE EXISTING SYSTEM

It appears to the pauper that the Government has undertaken to repeal, in his favour, the ordinary laws of nature; to enact that the children shall not suffer for the misconduct of their parents—the wife for that of the husband, or the husband for that of the wife: that no one shall lose the means of comfortable subsistence, whatever be his indolence, prodigality, or vice: in short, that the penalty which, after all, must be paid by some one for idleness and improvidence, is to fall, not on the guilty person or on his family, but on the proprietors of the lands and houses encumbered by his settlement. Can we wonder if the uneducated are seduced into approving a system which aims its allurements at all the weakest parts of our nature—which offers marriage to the young, security to the anxious, ease to the lazy, and impunity to the profligate?

p. 34

What motive has the man who is to receive 10s. every Saturday, not because 10s. is the value of his week's labour, but because his family consists of five persons, who knows that his income will be increased by nothing but by an increase of his family, and diminished by nothing but by a diminution of his family, that it has no reference to his skill, his honesty, or his diligence—what motive has he to acquire or to preserve any of these merits? Unhappily, the evidence shows, not only that these virtues are rapidly wearing out, but that their place is assumed by the opposite vices; and that the very labourers among whom the farmer has to live, on whose merits as workmen, and on whose affection as friends, he ought to depend, are becoming not merely idle and ignorant and dishonest, but positively hostile; not merely unfit for his service and indifferent to his welfare, but actually desirous to injure him.

p. 39

But though the injustice perpetrated on the man who struggles, as far as he can struggle, against the oppression of the system, who refuses, as far as he can refuse, to be its accomplice, is at first sight the most revolting, the severest sufferers are those that have become callous to their own degradation, who value parish support as their privilege, and demand it as their right, and complain only that it is limited in amount, or that some sort of labour or confinement is exacted in return. No man's principles can be corrupted without injury to society in general; but the person most injured is the person whose principles have been corrupted. The constant war which the pauper has to wage with all who employ or pay him, is destructive to his honesty and his temper; as his subsistence does not depend on his exertions, he loses all that sweetens labour, its association with reward, and gets through his work, such as it is, with the reluctance of a slave. His pay, earned by importunity or fraud, or even violence, is not husbanded with the carefulness which would be given to the results of industry, but wasted in the intemperance to which his ample leisure invites him. The ground on which relief is ordered to the idle and dissolute is, that the wife and family must not suffer for the vices of the head of the family; but as that relief is almost always given into the hands of the vicious husband or parent, this excuse is obviously absurd. It appears from the evidence that the great supporters of the beer-shops are the paupers. 'Wherever,' says Mr. Lawrence, of Henfield, 'the labourers are unemployed, the beer-shops of the parish are frequented by them.' And it is a striking fact, that in Cholesbury, where, out of 139 individuals, only 35 persons, of all ages, including the clergyman and his family, are supported by their own exertions, there are two public-houses. . . .

p. 49

LESS ELIGIBILITY

From the evidence collected under this Commission, we are induced to believe that a compulsory provision for the relief of the indigent can be generally administered on a sound and well-defined principle; and that under the operation of this principle, the assurance that no one need perish from want may be rendered more complete than at present, and the mendicant and vagrant repressed by disarming them of their weapon—the plea of impending starvation.

It may be assumed, that in the administration of relief, the public is warranted in imposing such conditions on the individual relief, as are conducive to the benefit either of the individual himself or of the country at large, at whose expense he is to be relieved.

The first and most essential of all conditions, a principle which we find universally admitted, even by those whose practice is at variance with it, is, that his situation on the whole shall not be made really or apparently so eligible as the situation of the independent labourer of the lowest class. Throughout the evidence it is shown, that in proportion as the condition of any pauper class is elevated above the condition of independent labourers, the condition of the independent class is depressed; their industry is impaired, their employment becomes unsteady, and its remuneration in wages is diminished. Such persons, therefore, are under the strongest inducements to quit the less eligible class of labourers and enter the more eligible class of paupers. The converse is the effect when the pauper class is placed in its proper position, below the condition of the independent labourer. Every penny bestowed, that tends to render the condition of the pauper more eligible than that of the independent labourer, is a bounty on indolence and vice. We have found, that as the poor's-rates are at present administered, they operate as bounties of this description, to the amount of several millions annually.

The standard, therefore, to which reference must be made in fixing the condition of those who are to be maintained by the public, is the condition of those who are maintained by their own exertions. But the evidence shows how loosely and imperfectly the situation of the independent labourer has been inquired into, and how little is really known of it by those who award or distribute relief. It shows also that so little has their situation been made a standard for the supply of commodities, that the diet of the workhouse almost always exceeds that of the cottage, and the diet of the gaol is generally more profuse than even that of the workhouse. It shows also, that this standard has been so little referred to in the exaction of labour, that commonly the work required from the pauper is inferior to that performed by the labourers and servants of those who have prescribed it: So much and so generally inferior as to create a prevalent notion among the agricultural paupers that they have a right to be exempted from the amount of work which is performed and indeed sought for by the independent labourer.

We can state, as the result of the extensive inquiries made under this Commission into the circumstances of the labouring classes, that the agricultural labourers when in employment, in common with the other classes of labourer throughout the country, have greatly advanced in condition; that their wages will not produce to them more of the necessaries and comforts of life than at any former period. These results appear to be confirmed by the evidence collected by the Committees of the House of Commons appointed to inquire into the condition of the agricultural and manufacturing classes, and also by that collected by the Factory Commissioners. No body of men save money whilst they are in want of what they deem absolute necessaries. No common man will put by a shilling whilst he is in need of a loaf, or will save whilst he has a pressing want unsatisfied. The circumstance of there being nearly fourteen millions in the savings banks, and the fact that, according to the last returns, upwards of 29,000 of the depositors were agricultural labourers, who, there is reason to believe, are usually the heads of families, and also the fact of the reduction of the general average of mortality, justify the conclusion, that a condition worse than that of the independent agricultural labourer, may nevertheless be a condition above that in which the great body of English labourers have lived in times that have always been considered prosperous. Even if the condition of the independent labourer were to remain as it now is, and the pauper were to be reduced avowedly below that condition, he might still be adequately supplied with the necessaries of life.

But it will be seen that the process of dispauperizing the able-bodied is in its ultimate effects a process which elevates the condition of the great mass of society.

In all the instances which we have met with, where parishes have been dis-pauperized, the effect appears to have been produced by the practical application of the principle which we have set forth as the main principle of a good Poor-Law administration, namely, the restoration of the pauper to a position below that of the independent labourer.

pp. 127–8

THE WORKHOUSE TEST

We therefore submit, as the general principle of legislation on this subject, in the present condition of the country:—

That those modes of administering relief which have been tried wholly or partially, and have produced beneficial effects in some districts, be introduced, with modifica-tions according to local circumstances, and carried into complete execution in all.

The chief specific measures which we recommend for effecting these purposes, are—

FIRST, THAT EXCEPT AS TO MEDICAL ATTENDANCE, AND SUBJECT TO THE EXCEPTION RESPECTING APPRENTICESHIP HEREIN AFTER STATED, ALL RELIEF WHATEVER TO ABLE-BODIED PERSONS OR TO THEIR FAMILIES, OTHERWISE THAN IN WELL-REGULATED WORKHOUSES (*i.e.*, PLACES WHERE THEY MAY BE SET TO WORK ACCORDING TO THE SPIRIT AND INTEN-TION OF THE 43d OF ELIZABETH) SHALL BE DECLARED UNLAWFUL, AND SHALL CEASE, IN MANNER AND AT PERIODS HEREAFTER SPECIFIED; AND THAT ALL RELIEF AFFORDED IN RESPECT OF CHILDREN UNDER THE AGE OF 16, SHALL BE CONSIDERED AS AFFORDED TO THEIR PARENTS.

It is true, that nothing is necessary to arrest the progress of pauperism, except that all who receive relief from the parish should work for the parish exclusively, as hard and for less wages than independent labourers work for individual em-ployers, and we believe that in most districts useful work, which will not inter-fere with the ordinary demand for labour, may be obtained in greater quantity than is usually conceived. Cases, however, will occur where such work cannot be obtained in sufficient quantity to meet an immediate demand; and when ob-tained, the labour, by negligence, connivance, or otherwise, may be made merely formal, and thus the provisions of the legislature may be evaded more easily than in a workhouse. A well-regulated workhouse meets all cases, and appears to be the only means by which the intention of the statute of Elizabeth, that all the able-bodied shall be set to work, can be carried into execution. . . .

And although we admit that able-bodied persons in the receipt of out-door allowances and partial relief, may be, and in some cases are, placed in a con-dition less eligible than that of the independent labourer of the lowest class; yet to persons so situated, relief in a well-regulated workhouse would not be a hardship: and even if it be, in some rare cases, a hardship, it appears from the evidence that it is a hardship to which the good of society requires the applicant to submit. The express or implied ground of his application is, that he is in danger of perishing from want. Requesting to be rescued from that danger out of the property of others, he must accept assistance on the terms, whatever they may be, which the common welfare requires. The bane of all pauper legislation has been the legislating for extreme cases. Every exception, every violation of the general rule to meet a real case of unusual hardship, lets in a whole class of fraudulent cases, by which that rule must in time be destroyed. Where cases of real hardship occur, the remedy must be applied by individual charity, a virtue for which no system of compulsory relief can be or ought to be a substitute.

pp. 146–7

1. The offer of relief on the principle suggested by us would be a self-acting test of the claim of the applicant.

It is shown throughout the evidence, that it is demoralizing and ruinous to offer to the able-bodied of the best characters more than a simple subsistence. The person of bad character, if he be allowed anything, could not be allowed less. By the means which we propose, the line between those who do, and those who do not, need relief is drawn, and drawn perfectly. If the claimant does not comply with the terms on which relief is given to the destitute, he gets nothing; and if he does comply, the compliance proves the truth of the claim—namely, his, destitution. If, then, regulations were established and enforced with the degree of strictness that has been attained in the dispauperized parishes, the workhouse doors might be thrown open to all who would enter them, and con-form to the regulations. Not only would no agency for contending against fraudulent rapacity and perjury, no stages of appeals, (vexatious to the appellants and painful to the magistrates,) be requisite to keep the able-bodied from the parish; but the intentions of the statute of Elizabeth, in setting the idle to work, might be accomplished, and vagrants and mendicants actually forced on the parish; that is, forced into a condition of salutary restriction and labour. It would be found that they might be supported much cheaper under proper regu-lations, than when living at large by mendicity or depredation.

p. 148

In the absence of fixed rules and tests that can be depended upon, the officers in large towns have often no alternative between indiscriminately granting or indiscriminately refusing relief. The means of distinguishing the really destitute from the crowd of indolent imposters being practically wanting, they are driven to admit or reject the able-bodied in classes. Now, however true it may be that the real proportion of cases which are found to have the semblance of being well founded may not exceed three or four per cent. of the whole amount of claims, yet since each individual thus rejected may possibly be one of that apparently deserving minority, such a rejection, accompanied by such a possibility, is at variance with the popular sentiment; and it is found that the great body of the distributors of relief do prefer, and may be expected to continue to prefer, the admission of any number of undeserving claims, to encountering a remote chance of the rejection of what may be considered a deserving case.

On the other hand, the belief which prevails that under the existing system some claims to relief *are* absolutely rejected, operates extensively and mis-chievously. It appears that this belief, which alone renders plausible the plea of every mendicant (that he applied for parochial relief, and was refused), is the chief cause of the prevalence of mendicity and vagrancy, notwithstanding the existence of a system of compulsory relief; a system which, if well administered, must immediately reduce and enable a police ultimately to extirpate all mendicity. If merit is to be the condition on which relief is to be given; if such a duty as that of rejecting the claims of the undeserving is to be performed, we see no possibility of finding an adequate number of officers whose character and decisions would obtain sufficient popular confidence to remove the impression of the possible rejection of some deserving cases; we believe, indeed, that a closer investigation of the claims of the able-bodied paupers, and a more extensive rejection of the claims of the undeserving, would, for a considerable time, be accompanied by an increase of the popular opinion to which we have alluded, and consequently by an increase of the disposition to give to mendicants.

We see no remedy against this, in common with other existing evils, except the general application of the principle of relief which has been so extensively tried and found so efficient in the dispauperized parishes. When that principle has been introduced, the able-bodied claimant should be entitled to immediate relief on the terms prescribed, wherever he might happen to be; and should be received without objection or inquiry; the fact of his compliance with the prescribed discipline constituting his title to a sufficient, though simple diet. The question as to the locality or place of settlement, which should be charged with the expense of his maintenance, might be left for subsequent determination.

pp. 152–3

2. Little need be said on the next effect of the abolition of partial relief (even independently of workhouse regulations) in drawing a broad line of distinction between the paupers and the independent labourers. Experience has shown, that it will induce many of those whose wants arise from their idleness, to earn the means of subsistence; repress the fraudulent claims of those who have now adequate means of independent support, and obtain for others assistance from their friends, who are willing to see their relations pensioners, but would exert themselves to prevent their being inmates of a workhouse.

3. It will also remove much of the evil arising from the situation of the distributors of relief.

It has been shown that destitution, not merit, is the only safe ground of relief. In order to enable the distributors to ascertain the indigence of the applicant, it has been proposed to subdivide parishes, and appoint to the subdivisions officers who, it is supposed, might ascertain the circumstances of those under their care. But when instances are now of frequent occurrence where a pauper is found to have saved large sums of money, without the fact having been known or suspected by the members of the same family, living under the same roof, how should a neighbour, much less a parish officer, be expected to have a better knowledge of the real means of the individual? We are not aware that our communications display one instance of outdoor pauperism having been permanently repressed by the mere exercise of individual knowledge acting on a limited area. What our evidence does show is, that where the administration of relief is brought nearer to the door of the pauper, little advantage arises from increased knowledge on the part of the distributors, and great evil from their increased liability to every sort of pernicious influence. It brings tradesmen within the influence of their customers, small farmers within that of their relations and connexions, and not unfrequently of those who have been their fellow workmen, and exposes the wealthier classes to solicitations from their own dependants for extra allowances, which might be meritoriously and usefully given as private charity, but are abuses when forced from the public. Under such circumstances, to continue out-door relief is to continue a relief which will generally be given ignorantly or corruptly, frequently procured by fraud, and in a large and rapidly increasing proportion of cases extorted by intimidation—an intimidation which is not more powerful as a source of profusion than as an obstacle to improvement. We shall recur to this subject when we submit the grounds for withdrawing all local discretionary power, and appointing a new agency to superintend the administration of relief.

pp. 154-5

1.2 Poor Law Amendment Act, 1834

After publication of the Report of the Royal Commission on the Poor Laws, the Whig Government lost little time in preparing and introducing the Bill which in due course became the Poor Law Amendment Act, 1834. In drafting the Bill the Cabinet had the help of two of the leading members of the Royal Commission, the economist Nassau Senior, and William Sturges Bourne, who with some assistance from Edwin Chadwick ensured that the Bill which Ministers took to Parliament embodied the principles and the chief recommendations of the Royal Commission. Opposition in Parliament and the Press was focused on the proposal to establish a central board to administer the New Poor Law, seen to involve a shift in power from the localities to the centre, an un-English 'centralization'. But the only important concession wrested from the Government was the limitation of the life of the Poor Law Commission to five years in the first instance, and the Bill passed through both Houses with large majorities. For most of the property owners, whether Whig or Tory, the Government's promise that the measure would halt and indeed reverse the steady rise in the poor rates was sufficient argument.

So the Commission was set up. Chadwick did not get a seat on the Commission itself, as he had expected; without aristocratic connections he had to be content with being appointed secretary, but with a curious and secret undertaking, which was to lead to trouble later, that he was to be regarded not merely as secretary to the Commission in the ordinary sense, but as a fourth commissioner. Chadwick and the three commissioners soon found themselves at loggerheads not only because of clashes of personality and the ambiguities of the secretary's position, but also because the commissioners wished to compromise when the Act proved unpopular, while Chadwick believed firmly that outdoor relief must be abolished as quickly as possible, as soon in fact as the workhouses were built and the workhouse test could be imposed.

Implementation of the Act started in the agricultural areas of the south, but resistance was particularly strong in the north of England, in the industrial areas. This, however, was not merely because the principles on which the Act was based took no account of the poverty which followed when trade depressions threw thousands of men out of work in a way that was beyond their control. It was indeed an implicit assumption of the New Poor Law that most able-bodied men would, for most of the time, be able to find work that would keep body and soul together if they tried hard enough, and that they would try hard enough if the alternative were sufficiently unpleasant. These assumptions were obviously not valid at times of widespread industrial recession, and at these times one would expect the inappropriateness and injustice of the workhouse test to be pointed out with some vigour, but in fact many of the anti-Poor Law riots and agitations occurred at times of industrial prosperity, and the fact that they occurred more in the industrial areas and in London rather than in the agricultural counties must be put down largely to the fact that the working classes in the towns were better educated, more articulate, better led and more politically conscious. The agricultural labourer did not accept the New Poor Law with passive acquiescence because he recognized in it an appropriate solution to the problem of rural poverty, but because he had not been taught to protest.

In many areas working-class suspicion of the New Poor Law and its 'Bastilles' was abetted by local officials who saw their vested interests threatened, for the old system was often wasteful and corrupt; by guardians who feared that a new workhouse would lead to higher rates; by local pride and resistance to dictation from London; and by local tradesmen who knew that if outdoor relief was given it would be spent in their shops, but if the destitute were taken into the workhouse this trade would be lost. To overcome resistance, to supervise the operation of the new law, and to decide when conditions were ripe for the imposition of the workhouse test in a particular area, the Poor Law Commission relied on a mere twenty or so assistant commissioners (by the 1840s these were reduced to nine), who were briefed to use persuasion whenever possible and to take every opportunity to expound the advantages of the new system. It is a measure of their achievement that in spite of noisy defiance in such places as Huddersfield, Bolton, London and parts of Wales, throughout the length and breadth of the country unions were formed, workhouses were constructed and the law was administered in a way that was acceptable to the commissioners. Nearly everywhere the assistant commissioners had the co-operation of men of substantial property, and these men reaped their reward when Chadwick's prophecies were fulfilled and the poor rates fell from the annual average of £6·7 million which had prevailed before 1834 to an annual average of £4·5 million in the nine years after 1834. Much of this reduction was achieved not by strict operation of the workhouse test, for more than 80 per cent of paupers continued to receive outdoor relief, but simply by better and more economical administration.

The Poor Law Commission set the pattern of central control over local administration that was followed, with variations, by a number of other specialized agencies of government during the Victorian era.Common to all these agencies—operating in fields as diverse as education, health, factories, mines and railways—was the idea of an inspectorate, and the power of report. Florence Nightingale some years later pointed out that 'Reports are not self-executive', but the reports made by government inspectors in the 1830s and 1840s were missionary documents designed to make converts to the policies of the central authorities, and the efforts of the inspectors were attended with a great deal of success. From 1848 onwards the newly appointed medical officers of health adopted a technique which they inherited from the poor law assistant commissioners and the education and factory inspectors, and used their power of report to expose intolerable sanitary conditions.

The Poor Law Commission was, however, exceptionally powerful and hedged around with fewer constraints than most of the other agencies of central government at that time. It had the power to issue general regulations which had the force of law; although these had to be sanctioned by the Home Office and laid before Parliament this was a stipulation easily evaded. A 'general regulation' was defined as one which applied to more than one union at a time, so all the commissioners had to do was to issue a series of special orders, in identical terms, to each board of guardians separately. Special orders did not require the sanction of the Home Office nor did they have to be laid before Parliament. The Commission could order rates to be raised for the building of a workhouse—taxation without representation with a vengeance. It had the power to confirm the appointments of local officials. The link between the Commission and the Government was through the Home Secretary, but it was by no means clear whether the Home Secretary was actually answerable to Parliament for the deeds of the Poor Law Commission or not. It had been intended that the Commission's quasi-independent status should give it immunity from day-to-day political interference, but the administration of the New Poor Law was a political issue and Parliament insisted on having its say. Ultimately the Commission was reconstituted as a board with a president fully answerable to Parliament, but this was in 1847, after the Andover inquiry had brought into the open the internal disputes between the commissioners and the secretary.

As the Act limited the life of the Poor Law Commission to five years in the first instance, Parliament had to be asked to renew its powers at the end of that period. From 1839 to 1842 the Commission's powers were renewed annually, but in 1842 it was given a further five-year term. In 1847 the Commission was replaced by the Poor Law Board, which in turn administered the Poor Law until 1871, when it was absorbed into the newly created Local Government Board.

1.3 Reports of the Royal Commission on the Poor Laws and Relief of Distress

Published: 1909

Chairman: *Rt Hon. Lord George Hamilton GCSI*

Members: *The Most Rev. Denis Kelly DD; Rt Hon. Sir Henry Robinson KCB; Sir Samuel B. Provis KCB; Frank Holdsworth Bentham JP; A. H. Downes MD; Rev. Thory Gage Gardiner MA; George Lansbury; C. Stewart Loch BA, LLD, DCL; J. Patten MacDougale CB; T. Hancock Nunn; Rev. L. R. Phelps MA; William Smart MA, DPhil, LLD; Rev. Prebendary H. Russell Wakefield MA; Mrs Bosanquet; Mrs Sidney Webb; Miss Octavia Hill; Francis Chandler; R. G. Duff (secretary)*

Terms of Reference (1905): *To inquire (1) into the working of the laws relating to the relief of poor persons in the United Kingdom; (2) into the various means which have been adopted outside of the Poor Laws for meeting distress arising from want of employment, particularly during periods of severe industrial depression; and to consider and report whether any, and if so, what, modifications of the Poor Laws or changes in their administration or fresh legislation for dealing with distress are advisable.*

The Royal Commission of 1905–9 was the first major inquiry into the whole operation of the Poor Laws since the Act of 1834, and the Royal Commission came into being because the Poor Law officials at the Local Government Board felt that the principles of 1834 had been eroded and ought to be re-established. They convinced their president, Gerald Balfour, that an inquiry was called for, and he persuaded his brother, the Prime Minister, to appoint the Royal Commission as one of the last acts of the Conservative government that in 1905 made way for the reforming Liberal administrations of Campbell-Bannerman and Asquith. The extent to which the officials were steeped in the principles of 1834 was made clear in the evidence offered by J. S. Davy, permanent head of the Poor Law Division, to the Royal Commission. The poor must, he argued, be deterred from applying for relief unless in dire necessity, by the threat of:

> firstly ... the loss of personal reputation (what is understood by the stigma of pauperism); secondly, the loss of personal freedom which is secured by detention in a workhouse; and thirdly, the loss of political freedom by suffering disfranchisement.

Davy believed there was no room for compromise in the principle of 'less eligibility' and in the administration of the workhouse test. In some ways he was more unyielding than Chadwick himself. If workhouse wards in which the aged were housed were made too comfortable, people would not save for old age. If homes for pauper children were too pleasant, parents would be encouraged to neglect their responsibilities and send their children away. Improvements in the workhouse infirmaries were a threat to the voluntary hospital system. The Poor Law officials were particularly unhappy about the Unemployed Workmen Act, 1905, which by-passed the Poor Law to assist the unemployed, whose numbers had risen steadily since the Boer War. Walter Long, the author of the Act and Gerald Balfour's predecessor at the local Government Board, had spoken of his feelings that it was right on this occasion to step outside the framework of the Poor Law.

> But for the other class—the men who want work and can't get it and have nobody to turn to for guidance—that these people should be manufactured into paupers seems to me to be a national crime.

J. S. Davy was not convinced. An unemployed man, he told the commissioners, 'must stand by his accidents; he must suffer for the general good of the body politic'.

The Royal Commission, however, did not prove as tractable as Davy and his colleagues had hoped. For one thing, Davy showed his hand too soon to Beatrice Webb, and she put her fellow commissioners on their guard. They refused to be spoon-fed with carefully chosen evidence to support the conclusions Davy wished them to reach, and insisted on mounting their own extensive inquiries. They wrote to boards of guardians throughout England and Wales inviting them to describe any serious defects in the existing Poor Law system and to suggest remedies. They received replies, many of them detailed, from 548 of the 645 unions. Similar inquiries were made in Scotland. Evidence was also sought from local distress committees (set up under the 1905 Unemployed Workmen Act), government departments, voluntary organizations, professional bodies, trade unions, friendly societies, employers, local authorities, and from numerous individuals with expert knowledge of the field of inquiry. The commissioners held 209 meetings, of which 159 were spent hearing the evidence of 452 witnesses who attended in person. Written evidence was received from about 900 more. In addition, the Royal Commission appointed a number of 'special investigators' to inquire into particular topics and report on them to the Commission. It was, however, never the intention that the position of these special investigators should be analogous to that of the assistant commissioners of 1832. As the Majority Report pointed out:

> To these Assistant Commissioners was practically delegated the whole responsibility for collecting the evidence upon which the Royal Commission should report. We felt that public opinion would not support us in so extensive a delegation of our responsibilities.

So the special investigators were kept on a tight rein and instructed to distinguish clearly in their reports between 'facts as ascertained by them, and ... such conclusions as might properly be drawn from the facts so ascertained'.

The commissioners themselves visited some 400 workhouses and other institutions in all parts of the United Kingdom, and some of them travelled through Europe to compare other systems of poor relief. Individual commissioners prepared papers on topics of which they had special knowledge, ranging from 'Poor Relief during the Period 1601–1834' (C. S. Loch) to 'The Medical Services of the Poor Law and the Public Health Departments of English Local Government' (Beatrice Webb). Statistical inquiries were mounted and actuaries were called in, while the help of the bishops was enlisted to collect information from every parish on the causes and extent of poverty, whether it was increasing or diminishing, and on various questions related to the administration of relief.

Much of the zeal for research and detailed factual information was contributed by Beatrice Webb and the six members who were associated with the Charity Organization Society—C. S. Loch, secretary of the COS, the Rev. T. G. Gardiner, T. H. Nunn, the Rev. L. R. Phelps, Mrs Bosanquet and Octavia Hill. But there were also four civil servants—including Sir Samuel Provis, permanent secretary of the Local Government Board—as well as a trade union official, Francis Chandler, and George Lansbury, who was later to hold office in the first Labour government. So it was hardly surprising that it proved impossible for the Commission to produce a unanimous report. The Minority Report was mainly the work of the Fabian Socialists, Sidney and Beatrice Webb. Sidney Webb was not a member of the Royal Commission, but that was a mere technicality. In all things the Webbs worked as a team. In signing the Minority Report, Beatrice Webb was joined by Lansbury, Chandler and Prebendary Wakefield.

There was a good deal of common ground between the Majority and Minority Reports. They agreed that the boards of guardians should be abolished; that the general mixed workhouse should go and be replaced by separate institutions for the able-bodied, the sick, the aged and children; that local administration should be brought under firmer central control; that outdoor relief should be more systematically administered; and that there should be machinery to coordinate charitable aid. The general mixed workhouse had, of course, been condemned by the 1834 commissioners, but seventy years later it was still very much in evidence. Both reports supported the introduction of old age pensions (which had taken place in 1908) and recommended state insurance schemes for sickness and unemployment. Neither group of commissioners felt the Act of 1905 to be a satisfactory solution to the problem of unemployment, although their own proposals in this respect differed widely.

Even those who at the beginning of the Commission's work were most inclined to defend the *status quo* were convinced by the end of the inquiry that the existing system would not do. The Majority Report argued that if the Poor Law had been undermined by the introduction of other forms of relief from public funds this was because the system of administration represented by the guardians no longer commanded public confidence. Poor Law administration stood 'in no organic relation to the rest of local government' and there was little interest in elections to boards of guardians. The majority commissioners therefore recommended that the administration of the Poor Law should be entrusted to the major local authorities, the county and county borough councils, which for this purpose should be known as public assistance authorities. In each authority there should be set up a statutory public assistance committee. The change of terminology from 'Poor Law' to 'public assistance' was an attempt to shake off some of the harsh associations of the former; similarly, the majority preferred the term 'necessitous' to 'destitute' as one which more accurately described the ground of entitlement to relief.

The majority argued that where indoor relief was granted, the workhouse regime should be 'as far as possible curative and restorative', while outdoor relief should be adequate in amount, awarded only after thorough investigation of the circumstances of the applicant, and accompanied by supervision designed to re-establish economic independence as soon as possible. The influence of the COS members was evident in the stress laid on the role of voluntary organizations in supplementing and supporting, by individual social casework and otherwise, the official provisions. In each area, it was suggested, a voluntary aid committee should be set up to co-operate closely with the public assistance authority. It was felt desirable that the two should have their offices in the same building.

The Royal Commission devoted a good deal of attention to the Poor Law medical services. The evidence showed that sickness was a chief cause of pauperism and the majority concluded that:

It is probably little, if any, exaggeration to say that, to the extent to which we can eliminate or diminish sickness among the poor, we shall eliminate or diminish one-half the existing amount of pauperism.

Nonetheless, the Majority Report expressed reservations about unhindered access to medical treatment for all.

> We do not pretend that the system we propose will realise the ideals of those enthusiasts who contemplate unfettered and unintermittent medical control, supervision and treatment of every human being from the cradle to the grave. A system which thus made every human life the helpless subject of relentless and aggressive medical inspection and, to some extent, of medical experiment, might tend to encourage morbidly some of the human ills it was designed to destroy. A race of hypochondriacs might be as useless to the State as a race of any other degenerates. Good health is no doubt a matter of the greatest importance to all, but it is not the sole aim in life, and it is possible to exaggerate the part it plays in the attainment of human welfare.

The majority therefore proposed limited reforms designed to promote closer co-operation between the various voluntary and statutory agencies providing medical services for the poor. Each public assistance authority should appoint a medical assistance committee, consisting of members of the health and public assistance committees together with representatives of the local branch or branches of the British Medical Association and of local hospitals, dispensaries and friendly societies. A system of provident dispensaries should be established and membership of this scheme should carry the right to medical treatment at a modest fee and to institutional treatment upon recommendation from the dispensary doctor. Necessitous persons would, however, receive medical treatment through the public assistance committee, although in certain cases, such as the aged and widows with young children, the public assistance committee might pay the necessary fees to enable them to become members of a provident dispensary. The Majority Report recommended that medical relief should not incur disenfranchisement.

To solve the unemployment problem the Majority Report recommended a national system of labour exchanges (introduced in 1909); a more vocational bias to education in the public elementary schools; a state system of unemployment insurance; and the timing of public works to coincide with periods of trade depression.

The Minority Report was a more radical document which demanded that the Poor Law should not be reformed, but swept away entirely, and its functions distributed among the several specialized committees of the major local authorities. The minority commissioners described the schemes they had rejected as:

> (i) The Continuance of a Denuded Destitution Authority alongside of other Local Authorities Providing for the Poor [this was how they saw the majority recommendations];

(ii) The Monopoly of Public Assistance by a Deterrent Destitution Authority;

(iii) The Extension of Public Assistance by a Disguised and Swollen Poor Law.

For their part they recommended that:

(1) the entire care of pauper children of school age should be entrusted to local education authorities under the supervision of the Board of Education;

(2) responsibilities relating to birth and infancy, the treatment of the sick and incapacitated, and institutional provision for the aged, should be transferred to the local health authorities;

(3) there should be local pensions, for the elderly not entitled to national pensions, administered by the local pensions committees set up under the Old Age Pensions Act, 1908;

(4) the care of all persons certified as of unsound mind (including mental defectives) should be the responsibility of asylums committees of the major local authorities.

In addition each county or county borough should appoint a registrar of public assistance to keep registers of all persons receiving any form of public assistance, to assess charges to be made to individuals or their relatives, and to coordinate the activities of the various committees dispensing assistance in one form or another.

Because of the split in the Royal Commission, this great inquiry had little immediate effect. Employment exchanges would have been introduced in 1909 and it is likely that the 1911 National Insurance Act would have taken much the form it did even if the Royal Commission had never sat. The Webbs conducted a well publicized campaign to secure acceptance of the Minority Report, but by the time war broke out in 1914 no legislative action had been taken on the major proposals of either report. In 1918 the Maclean Committee attempted to reconcile the views of the majority and the minority and between 1919 and 1921 Dr Christopher Addison, Britain's first Minister of Health, made several attempts to legislate for the break-up of the Poor Law. After Addison's resignation in 1921 the subject was dropped and was not raised again until 1924.

Reports of the Royal Commission on the Poor Laws and Relief of Distress, 1909

Majority Report

DEFECTS OF THE POOR LAW SYSTEM

The preceding pages of this Report, and the voluminous evidence we have collected, will have laid bare the main defects in our present system of Poor Law administration. They may be briefly summarised under the following heads:—

(i) The inadequacy of existing Poor Law areas to meet the growing needs of administration.

(ii) The excessive size of many Boards of Guardians.

(iii) The absence of any general interest in Poor Law work and Poor Law elections, due in great part to the fact that Poor Law work stands in no organic relation to the rest of local government.

(iv) The lack of intelligent uniformity in the application of principles and in general administration.

(v) The want of proper investigation and discrimination in dealing with applicants.

(vi) The tendency in many Boards of Guardians to give outdoor relief without plan or purpose.

(vii) The unsuitability of the general workhouse as a test or deterrent for the able-bodied; the aggregation in it of all classes without sufficient classification; and the absence of any system of friendly and restorative help.

(viii) The lack of co-operation between Poor Law and charity.

(ix) The tendency of candidates to make lavish promises of out-relief and of Guardians to favour their constituents in its distribution.

(x) General failure to attract capable social workers and leading citizens.

(xi) The general rise in expenditure, not always accompanied by an increase of efficiency in administration.

(xii) The want of sufficient control and continuity of policy on the part of the Central Authority.

These defects have produced, notably in urban districts, a want of confidence in the local administration of the Poor Law. They have also been mainly the cause of the introduction of other forms of relief from public funds which are unaccompanied by such conditions as are imperatively necessary as safeguards.

Any reform to be effective must be thorough. We will now state what portion of the old system we propose to sweep away, what to retain, and the conditions necessary in order to create for the future a trustworthy and elastic administrative system of Public Assistance.

Part IX paras. 1–2

PUBLIC ASSISTANCE

It has been impressed upon us in the course of our enquiry that the name 'Poor Law' has gathered about it associations of harshness, and still more of hopelessness, which we fear might seriously obstruct the reforms which we desire to see initiated. We are aware that a mere change of name will not prevent the old associations from recurring if it does not represent an essential change in the spirit of the work. But in our criticism and recommendations we hope to show the way to a system of help which will be better expressed by the title of Public Assistance than by that of Poor Law.

We therefore recommend that the new Local Authority shall be known as the Public Assistance Authority, and that the Committees which will carry on its work locally shall be known as the Public Assistance Committees. The name is not intended to disguise the fact that those who come within the scope of the operations of the new authority are receiving help at the public expense; but it is intended to emphasise the importance of making that help of real assistance. We hope also that the change may make it easier for those directly engaged in administrating relief to build up new traditions, and to carry on their work with a higher aim before them.

The principles dominating the spirit of the existing English Poor Law, so far as they determine the definition of those qualified for relief, seem to us both sound and humane. They contain a positive and a negative element; to relieve those who are qualified for public relief, and to discourage those who do not legitimately come within this category from becoming a public burden. The conditions under which relief is given ought to be prescribed, not by the applicant, but by the authority that relieves the applicant. We do not recommend any alteration of the law which would extend the qualification for relief to individuals not now entitled to it, or which would bring within the operation of assistance from public funds classes not now legally within its operation. The term 'destitute' is now in use to describe those entitled to claim relief. . . .

We prefer the term 'necessitous,' for we believe that it more accurately describes those who are at present held to be qualified for relief. We recommend, therefore, that the term 'necessitous' take the place of 'destitute.'

Those, however, who are now qualified for relief by coming within the definition of destitution, fall into many classes, and the treatment of each class, and of each individual within that class, should be governed by the conditions surrounding the class or the individual. Help, prevention, cure, and instruction, should each find its place within the processes at the disposal of the new authorities. Too much importance cannot be attached to the organisation to which the selection of the appropriate treatment is to be entrusted.

Part IX paras. 3–4

UNIT OF ADMINISTRATION

. . . We propose that in future the unit of administration shall be the County and the County Borough. In view of the strength of sentiment as regards areas, we have thought it better to adopt an existing area. We are well aware that objections may be made to it, but the fact that it is already recognised and familiar has had great weight with us.

The main objection urged against any enlargement of area, and the association under one authority of institutions distant from one another, is that some of the recipients of institutional relief may be so far away from their friends and relatives as to make visits to them difficult. We believe that any such inconvenience

is greatly exaggerated. Communication has been so far facilitated and cheapened
that the several parts of a county are now, for practical purposes, no more
distant from one another than were the individual parishes of a union in 1834.
Moreover, analysis of the inmates of a country workhouse shows that the greater
proportion of the adults so relieved are infirm or old persons. We have recommended that the old shall in future be cared for in small homes, and these would
be available in different parts of the county. For those needing special care, we
think that the superior treatment offered in a county institution would far outweigh any inconvenience to relatives and friends. In pursuance of our proposals
we would therefore lay down the following principles as governing the re-
adjustment of areas:—

(a) That the area of the Public Assistance Authority shall be coterminous
with the area of the county or county borough, and that no exception from this
principle shall be permissible unless the Local Government Board is satisfied
that such exception would, in each particular case, be in the best interests of
administration.

(b) Any union area, which at present overlaps a county or county borough,
shall be divided up so that each part of it will be attached for Public Assistance
purposes to the county or county borough within the boundaries of which such
part is at present situated.

(c) Any injustice or anomaly arising from this arrangement may be remedied
subsequently by the ordinary procedure for altering county or county borough
boundaries, supplemented, if necessary, by further powers to the Local Government Board.

(d) Financial adjustments necessitated by the partition of a union area shall
be determined by agreement between the authorities concerned, and, failing
agreement, by arbitration as under Section 62 of the Local Government Act,
1888.

It remains to determine the area of charge. The Royal Commissioners of 1832
found that under the 43rd Eliz. the area of charge was the parish. The changes
which they proposed necessitated its enlargement, and by successive Acts of
Parliament, the Union was gradually substituted for the parish. In view of the
fresh changes which we suggest, we have been led to the conclusion that the area
must be once more enlarged. If the classification of institutions which we propose
is adopted, it will logically follow that the area of charge should coincide with
the area of administration. It may well be that some new institutions will be
required, and that some of the old can be dispensed with. But however that may
be, it would clearly be difficult or impossible for the new Authority to enforce
a common standard of efficiency in the institutions in their area, unless the cost
of maintaining such institutions was a charge common to the whole area. And
with regard to out-relief, or, as we shall call it, home assistance, the same holds
good. We anticipate that the Public Assistance Authority of the future will
supervise the work of its Committees. If this supervision is to be thorough and
effective, the Committees must be dependent upon the Authority for the necessary funds. We propose therefore that the cost of Public Assistance, so far as its
incidence remains local, shall be borne by a County or County Borough rate.

Part IX paras. 6–8

BREAKING UP THE POOR LAW

There was a scheme brought to our notice known as the 'Breaking up of the Poor Law.' Its ideas appear to be the foundation of the alternative proposals recommended by certain of our colleagues who dissent from our Report. Under this scheme the whole existing machinery of Poor Law administration would disappear with the abolition of the Guardians, and the work previously performed by them would be broken up into sections and transferred to existing Committees of County and County Borough Councils.

Though we have had the scheme fully before us, we do not propose to criticise it in detail. It seems clear to us that the idea upon which it is founded is faulty and unworkable. The question at issue is whether the work of maintaining those members of the community who have lost their economic independence can be safely entrusted to authorities whose primary duty is something quite distinct— such as that of Education or Sanitation—or whether it is essential that there should be an authority devoting itself entirely to the work. We consider that the many and subtle problems associated with Public Assistance, especially when it is a family rather than an individual that requires rehabilitation, cannot be solved by the simple process of sending off each unit to a separate authority for maintenance and treatment. What is needed is a disinterested authority, practised in looking at all sides of a question and able to call in skilled assistance. The specialist is too apt to see only what interests him in the first instance and to disregard wider issues.

Moreover, the existing educational and sanitary authorities ought not, in our judgment, to be converted into agencies for the distribution of relief; and the less their functions are associated with the idea of relief, the better will they perform the public work for which they were specially called into existence. To thrust upon those Authorities, while their work is still incomplete, the far more difficult and delicate duties of dealing with families which have already broken down, would be to court failure in both directions—that of prevention and that of cure.

There are further difficulties which would inevitably arise from this multiplication of agencies authorised to grant public relief. Whilst a combination of incompatible duties is imposed upon the Education and the Health Committees by the scheme, its operation in another direction is to dislocate and separate work which cannot be effectively discharged unless it is combined and under the control of one authority or committee. The functions of granting relief, and of the recovery of the cost either from the recipients or those legally liable for them, should be in the hands of one body and not divided between two or more organisations with separate staffs, and methods of investigation. Such a separation must result in a multiplication of inquiries and visitations, causing annoyance and waste of time and money. The same criticism applies to domiciliary and institutional relief. Being the two recognised methods of Public Assistance they should be utilised together as one system under one supervision. Their disconnection by being placed under two tribunals must lead to administrative inefficiency and confusion. Whilst a multiplication of authorities and organisations for the discharge of local duties is to be deprecated as tending to delay and friction, care must be taken not to run to the other extreme by the abolition of organisations specially qualified for a certain class of work and the transfer of such work to existing bodies who are not specially qualified for its discharge.

Part IX paras. 12–14

Minority Report

THE SCHEME OF REFORM

The state of anarchy and confusion into which has fallen the whole realm of relief and assistance to the poor and to persons in distress, is so generally recognised that many plans of reform have been submitted to us, each representing a section of public opinion. In fact, throughout the three years of our investigations we have been living under a continuous pressure for a remodelling of the Poor Laws and the Unemployed Workmen Act, in one direction or another. We do not regret this peremptory and insistent demand for reform. The present position is, in our opinion, as grave as that of 1834, though in its own way. We have, on the one hand, in England and Wales, Scotland and Ireland alike, the well-established Destitution Authorities, under ineffective central control, each pursuing its own policy in its own way; sometimes rigidly restricting its relief to persons actually destitute, and giving it in the most deterrent and humiliating forms; sometimes launching out into an indiscriminate and unconditional subsidising of mere poverty; sometimes developing costly and palatial institutions for the treatment, either gratuitously or for partial payment, of practically any applicant of the wage-earning or of the lower middle class. On the other hand, we see existing, equally ubiquitous with the Destitution Authorities, the newer specialised organs of Local Government—the Local Education Authority, the Local Health Authority, the Local Lunacy Authority, the Local Unemployment Authority, the Local Pension Authority—all attempting to provide for the needs of the poor, *according to the cause or character of their distress*. Every Parliamentary session adds to the powers of these specialised Local Authorities. Every Royal Commission or Departmental Committee recommends some fresh development of their activities. Thus, even while our Commission has been at work, a Departmental Committee has reported in favour of handing over the Vagrants and what used to be called the 'Houseless Poor,' to the Local Police Authority, as being interested in 'Vagrancy as a whole,' apart from the accident of a Vagrant being destitute. The Royal Commission on the Care and Control of the Feeble-minded has recommended that all mentally defective persons now maintained by the Poor Law should be handed over to the Local Authority specially concerned with mental deficiency, whether in a destitute, or in a non-destitute person. The increasing activities of these specialised Local Authorities, being only half-consciously sanctioned by public opinion, and only imperfectly authorised by statute, are spasmodic and uneven. Whilst, for instance, the Local Education Authorities and the Local Health Authorities are providing, in some places, gratuitous maintenance and medical treatment, for one set of persons after another, similar Authorities elsewhere are rigidly confining themselves to a bare fulfilment of their statutory obligations of schooling and sanitation. Athwart the overlapping and rivalry of these half a dozen Local Authorities that may be all at work in a single district, we watch the growing stream of private charity and voluntary agencies—almshouses and pensions for the aged; hospitals and dispensaries, convalescent homes and 'medical missions' for the sick; free dinners and free boots, country holidays and 'happy evenings' for the children; free shelters and soup kitchens, 'way tickets' and charitable jobs for the able-bodied, together with uncounted indiscriminate doles of every description—without systematic organisation and without any co-ordination with the multifarious forms of public activity. What the nation is confronted with today is, as it was in 1834, an ever-growing expenditure from public and private funds, which results, on the one hand, in a minimum of prevention and cure, and on the other in far-reaching demoralisation of character and the continuance of no small amount of unrelieved destitution.

pp. 384–5

THE SUPERSESSION OF THE DESTITUTION AUTHORITY

We think that the time has arrived for the abolition of the Boards of Guardians in England, Wales and Ireland; and, so far as any Poor Law duties are concerned, of the Parish Councils in Scotland. We come to this conclusion not from any lack of appreciation of the devoted public service gratuitously rendered on these Boards of Guardians and Parish Councils by tens of thousands of men and women of humanity, ability, and integrity, which, we feel, has never received adequate recognition. But it has become increasingly plain to us in the course of our inquiry—it is, in fact, recognised by many of the members of these bodies themselves—that the character of the functions entrusted to the Poor Law Authorities is such as to render their task, at best, nugatory; and, at worst, seriously mischievous. The mere keeping of people from starving—which is essentially what the Poor Law sets out to do—may have been useful as averting social revolution; it cannot, in the twentieth century, be regarded as any adequate fulfilment of social duty. The very conception of relieving destitution starts the whole service on a demoralising tack. An Authority having for its function merely the provision of maintenance for those who are starving is necessarily limited in its dealings to the brief periods in each person's life in which he is actually destitute; and has, therefore, even if it could go beyond the demoralising dole—too bad for the good, and too good for the bad—no opportunity of influencing that person's life, both before he becomes destitute and after he has ceased to be destitute, in such a way as to stimulate personal effort, to strengthen character and capacity, to ward off dangers, and generally to keep the individual on his feet. As regards the effect on individual character and the result in enforcing personal and family responsibilities, of the activities of the Destitution Authority on the one hand, and those of the Local Education Authority and the Local Health Authority on the other—even where these latter give food as well as treatment—there is, as all our evidence shows, no possible doubt on which side the advantage lies. Yet if a Poor Law Authority attempts to do more than provide bare subsistence for those who are actually destitute, for the period in which they are destitute; if it sets itself to give the necessary specialised treatment required for birth and infancy; if it provides education for children, medical treatment for the sick, satisfactory provision for the aged, and specialised compulsion for the able-bodied, it ceases to be an '*ad hoc*' Authority, with a single tradition and a single purpose, and becomes a 'mixed' Authority, without either the diversified professional staff, the variety of technical experience, or even a sufficiency and continuity of work in any one branch to enable it to cope with its multifarious problems. Moreover, as has been abundantly demonstrated by experience, every increase in the advantageousness of the 'relief' afforded by the Destitution Authority, and every enlargement of its powers of compulsory removal and detention, brings it into new rivalry with the other Local Authorities, and drags into the net of pauperism those who might otherwise have been dealt with as self-supporting citizens. If, as it seems to us, it has become imperative to put an end to the present wasteful and demoralising overlapping between Local Authorities, it is plain that it is the Destitution Authority—already denuded of several of its functions—that must give way to its younger rivals.

pp. 396–7

1.4 Local Government Act, 1929

In 1924 a Conservative Government under Stanley Baldwin succeeded the short-lived first Labour Government and Neville Chamberlain returned to the post which he had formerly held at the Ministry of Health. In this term of office he determined to tackle the problem of Poor Law reform. Chamberlain was above all a gifted administrator, who was appalled by the waste and inefficiency he saw in the existing system. In 1925 he tightened central control over boards of guardians by taking power in the Boards of Guardians (Default) Act to dismiss a board that did not abide by his instructions and to replace it with his own nominees. These powers were used at West Ham and Chester-le-Street in 1926 and at Bedwellty in South Wales in 1927, and the threat of their use was held over the heads of other unions that were pursuing policies likely to outrun their resources. This was the time when Poor Law finances were under strain from rising unemployment figures, and also from the payment of relief either to men on strike or to their families in the mining areas. The Government were quick to react to any suspicion of unduly lavish administration of poor relief such as had brought the central authority into collision with the Poplar guardians in 1921.

Chamberlain's next step was the consolidation of over 100 Poor Law statutes in the Poor Law Act of 1927, and then he was ready to abolish the boards of guardians and transfer their powers to the major local authorities. The Local Government Act of 1929 did not break up the Poor Law but this was not Chamberlain's intention. He saw the question as one mainly of improving administrative efficiency. Introducing the Bill late in 1928, he spoke of the confusion, waste and inefficiency resulting from the continued existence of boards of guardians alongside other local authorities with overlapping functions and areas. Both the major local authorities and the guardians provided services for the tuberculous and the mentally ill, for maternity care and child welfare, and whether a person received treatment at the hands of the local authority or of the guardians depended not on the nature of his need but on whether he was destitute or not. The Minister went on to refer to the continued scandal of the mixed workhouse and quoted one with seven inmates who were acutely sick, fifty-five who were infirm and senile, six who suffered from epilepsy, eight who were certified lunatics, eighteen certified mental defectives and nine uncertified mental defectives. There was also one able-bodied man and three healthy infants.

Part I of the Act transferred the functions of the Poor Law authorities to county and county borough councils, and included provision for combining neighbouring authorities for Poor Law purposes by the establishment of a joint committee, either on the initiative of the authorities themselves, or by order of the Minister where combination 'would tend to diminish expense, or would otherwise be of public or local advantage'. Councils were called upon to prepare schemes for the discharge of their Poor Law functions and to submit them to the Minister within six months of the passage of the Act. S.5 laid down that 'A council in preparing an administrative scheme shall have regard to the desirability of securing that, as soon as circumstances permit, all assistance which can lawfully be provided otherwise than by way of poor relief shall be so provided . . .' Where authorities had powers to grant assistance under the Public Health, Mental Deficiency, Education, Maternity and Child Welfare and other Acts they were enjoined to use these powers rather than their Poor Law powers.

Each council was required to set up a public assistance committee, although it was left open to local authorities to designate any of their existing committees to act as the public assistance committee if they wished. Thus some councils discharged their functions relating to health and public assistance through the same committee. All matters relating to poor relief, except the raising of a rate or the borrowing of money, were to stand referred to the public assistance committee.

In counties the Act required that there should be a subcommittee of the public assistance committee set up for each area, consisting of one or more county districts, to be known as the guardians committee and to be responsible for dealing with individual applications for relief, and the visiting, inspection and, in some cases, management of public assistance institutions. By virtue of the Act, the workhouse infirmaries were of course transferred to the major local authorities along with the workhouses proper. In this way the local authorities acquired a number of general hospitals and hospitals for the chronic sick to add to their existing hospitals built under their public health powers. The 1929 Act laid on local authorities the duty of consulting with voluntary hospitals in their areas when making provision for hospital accommodation. They were to consult both with the governing bodies and with the medical and surgical staffs of these hospitals 'as to the accommodation to be provided and as to the purposes for which it is to be used'.

Certain local authorities, notably London County Council, seized the opportunity they had been given to develop a first-class municipal hospital system, but others, the majority, showed little interest in the newly acquired infirmaries or lacked the resources in the economic climate of the early 1930s to do much about developing them and raising their standards. The outbreak of war in 1939 came too soon after the transfer and too soon after the great slump for the local authorities to have had a fair chance to show what they could do in this respect. The war years were abnormal in every way and immediately afterwards local authorities lost their hospitals to the newly constituted National Health Service authorities.

Part II of the Act dealt with registration of births, deaths and marriages; Part III with roads and town planning; Part IV with miscellaneous local government provisions, such as the rearrangement of county districts and the review of electoral divisions. S.58 laid on county councils the duty of ensuring, if necessary by combination of districts, that medical officers of health to county districts were able to devote their full time to public health matters and were prohibited from the private practice of medicine. Many medical officers of health at this time combined a part-time appointment with general medical practice. S.63 required county councils to ensure the provision of adequate hospital accommodation for the treatment of infectious diseases in the county as a whole, and where necessary hospitals provided by district councils were to be made available to the inhabitants of other districts as well.

Part V dealt with rating and valuation; Part VI with exchequer grants and other financial provisions; and Part VII with property, liabilities and officers, including the transfer of officers from Poor Law authorities to the county and county borough councils. Part VIII included other provisions of a general or technical nature.

2 Public Health and Community Health Services

Introduction

If we want to know why people talked in the nineteenth century of public health, and in the third quarter of the twentieth century of community medicine, or social medicine, it will not be much help to consult a dictionary. Those who read through this section will, however, be conscious of a shift of emphasis that corresponds to the change of usage. The great Public Health Acts of 1848 and 1875 were directed at environmental threats to health, faulty sanitation and defective water supplies that produced epidemics of cholera and smallpox, typhus and typhoid. King Cholera was conquered by 1890, and he was conquered as much by the engineers as the doctors. The doctors played the major part in the control of smallpox. In the case of many other diseases which spread in conditions of squalor, filth and overcrowding, doctors, legislators and sanitary engineers all deserve their share of the credit. In the twentieth century the partnership continued, with the importance of a healthy environment fully recognized, and with vaccination and immunization the main weapons in the hands of the doctors until the introduction of sulphonamides and antibiotics from the 1930s onwards. The last of the infectious diseases to represent a major threat to life in Britain was tuberculosis, and it yielded to streptomycin and other antituberculous drugs in the 1950s. By this time local authorities had extensive powers, under the 1936 Public Health Act, to control environmental threats to health, and the old controversies about the vesting of what were at one time considered to be dictatorial powers in the hands of the medical officer of health were long forgotten.

To discover the full story of the nineteenth-century struggle for a healthy environment it would be necessary to examine, in addition to the documents outlined here, the Public Health Acts of 1858 and 1859 which took John Simon from the Medical Officership of the City of London to the newly created post of Medical Officer to the Privy Council; the Sanitary Act of 1866, which Simon declared would make 'an almost incredible difference to human life in this country', but which so cruelly disappointed his hopes; and the Local Government Board Act of 1871 which brought Simon into conflict with the Poor Law officials and led to his premature retirement from the public service. There was also the 1869 Report of the Royal Commission on Sanitary Conditions in England and Wales and in the mid-1860s the two Contagious Diseases Acts ('contagious diseases' being a Victorian euphemism for venereal diseases) which gave rise to a celebrated early manifestation of Women's Lib.

With more general threats to health reasonably under control, attention turned to matters of organization, to the problems of particular groups in the population, and to education in healthy living. There was still, however, some tidying up to be done. The Clean Air Act of 1956 could reasonably be regarded as a belated piece of Victorian sanitary reform. The Noise Abatement Act of 1960 could perhaps be regarded in the same light. But consciousness that the public health scene was changing was shown in many reports and publications during the first twenty years of the health service. The Jameson Report reviewed the functions of the health visitor. The previous year the Armer Report had looked at the training of district nurses. The Cohen Report on Health Education was published in 1964 and the Sheldon Report on Child Welfare Centres in 1967. There was a general sense that ground gained in the past could easily be lost if too much was taken for granted, but that with a changing population structure, changing beliefs, and greater affluence, new problems were coming to the fore.

The Family Planning Act and the Abortion Act of 1967 showed a society that was beginning to be able to apply some measure of rationality to the discussion of sexual matters—though there are still times when perusal of the correspondence columns of the newspapers makes this seem too strong a claim—and the Chronically Sick and Disabled Persons Act showed a society increasingly sensitive to the claims of underprivileged minorities.

2.1 Report to Her Majesty's Principal Secretary of State for the Home Department from the Poor Law Commissioners on an Inquiry into the Sanitary Condition of the Labouring Population of Great Britain

Published: 1842

By Edwin Chadwick

Chadwick's great Sanitary Report of 1842, which led to the appointment by Peel's Tory Government in the following year of the Health of Towns Commission, and ultimately to the Public Health Act of 1848, bears his name and his alone because although it was written in the discharge of his duties as secretary to the Poor Law Commission, when the commissioners saw what he had produced they refused to accept responsibility and put their names to it. The background to this was a long drawn-out dispute between Chadwick and his nominal masters about the interpretation and enforcement of the 1834 Poor Law Amendment Act and about the conduct of the business of the Poor Law office. His enemies on the Commission had eventually succeeded in excluding him from meetings and in leaving him virtually without employment in poor law matters—though he clung tenaciously to his office as secretary. It was in these circumstances that he was able to devote his great energies and abilities to an examination of the public health problems which he was persuaded were intimately linked with the problems of poverty. When in 1841 Chadwick was passed over for a vacancy on the Poor Law Commission itself, the Home Secretary whose hostility had dealt him this snub attempted to soften the blow by asking him to renew work on his sanitary report, which had been set on one side a few months earlier when it seemed the previous Whig Government would be introducing a sanitary reform bill without waiting for Chadwick's report.

The report was based on detailed inquiries in every part of the country, using the machinery of the Poor Law to collect information from poor law medical officers, local relieving officers, boards of guardians and others with special knowledge and experience of the living conditions of the working classes. Most of this information was collated and forwarded to Chadwick by the assistant commissioners, officials whose job it was to represent the Poor Law Commission throughout the length and breadth of the country, to enforce its policies, and to act as its eyes and ears. Chadwick prepared detailed notes of guidance and questionnaires to assist those collecting the information he required, and systematically followed up any points that were not clear to him in the reports he received. Wherever possible independent verification was sought when statements were disputed or seemed open to doubt. All this information was supplemented by statistical material from the files of the Poor Law Commission and the office of the Registrar-General (registration of births and deaths had been introduced in 1837), and by wide reading of the relevant literature, including a great deal that had been published on the Continent. Chadwick's controversial reputation as an administrator has perhaps obscured his contribution to the technique of social inquiry, but if at times wrongheaded he was thorough in all things and spared no pains to get what he could regard as reliable information on the matters with which he was concerned.

The Sanitary Report described to legislators the living conditions of the poor, it showed that insanitary conditions, defective drainage, inadequate water supply and overcrowding were invariably associated with disease, high mortality rates and low expectation of life; that the economic cost of ill-health—computed by such means as taking into account the cost of maintaining widows and orphans—was impressive, but that the damage to the fabric of society went far beyond what could be measured in financial terms; that existing authorities and legislation were quite inadequate for the purpose of improving the sanitary conditions and health of the population; and that both reform of the law and the setting up of adequate administrative machinery were called for.

The report did not make detailed recommendations as to the form legislation might take. Chadwick rather expected that after the presentation of his report he might be asked to draft a Bill, but in the event the working out of detailed proposals was left to a Royal Commission under the chairmanship of the Duke of Buccleuch. There is much in the report that is revealing of the man, as well as of his times, but comparison of this report with some of his earlier work shows also how much he had learned and how much his sympathies had widened in the course of the inquiries which formed its basis.

It was characteristic of Chadwick that he attached great importance to showing the economic cost of ill-health, but in the final version of the report this aspect was dismissed in a mere twenty pages, utterly overshadowed by arguments of a social and humanitarian nature. Chadwick's paternalism comes out again and again. He pointed out how much in the way of sanitary improvement could be achieved with what the poor spent on drink. He devoted an important section to illustrations of the good that employers and landlords could do to both the health and the morals of their employees and tenants by providing enlightened working and living conditions. (This section was in fact a pioneering contribution to the science of occupational health.) He was concerned that high death rates among the older working men removed their steadying influence on the young and provided a threat to law and order.

Chadwick the administrator is to be seen in the emphasis on having properly qualified engineers and doctors to enforce new measures, and on the need to consolidate the duties of the many existing *ad hoc* authorities for water, drainage, paving, lighting and sanitation. He appealed extensively to the experience of the army and navy in sanitary regulation and contrasted the qualifications of the army engineers with those commonly considered to be necessary to superintend schemes of drainage and sewerage in civilian life.

This was of course an area where Chadwick had his own pet theories, theories which were later at the General Board of Health to lead him into headlong collision both with the London sanitary authorities and the civil engineering profession. In the report he was anxious to show that sewage could be turned into an economic asset by sprinkling it in diluted form over the countryside as manure. Because his theories on the causes of disease led him to regard smells and vapours arising from sewage as the chief danger, he was very much more concerned with getting it away from dwelling-places by improved systems of drainage than he was with what happened to it afterwards. He was not to be blamed for failing to anticipate such discoveries as the germ theory of disease and the water-borne nature of cholera, but it is an indication of his temper that he was prepared to be quite dogmatic on such matters and to consider that he had as good a right as any member of the medical profession to hold opinions on them.

However, in the arguments he put forward for having sewage carried away by a constant flow of water he was on sure ground, endorsed by posterity. Few towns at that time had a water supply adequate for this purpose, but there were a number of other grounds for urging a high priority for improvements in this respect. Once again, Chadwick was careful to point out the relative cheapness as well as the greater efficacy of constant, as opposed to intermittent, water supply.

The original report is no longer easily obtainable. The fact that it was published as a House of Lords paper, rather than a House of Commons paper, has contributed to this. The page numbers of the following extracts are therefore those of the edition published in 1965 by Edinburgh University Press and edited by M. W. Flinn.

Report on the Sanitary Condition of the Labouring Population of Great Britain, 1842

INSANITARY CONDITIONS IN WINDSOR

The state of Windsor affords an example that the highest neighbourhoods in power and wealth do not at present possess securities for the prevention of nuisances dangerous to the public health. *Mr. Parker*, in his report on the condition of his district, states:

'With regard to the drainage of the towns in the counties of Buckingham, Oxford, and Berks, it may be observed that there is no town in which great improvements might not be effected. In Reading there are commissioners appointed under a local Act to make provision for cleansing the town and removing nuisances; but their duties do not appear to be performed with due regard to the importance of the trust, for the Board of Guardians of the Reading union, by resolutions entered in their minutes, frequently point out nuisances, and remind the commissioners of the filthy condition of many of the courts and back streets. But extensive as the improvements in the state of the drainage of almost every town in these counties might be, there is no town amongst them in which there is so wide a field for improvement as Windsor, which, from the contiguity of the palace, the wealth of the inhabitants, and the situation, might have been expected to be superior in this respect to any other provincial town. Such, however, is not the case; for of all the towns visited by me, Windsor is the worst beyond all comparison. From the gas-works at the end of George-street a double line of open, deep, black, and stagnant ditches extends to Clewer-lane. From these ditches an intolerable stench is perpetually rising, and produces fever of a severe character. I visited a cottage in Clewer-lane in which typhus fever had existed for some time, and learnt from a woman who had recently lost a child the complaint was attributable to the state of these ditches. Mr. Bailey, the relieving officer, informs me that cases of typhus fever are frequent in the neighbourhood; and observes that there are now seven or eight persons attacked by typhus in Charles-street and South-place. He considers the neighbourhood of Garden-court in almost the same condition. "There is a drain," he says, "running from the barracks into the Thames across the Long Walk. That drain is almost as offensive as the black ditches extending to Clewer-lane. The openings to the sewers in Windsor are exceedingly offensive in hot weather. The town is not well supplied with water, and the drainage is very defective." The ditches of which I have spoken are sometimes emptied by carts; and on the last occasion their contents were purchase for the sum of 15*l*. by the occupier of land in the parish of Clewer, whose meadows suffered from the extraordinary strength of the manure, which was used without previous preparation.'

pp. 87–8

DRAINS AND SEWERS

The local arrangements for the cleansing and drainage of towns, &c., generally present only instances of varieties of grievous defects from incompleteness and from the want of science or combination of means for the attainment of the requisite ends. Thus the local reports abound with instances of expensive main-drains, which from ignorant construction as to the levels, do not perform their office, and do accumulate pestilential refuse; others, which have proper levels, but from the want of proper supplies of water do not act; others, which act only partially or by surface drainage, in consequence of the neglect of communication from the houses to the drains; others, where there are drains communicating from the houses, but where the house-drains do not act, or only act in spreading the surface of the matter from cess-pools, and increasing the fœtid exhalations from it in consequence of the want of supplies of water; others again, as in some of the best quarters of the metropolis, where the supplies of water are adequate, and where the drains act in the removal of refuse from the house, but where from want of moderate scientific knowledge or care in their construction, each drain acts like the neck of a large retort, and serves to introduce into the house the subtle gas which spreads disease from the accumulations in the sewers. Other districts there are where their structural arrangements may be completed, and water supplied, and the under drainage in action, and yet pestilential accumulations be found spread before the doors of the population in consequence of the defective construction, and the neglect of the surface-cleansing of the streets and roads. Recently a remonstrance was made to an able and active member of a Commission of Sewers, for taking no steps to extend the drainage in a wretched district of the metropolis. The reply was, a statement, that a drain had been cut through a portion of it, but that it had done no good; and the remonstrant was invited to inspect the district himself, and judge whether, with streets that were unpaved and uncleansed, wet and miry, with deep holes full of refuse, it were possible by any under drainage to remove the evil complained of. Other districts there are in which the Road Commissioners or the Paving Board appears to have done their duty; but the benefit is prevented, and the road is kept continually out of repair by the neglect of the service of scavengers.

All these local defects again are referred back to the defective construction of the Acts of Parliament,—which generally either presume that no science, no skill is requisite for the attainment of the objects, or presume both to be universal,—which in some instances actually prohibit the only effectual mode of drainage, namely, that from the houses into the main-drains; and in others, prescribe cleansing by house-drains without supplies of water; or prescribe the construction of roads independently of drains, and direct the execution of only part of the necessary means, leaving other essential parts to the discretion of individuals.

pp. 109–10

CLASS AND THE EXPECTATION OF LIFE

It is proper to observe, that so far as I was informed upon the evidence received in the Factory Inquiry, and more recently on the cases of children of migrant families, that opinion is erroneous which ascribes greater sickness and mortality to the children employed in factories than amongst the children who remain in such homes as these towns afford to the labouring classes. However defective the ventilation of many of the factories may yet be, they are all of them drier and more equably warm than the residence of the parent; and we had proof that weakly children have been put into the better-managed factories as healthier places for them than their own homes. It is an appalling fact that, of all who are born of the labouring classes in Manchester, more than 57 per cent. die before they attain five years of age; that is, before they can be engaged in factory labour, or in any other labour whatsoever.

Of 4,629 deaths of persons of the labouring classes who died in the year 1840 in Manchester, the numbers who died were at the several periods as follows:

Under 5 years of age	2,649 or 1 in $1\frac{7}{10}$
Above 5 and under 10	215 or 1 in 22
Above 10 and under 15	107 or 1 in 43
Above 15 and under 20	135 or 1 in 34

At seven, eight, or nine years of age the children of the working classes begin to enter into employment in the cotton and other factories. It appears that at the period between 5 and 10 years of age the proportions of deaths which occur amongst the labouring classes, as indicated by these returns, are not so great as the proportions of deaths which occur amongst the children of the middle classes who are not so engaged. Allowing for the circumstance that some of the weakest of the labourers' children will have been swept away in the first stage, the effect of employment is not shown to be injurious in any increase of the proportion who die in the second stage.

In a return obtained from a district differently situated (Bethnal Green, where the manufactory is chiefly domestic) it appears that of 1,268 deaths amongst the labouring classes in the year 1839, no less than 783, or 1 in $1\frac{4}{7}$, died at their own residences under 5 years of age. One in 15 of the deaths occurred between 5 and 10, the age when employment commences. The proportion of deaths which occurred between 10 and 15, the period at which full employment usually takes place, is 1 in 60 only.

In that district the average age of deaths in the year 1839 was as follows, in the several classes, from a population of 62,018:

No. of Deaths	BETHNAL GREEN	Average Age of Deceased
101	Gentlemen and persons engaged in professions, and their families	45 years
273	Tradesmen and their families	26
1,258	Mechanics, servants, and labourers, and their families .	16

The mean chances of life amongst the several classes in Leeds appear from the returns to the Registrar-general generally to correspond with the anticipations raised by the descriptions given of the condition of the labouring population.

No. of Deaths	LEEDS BOROUGH	Average Age of Deceased
79	Gentlemen and persons engaged in professions, and their families	44 years
824	Tradesmen, farmers, and their families . . .	27
3,395	Operatives, labourers, and their families . . .	19

But in Liverpool (which is a commercial and not a manufacturing town) where, however, the condition of the dwellings are reported to be the worst, where, according to the report of Dr. Duncan, 40,000 of the population live in cellars, where 1 in 25 of the population are annually attacked with fever,—there the mean chances of life appear from the returns to the Registrar-general to be still lower than in Manchester, Leeds, or amongst the silk weavers in Bethnal Green. During the year 1840, the deaths, distinguishable in classes, were as follows:

No. of Deaths	LIVERPOOL, 1840	Average Age of Deceased
137	Gentry and professional persons, &c. . . .	35 years
1,738	Tradesmen and their families	22
5,597	Labourers, mechanics, and servants, &c. . . .	15

Of the deaths which occurred amongst the labouring classes, it appears that no less than 62 per cent. of the total number were deaths under five years of age. Even amongst those entered as shopkeepers and tradesmen, no less than 50 per cent. died before they attained that period. The proportion of mortality for Birmingham, where there are many insalubrious manufactories, but where the drainage of the town and the general condition of the inhabitants is comparatively good, was, in 1838, 1 in 40: whilst in Liverpool it was 1 in 31.

I have appended the copy of a map of Bethnal Green, made with the view of showing the proportions in which the mortality from epidemic diseases and diseases affected by localities, fell on different classes of tenements during the same year. The localities in which the marks of death (×) are most crowded are the poorest and the worst of the district; where the marks are few and widely spread, the houses and streets, and the whole condition of the population, is better. By the inspection of a map of Leeds, which Mr. Baker has prepared at my request, to show the localities of epidemic diseases, it will be perceived that they similarly fall on the uncleansed and close streets and wards occupied by the labouring classes; and that the track of the cholera is nearly identical with the tract of fever. It will also be observed that in the badly cleansed and badly drained wards to the right of the map, the proportional mortality is nearly double that which prevails in the better conditioned districts to the left.

To obtain the means of judging of the references to the localities in the sanitary returns from Aberdeen, the reporters were requested to mark on a map the places where the disease fell, and to distinguish with a deeper tint those places on which it fell with the greatest intensity. They were also requested to distinguish by different colours the streets inhabited by the higher, middle, and lower classes of society. They returned a map so marked as to disease, but stated that it had been thought unnecessary to distinguish the streets inhabited by the different orders of society, as that was done with sufficient accuracy by the different tints representing the degrees of intensity of the prevalence of fever.

pp. 223–6

LAW AND ORDER

Whenever the adult population of a physically depressed district, such as Manchester, is brought out on any public occasion, the preponderance of youth in the crowd, and the small proportion of aged, or even of the middle-aged, amongst them is apt to strike those who have seen assemblages of the working population of other districts more favourably situated.

In the course of some inquiries under the Constabulary Force Commission as to the proportions of a paid force that would apparently be requisite for the protection of the peace in the manufacturing districts, reference was made to the meetings held by torchlight in the neighbourhood of Manchester. It was reported to us, on close observation by peace-officers, that the bulk of the assemblages consisted of mere boys, and that there were scarcely any men of mature age to be seen amongst them. Those of mature age and experience, it was stated, generally disapproved of the proceedings of the meetings as injurious to the working classes themselves. These older men, we were assured by their employers, were intelligent, and perceived that capital, and large capital, was not the means of their depression, but of their steady and abundant support. They were generally described as being above the influence of the anarchical fallacies which appeared to sway those wild and really dangerous assemblages. The inquiry which arose upon such statements was how it happened that the men of mature age, feeling their own best interests injured by the proceedings of the younger portion of the working classes, how they, the elders, did not exercise a restraining influence upon their less experienced fellow-workmen? On inquiring of the owner of some extensive manufacturing property, on which between 1000 and 2000 persons were maintained at wages yielding 40s. per week per family, whether he could rely on the aid of the men of mature age for the protection of the capital which furnished them the means of subsistence? he stated he could rely on them confidently. But on ascertaining the numbers qualified for service as special constables, the gloomy fact became apparent, that the proportion of men of strength and of mature age for such service were but as a small group against a large crowd, and that for any social influence they were equally weak. The disappearance by premature deaths of the heads of families and the older workmen at such ages as those recorded in the returns of dependent widowhood and orphanage must to some extent practically involve the necessity of supplying the lapse of staid influence amidst a young population by one description or other of precautionary force.

p. 266

NEED FOR QUALIFIED ENGINEERS

It has been shown, in respect to drainage as well as road construction, that the economy and efficiency of the works will be according to the qualifications, the powers, and responsibilities of the officers appointed to execute them, secured by legislative means, and that new labour on the old condition, without skill, will be executed in the old manner, extravagantly and inefficiently. But engineers or properly qualified officers having the science of civil engineering could not be procured for every separate purpose in every part of the country, as is generally assumed in Acts of Parliament for effecting particular objects. When such connected work is divided and separated, the remuneration necessary to obtain properly qualified officers to attend to the fragment of service is too high; the separation, therefore, in most places, amounts to the exclusion of science from public work, or, in other words, to its degradation. It will be found, when the works of draining and road making and maintenance are examined, that the common practice of making sewers on plans independently of the construction of roads, and roads independently of the arrangements for cleansing and keeping them dry, is always to the disadvantage of the work and to the public. The same surface levels and surveys serve for drainage and for road construction. The construction of the drains for roads and streets, and the maintenance of them, are the primary and most important works; the construction and maintenance of the surface of the road is a connected work, subsequent in order, and can be best superintended by the same officer. In every part of the country inconveniences and losses are experienced from the separation of such work on almost every occasion where repair or new construction is needed. In the towns a road is broken up by the bursting of a sewer or the necessity of cleansing or repairing it; the sewer is repaired, but the road is left broken, because the road surveyor and his separate set of workmen are engaged in some other work. In the metropolis, the breaches left in the roads by the delay and want of concert amongst the various officers are a source not only of great obstruction but of frequent accidents. In replacing the pavements the water and the gaspipes are not unfrequently put out of order, and these again occasion another opening and another expense to the public, for repairs. In the rural districts a road is out of repair, but the first remedy is drainage; the road surveyor cannot proceed because the sewers' surveyor has his men elsewhere occupied. In various other particulars the consolidation of the same work under the same officer, acting with a combined staff of foremen and workmen, is attended with advantages in efficiency and economy to which it were unnecessary to advert, if the opposite arrangements were not the most frequent. In the few instances that have taken place of a combination of duties, the experience of the advantages of the combination would occasion a proposal for separating them to be viewed as an increase of trouble and expense, and a hindrance to the proper execution of the work.

In the districts where the greatest defects prevail, we find such an array of officers for the superintendence of public structures as would lead to the *a priori* conclusion of a high degree of perfection in the work from the apparent subdivision of labour in which it is distributed. In the same petty districts we have surveyors of sewers appointed by the commissioners of sewers, surveyors of turnpike-roads appointed by the trustees of the turnpike trusts, surveyors of highways appointed by the inhabitants in vestry, or by district boards under the Highway Act; paid district surveyors appointed by the justices, surveyors of paving under local Acts, surveyors of building under the Building Act, surveyors of county bridges, &c.

The qualifications of a civil engineer involve the knowledge of the prices of the materials and labour used in construction, and also the preparation of surveys, and the general qualifications for valuations, which are usually enhanced by the extent of the range of different descriptions of property with which the valuator is conversant. The public demands for the services of such officers as valuators are often as mischievously separated and distributed as the services for the construction and maintenance of public works. Thus we have often, within the same districts, one set of persons appointed for the execution of valuations and surveys for the levy of the poor's rates; another set for the surveys and valuations for the assessed taxes; another for the land tax; another for the highway rates; another for the sewers' rates; another for the borough rates; another for the church rates; another for the county rates, where parishes neglect to pay, or are unequally assessed, and for extra-parochial places; another for tithe commutation. And these services are generally badly rendered separately at an undue expense.

pp. 382–4

The high rates of remuneration ordinarily given for fragments of practically irresponsible service, would not only serve to defray the expense of direction by scientific officers, but of execution by trained subordinate officers.

p. 389

2.2 Public Health Act, 1848

The Public Health Act of 1848 was the culmination of a long campaign in which Chadwick's 1842 *Report on the Sanitary Conditions of the Labouring Population of Great Britain*, the agitation of the Health of Towns Association, and the two Reports, 1844 and 1845, of the Royal Commission on the Health of Towns were the crucial factors. The Act, known in its original form as the Health of Towns Bill, had a troubled passage through Parliament, partly because it threatened the powers of the Sewage Commissioners who were responsible for drainage and sewerage in London, and partly because of general opposition to its 'centralizing' tendencies. Lord Morpeth, who as First Commissioner of Woods and Forests was responsible for the Bill, withdrew his first version in 1847 and his second draft left London to be dealt with by separate legislation. On this occasion he had an unwelcome ally, the threat of cholera, the reappearance of which in Europe (from May onwards) underlined the need for sanitary reform.

The Act set up a General Board of Health, with the First Commissioner of Woods and Forests as its President, and two other members, one of whom was to be paid. Edwin Chadwick was appointed as the paid member, and Lord Ashley, later Lord Shaftesbury, as the other. The likelihood that a cholera epidemic was imminent had persuaded Chadwick, during the passage of the Public Health Bill, to agitate for the Board to be given powers to control the precautions against epidemics that were then in the hands of the Privy Council. It was decided that to insert new clauses in the Bill would delay and possibly jeopardize its passage, so a separate Bill was prepared and passed as the Nuisances Removal Act, 1848. This required an Order in Council to bring it into force, but when cholera broke out in Sunderland in September 1848, the necessary Order was obtained, the Act brought into operation and its provisions used to secure the appointment of a doctor, Southwood Smith, as a fourth member of the General Board. His appointment at this time was a temporary one and only became permanent under the Burials Act of 1852, when the General Board were waging a campaign to close down congested graveyards and to stop burials in built-up areas.

It is significant that the appointment of a doctor to the General Board appears almost an afterthought, because Chadwick, at this time probably at the peak of his influence as a sanitary reformer, undoubtedly believed that engineers and legislators had more to contribute to the health of towns than doctors. The Board was soon in headlong collision with the Royal College of Physicians on the subject of precautions against cholera. The College resented the fact that a predominantly lay body should presume to give advice on matters which lay within its province.

In addition to setting up the General Board the Public Health Act of 1848 provided for the creation of local boards of health in places where either one-tenth of the ratepayers petitioned for the Act to be applied, or the average death rate exceeded 23 per 1,000. In the latter case the General Board could act on its own initiative, and apply the Act even against the wishes of the local ratepayers, by securing an Order in Council. When a petition was received the General Board sent down an inspector, who held a public inquiry, and the Board could apply the Act by making a Provisional Order which could, however, later be challenged in Parliament.

As soon as it was created, therefore, the General Board not only had to organize the nation's defences against cholera, but to deal with the petitions that came flooding in for the application of the Act to particular towns and districts. A district where the Act was applied received at very small cost all the powers to deal with nuisances and improve sanitation that had previously only been obtainable through a local Act of Parliament, a troublesome and costly procedure which few localities were prepared to contemplate. Three days after the Board's first meeting, in November 1848, sixty-two petitions had been received and for some time the Board was too busy dealing with these and others which followed to make extensive use of its powers to deal with places where the local mortality rate was excessive. Not until July 1852 did the Board start totting up the places where the mortality exceeded 23 per 1,000 and the Act had not been applied, with a view to taking action against them.

Each of the local boards of health—and nearly 200 were created between 1848 and 1856—were empowered to appoint as an 'officer of health' 'a legally qualified medical practitioner or member of the medical profession', a phrase which was not intended, as the *Lancet* feared, to enable any unqualified quack to be appointed, but merely to get round the fact that at that time some doctors with perfectly respectable qualifications were not legally permitted to practise in London, a legacy of the ancient monopoly of practice in London which had formerly been enjoyed by the Royal College of Physicians.

The post of medical officer of health, as it soon came to be called, was not created by the Public Health Act. The pioneers, William Duncan in Liverpool and John Simon in the City of London, were appointed under local Acts, and the General Board was soon turning to Duncan for advice in the framing of its guidance to local boards on the duties of the medical officer of health. Although boards were empowered to appoint a MOH, they were not obliged to do so, and many of them did not. Again, many of the appointments were temporary, perhaps to deal with a local epidemic, and in the early years nearly all of them were part-time. Some were salaried, others were not. All appointments had, however, to be approved by the General Board.

The policy of the General Board was to press for full-time appointments which precluded private practice, but normally it had to give way on this. In its memorandum of 1851 on the duties of the MOH, it required that the medical officer's annual and quarterly reports should be printed and widely circulated. This, as John Simon had already demonstrated in London, was to place in the hands of the MOH a very powerful weapon, enabling him to expose publicly the vested interests that opposed improved sanitation and other measures to improve the health of the population, and enabling the General Board to bring pressure to bear on local boards when it appeared that the advice of the medical officer was being disregarded.

In its early days the General Board reaped prestige from its fight against the cholera epidemic, and against the vested interests and apathetic Boards of Guardians who sought to hinder it in its work. The reluctance of some of the guardians to incur expense at this time was almost unbelievable; 14,000 people perished from cholera in London alone, yet the authorities were only complying sulkily and half-heartedly with the General Board's measures. Nonetheless, the prestige that the Board gained at this time was soon dissipated. Chadwick, who dominated the Board, was a man with a massive contempt for public opinion and vested interests alike. He claimed a wide scope for state action in an age when the doctrine of *laissez faire* held sway. He held that civil servants generally knew better than politicians, and this led to trouble when Lord Morpeth was succeeded as President of the General Board by Lord Seymour, with whom Chadwick did not see eye to eye. Chadwick made enemies of the London vestrymen through his sweeping schemes of sanitary reform for the metropolis, he made enemies of the civil engineers whose drainage and sewerage schemes he derided. The General Board got into difficulties over a grandiose scheme devised by Chadwick for securing a State monopoly of all burials in the metropolis, and again in London the Board met with defeat in its scheme to reform the water supply.

When the time came to renew the powers of the General Board, in 1854, the opposition seized its opportunity. In Parliament and in the press Chadwick himself was subjected to sustained personal attack. His health had suffered from the strain of the constant struggles of the last five years and he prepared to resign. In the event the opponents of the

General Board ambushed the government in the House of Commons and in a vote that Palmerston described as 'the foulest vote I have ever known in all my parliamentary experience', forced the complete reconstitution of the Board. The new Board was a Board only in name, with a President who accepted full ministerial responsibility for the work of a salaried staff directly accountable to him. In this form, the Board lasted until 1858, when its functions were divided between the Poor Law Board and the Privy Council.

The Public Health Act of 1848 was possibly the most significant piece of health legislation in the nineteenth century. It marked the first clear acceptance by the State of responsibility for the health of the people. In 1805 a Central Board of Health had been created to deal with the threat of a yellow fever epidemic, but once the threat had passed the Board was wound up. Again in 1831 a Central Board was set up to supervise precautions against cholera, and 1,200 local boards were brought into being to act under its supervision. Three years later the Central Board was dissolved and the local boards simply faded away. But the machinery inaugurated in 1848 was intended to be permanent and not simply to meet a particular emergency. Therein lies its significance.

2.3 Public Health Act, 1875

The Public Health Act of 1875 was the last legislative fruit of the work of the Royal Sanitary Commission and it stood as the basis of English public health administration until it was superseded by the equally wide-ranging Act of 1936. The 1875 Act consolidated the provisions of twenty-nine existing pieces of legislation, codifying the law rather than extending it to any great extent. Many of the definitions and provisions were taken almost verbatim from earlier Acts; for example the powers bestowed on sanitary authorities to provide infectious diseases hospitals, taken from the Act of 1866. But for the first time the Act provided a complete statement of the powers and duties of local sanitary authorities, setting out their responsibilities for sewerage and drainage, scavenging and water supply; their powers to provide public lavatories, to control nuisances and offensive trades; and their rights to stop the building of houses without privy accommodation, to inspect and destroy unsound food, to cleanse and disinfect, or destroy, infected bedding, and to provide hospitals. This was clearly the age when the health of the people was to be improved through control of the environment, a necessary stage before any meaningful attempt could be made to influence more personal factors relevant to health, and a stage which reflected both existing disease patterns and the current state of scientific knowledge. Bacteriology was in its infancy and one death in three between 1848 and 1872 was due to infectious disease; there were recurrent epidemics of cholera and smallpox.

In the last quarter of the nineteenth century the situation improved dramatically, and although the causes of this improvement are likely to have been complex and multiple, substantial credit at least must go to the system of sanitary control embodied in—though not, as has been said, inaugurated by—the Act of 1875. Between 1875 and 1900 the mean annual death rate fell from 23·3 to 18·8 per 1,000 population for males; and from 20·7 to 16·6 for females. The last serious epidemic of cholera was in 1866—and this was undoubtedly the disease which had given more impetus than any other to the sanitary movement; the last serious epidemic of smallpox was in 1871. Death rates from typhus, typhoid, scarlet fever and tuberculosis all fell markedly in the last quarter of the nineteenth century.

The chief extensions to existing law which were introduced in the 1875 Act were to increase the powers of local authorities over gas and water supply, the inclusion of houses occupied by a single family in the provisions relating to overcrowding, and provisions to remedy some of the defects of the 1872 Act by enabling the Local Government Board to combine districts and create machinery to maintain full-time medical officers of health to serve the combined districts.

In its form, logical, coherent and lucid, the Act owed much to the draft Bill which had been prepared by the Royal Sanitary Commission, but even more perhaps to patient work by John Simon, medical officer to the Local Government Board, and the government lawyers. Simon did not get all his own way, and in certain respects the Act was less innovatory than he wished—for example he was anxious to establish at this time the national system for notification of infectious diseases which only came into being much later—so he did not attach the importance which later generations have attached either to the Act or his own work on it. In the following year, disappointed and frustrated in his work at the Local Government Board at the subordination of the medical department to the administrators, and of medical science to the traditions of Poor Law administration, John Simon left the public service. Full official recognition of his work as medical officer did not come until 1887, when he was awarded the KCB.

The marriage of public health administration to the Poor Law was not, even allowing for the understandable bitterness of Simon, an entirely happy one. Much was indeed accomplished under the supervision of the Local Government Board, but dominated as it was by ex-Poor Law officials, its interpretation of the law was often narrow and legalistic. Local authorities were slow to take advantage of the opportunities given them in the Acts of 1866 and 1875 to build hospitals outside the provisions of the Poor Law, and so patients with infectious diseases who were by no means paupers in many cases had to be admitted to Poor Law infirmaries, which meant, for those entitled to vote, automatic disenfranchisement. The officials of the LGB stuck stubbornly to the letter of the law until it was changed in 1885, and some of them were still lamenting the change twenty years later when they gave evidence to the Royal Commission on the Poor Laws. Similarly the LGB withheld permission from a local authority to build a maternity hospital because although the 1875 Act had authorized the building of hospitals for the sick, childbirth was not sickness 'within the meaning of the Act'.

2.4 Public Health Act, 1936

The 1875 Act stood as the basic public health legislation for sixty years, but by the 1930s there was again a need for consolidation, and in 1930 a departmental committee was set up by the Minister of Health, Mr Greenwood, to consider the whole field of public health law. The committee sat for five years under the chairmanship first of Lord Chelmsford and later of Lord Addington, and produced recommendations which were incorporated in the Public Health Act of 1936. This Act was essentially a work of consolidation and codification, and attracted little controversy in Parliament or the press as it passed through the two Houses. The Act was accompanied by a separate Act dealing with London, but otherwise, with certain minor exceptions, applied to the whole of England and Wales.

This measure consolidated into its 356 sections some 600 sections from fifty-five previous Acts and served in its turn as the basic public health legislation up to the present time. Most of the changes made in the process of consolidation were minor ones designed to bring about some uniformity between the powers of different local authorities. In addition a number of adoptive Acts were incorporated into general law, and thus applied to the country as a whole and not merely to those localities that chose to adopt them.

However, while the 1936 Act marked no new departure of principle, its wide coverage provides the opportunity to indicate the scope of the powers and interests in the public health field that local authorities had by then acquired.

Part I dealt with local administration and the powers of local health authorities. Part II covered sanitation and buildings, including sewerage and sewage disposal, building standards, fire precautions, the removal of refuse, public conveniences, and provisions enabling local authorities to take action against filthy or verminous premises. In 1961 greater uniformity was introduced in the administration of these provisions through the introduction of regulations made under the Public Health Act of that year in place of by-laws made locally under the Act of 1936.

Part III dealt with nuisances and offensive trades, including smoke nuisance, but powers to deal with and to prevent atmospheric pollution were greatly extended under the Clean Air Act of 1956, which implemented the recommendations of the Beaver Committee on Air Pollution, 1953-4. The Noise Abatement Act, 1960, provided that noise or vibration might be a statutory nuisance under the 1936 Act.

Part IV was devoted to water supply, and included clauses on waterworks and other sources of supply, public wells, pumps etc., the prevention of waste of water, charges for water, the powers of local authorities to require homes to be supplied with water, and the protection of the public from polluted water. This part was in due course amended by the Water Act of 1945, which made further provision for the conservation and use of water supplies.

Part V provided for the prevention, notification and treatment of infectious diseases and also included provisions with respect to the blind. Part III of the Public Health Act, 1961, further strengthened the powers of medical officers of health to control the spread of infectious diseases.

Part VI dealt with hospitals and nursing homes and under this part local authority hospitals were for the first time given specific authority to provide outpatient departments. Lack of this specific authority had not prevented nearly 1,500,000 outpatient consultations from taking place in local authority hospitals in 1935, but many of these would have been former in-patients being seen for follow-up purposes. After 1936 there was a marked expansion in outpatient services in local authority hospitals. Further controls over nursing homes were enacted in the Nursing Homes Act of 1963 and power given to local authorities to prosecute for breaches of regulations under this Act repaired a serious loophole in the 1936 Act.

Part VII consolidated provisions relating to the notification of births, maternity and child welfare, and child life protection; while Part VIII regulated baths, washhouses and bathing places. Part IX dealt with common lodging houses, Part X with canal boats, and Part XI with such miscellaneous topics as watercourses, ditches, ships and boats, tents, vans, sheds, and the health of hop-pickers. Part XII included various clauses relating to administration, enforcement and interpretation.

Some of the examples quoted illustrate how this massive piece of legislation, while acting as the basis of health authorities' powers to deal with environmental threats to health, has subsequently been added to or strengthened by further legislation. There is no sign at the time of writing that the Act has outlived its usefulness, although with the reorganization of the health service and of local government in 1974 it has obviously been necessary to transfer many of the powers granted to local authorities in 1936 to the new health authorities. This has not invariably been the case, however, for the new local authorities themselves retain important responsibilities for environmental control, as distinct from personal health services.

2.5 An Inquiry into Health Visiting (Jameson Report)

Report of a Working Party

Published: 1956

Chairman: *Sir Wilson Jameson GBE, KCB, MD, FRCP*

Members: *A. Beauchamp OBE, MB, ChB, MRCS, LRCP; Alderman Mrs M. Chambers CBE, LLD, JP; Miss E. W. Himsworth RGN, SCM, QN, HV Cert; Miss E. Stephenson SRN, RFN, SCM, HV Cert; J. F. Warin MD, DPH; R. Pronger and M. H. Cook (joint secretaries)*

Terms of Reference (1953): *To advise on the proper field of work, the recruitment and training of health visitors in the National Health Service and School Health Service.*

Health visiting started in the north of England, when in 1862 the Ladies' Sanitary Reform Association of Manchester and Salford employed women to visit working class homes and teach the rudiments of hygiene and child-rearing. By 1890 the experiment had sufficiently proved its value to persuade Manchester Corporation to pay the salaries of some of the visitors. Buckinghamshire County Council, encouraged by Florence Nightingale, engaged women to do similar work in 1892, and other authorities soon followed. The Maternity and Child Welfare Act of 1918 confirmed the tendency of health visitors to concentrate their attention on families with young children, and this bias was clear in the early training schemes. In 1919 the newly established Ministry of Health and the Board of Education jointly sponsored a two-year course of training, but laid it down that trained nurses, graduates and women with three years' experience of health visiting might take a one-year course. Many of the early health visitors had been women sanitary inspectors, some even women doctors.

In 1925 the Royal Sanitary Institute (later Royal Society for the Promotion of Health) became the central examining body and trained nurses were allowed to qualify as health visitors in six months, provided they were also trained midwives (the length of the midwifery course was then also six months for trained nurses). Between the wars the pattern became firmly established whereby a health visitor was a trained nurse and midwife who had undergone a further six-month training in public health. All other avenues of entry to the profession became exceptional. When midwifery training for registered nurses was extended to one year, divided into two six-month parts, in 1938, it was laid down that Part 1 (the hospital-based part) was sufficient for entry to health visitor training.

The start of the National Health Service brought two major developments in health visiting. All health visitors were now required to be qualified—previously many of those working for voluntary associations (and some local authorities contracted with voluntary organizations to provide health visiting and district nursing services) had had no formal training. Secondly, the National Health Service Act widened the scope of the health visitor's work by requiring her to give 'advice as to the care of persons suffering from illness and as to measures necessary to prevent the spread of infection'. In a circular the Ministry emphasized that after the appointed day the health visitor would be concerned with the health of the household as a whole. This perhaps was not so very different from the role that had been envisaged for the health visitor in Salford in the 1860s or in Buckinghamshire in the 1890s, but the emphasis it was necessary to lay on the wording of the Act was a mark of the extent to which the health visiting profession had become almost exclusively concerned— with the exception of some specialist workers, such as TB visitors—with the welfare of mothers and young children. It was to be some years before this shift of emphasis actually became evident in the day-to-day work of any large number of health visitors.

By the early 1950s there were more than 6,000 health visitors employed in England and Wales. Since many of these worked part-time, this made the equivalent of rather more than 4,000 full-time workers. In rural areas the same person often combined the duties of health visitor, district nurse, school nurse and midwife. This degree of versatility was not often required of the urban health visitor, but it was the policy in a number of urban authorities to combine the duties of school nurse and health visitor. The health visitor as such still spent more time on duties related to maternal and child welfare than on any other type of duty and divided her time for the most part between clinic duties and visiting mothers and children at home.

The Jameson Report defined the function of the health visitor as 'primarily . . . health education and social advice', but with the emphasis firmly on health education. The health visitor should continue, the report said, to keep contact with all families where there were children, but should be prepared to extend her role to become a general family visitor.

She had an important contribution to make in such fields as mental health, hospital after-care and the care of the aged. She could provide a link to a wide variety of more specialized services and workers when required. Since the working party suggested 2,000 visits a year as a suitable work-load for one health visitor it was clear that it was not envisaged she would ever undertake case-work in depth.

Specialization in a particular aspect of health visiting was deprecated, but the combination of health visiting with other public health nursing duties was accepted as for the time being inevitable in areas where other-wise the service could not be adequately or economically staffed. It was, however, felt that even in such areas health visiting would in the future need to be a full-time job if it were to develop on the lines suggested. The introduction of a new grade of health visitor, the 'group adviser', between the field workers and the administrative staff, was suggested as a way of creating posts in which experienced health visitors with further training could give close support to less experienced staff, who could if necessary refer particularly difficult cases to them. The further develop-ment of health visiting envisaged by the working party would, it was thought, require the recruitment of an additional 3,500 health visitors over the next ten years. To reach and maintain this figure it would be necessary to increase the number of new health visitors trained annually from 640 to 1,100.

The working party recommended that registration as a nurse should continue to be a prerequisite for training as a health visitor, but did not consider that Part 1 of the midwifery certificate provided suitable training in maternity care for future domiciliary workers. They therefore recom-mended that intending health visitors should either be fully qualified midwives, having done both parts of the midwifery training, or have undergone a special three-month course in aspects of midwifery relevant to health visiting. The report expressed interest in the development of integrated courses embodying general nursing, maternity and public health training, which would appeal to those who knew at an early stage that health visiting would be their chosen field of work.

The other principal recommendation was that a new central training body should be set up (for England and Wales; Scotland would have its own), with representation of professional interests, employing authorities, and educational interests, to devise a national syllabus, approve courses and appoint examiners.

The Jameson Report was followed in due course by the Health Visiting and Social Work (Training) Act, 1962, which set up the Council for the Training of Health Visitors on the lines recommended in the report. When the General Nursing Council introduced a three-month obstetric nursing course as an optional element in general nurse training, this was accepted as providing a satisfactory basis for the intending health visitor.

The grade of group adviser was introduced and the numbers of training places were expanded. During the 1960s health visiting in many areas moved towards a far closer relationship with general medical practice than had been envisaged by the Jameson working party. The working party had emphasized the need for good relationships and co-operation between health visitors and general practitioners, but felt this situation could best be achieved by organizing health visitors' work on an area basis, with clearly defined arrangements for liaison with practices in the area.

What in fact developed was the system, pioneered in the City of Oxford, of attaching health visitors (and in some areas home nurses and midwives also) to particular practices—it was easier where doctors worked in groups—so that instead of visiting families in a defined geographical area they visited families whose members were patients of the practice, wherever they happened to live. The Jameson working party seemed to have hardly considered this possibility, commenting briefly: 'It will often not be possible to make Health Visitors' areas and doctors' practices coincide. One team of Health Visitors may well be working with a number of doctors, but the fact that areas of operation do not coincide should present no insuperable difficulties.'

Less than fifteen years later it was generally accepted that where it was at all practicable, attachment to a group general practice was the most fruitful way of using a health visitor's skills. By that time, too, the employment of an increasing number of ancillary workers, clinic nurses, clerks etc., in the public health service was helping local authorities to meet some of the criticisms the Jameson Report had made of the wasteful use of health visitors to do work that did not require their degree of skill.

Jameson Report, 1956

THE WORK OF THE HEALTH VISITOR

Health Visiting emerged in the first decades of this century from the activities of a variety of public health workers as specialised health education directed to mothers and young children in their own homes. Having its origins in voluntary effort, it is now almost exclusively a public service. Its object has been primarily to persuade, guide, advise, direct mothers in ways of health and it undoubtedly has had great success. The same kind of need for health education has been manifest in the schools and school nurses who undertake such work are expected to be qualified Health Visitors. In these, the main fields of employment, the Health Visitor is primarily concerned with the healthy and her object is to preserve health and watch for early signs of departure from the normal; she visits her families at intervals and is not associated necessarily with crisis. Health Visitors also have, however, responsibilities in relation to communicable diseases generally, and in particular for the tuberculosis visiting service. Here they are concerned with the situation produced by an illness; they come on the scene when help is required and leave it when help is no longer needed. In addition, a small proportion of all Health Visitors act, in country areas—especially in Scotland—as nurses and midwives, or, more accurately, the latter act as Health Visitors. Though the Health Visiting functions of such workers are fairly distinct, their relationships with clients and colleagues are also rather different from those of the full-time Health Visitor. No objective study of the relative effectiveness of these varying types of workers has been made, and it would present great difficulties. Policy is determined by local opinion and experience.

A general improvement in the physical health of the population, and especially in the health of mothers and children, must necessarily affect the Health Visitor in her role as health educator. It would be claimed by some that the need for attention to the healthy has diminished. The work is affected in another way. Mothers with their children now have the opportunity for free consultation with a family doctor. It may be expected that doctors will be increasingly concerned with child welfare and that the Health Visitor will necessarily be associated with them.

Besides being a health educator, the Health Visitor has always obviously been faced with the necessity for giving social advice and taking social action to make effective the health education that is her primary concern. Dirt, squalor, neglect and illness can hardly be remedied by education only; the Health Visitor has always had to 'pitch in' and find some way of helping clients to better material standards. The Health Visitor has always, however, been expected to carry a large case-load and much of her work is concerned with people not in social need. Except in times of crisis, it can be assumed that social action could only have been secondary to her main task. The war and the period of reconstruction have been times of great social change. Social welfare legislation has created or developed services which offer increasing opportunities of service to a variety of social workers. We can safely assume that the social aspects of Health Visitors' work have reflected the new situation. Our studies—limited as they were—suggest strongly that the purely social element in visiting for health purposes has increased and is larger than many suppose. It still does not, however, constitute more than an incidental aspect of the main purpose; Health Visitors go to their clients for health education purposes, not primarily to remedy social difficulties. Social welfare as a whole is highly complex and many branches of it call for expert knowledge. Even if this were not so, the shortage of Health Visitors, concentration on the purpose of health education and the great variety of problems thrown up by the Health Visitor's peculiarly extensive clientele would have prevented much more from being done. In the event, other and 'non-medical' workers have been developed or created to do this work, which may arise both with families where there are mothers and children and with other families. These workers are usually specialised in the sense that they are concerned with one aspect of service or one relatively limited class of clientele in need, but they may be non-specialised in the sense that they may organise for their limited clientele a very wide range of services and facilities. They thus contrast with the Health Visitor, with her fairly narrow *main* purpose directed to a very wide and actively visited clientele not necessarily in obvious social or economic need.

The nature of the problems which face all concerned with medico-social problems seems also to be affected by marked improvements in material conditions. Problems overlaid while material improvement was of first urgency are now thrown into relief. The general raising of standards, for example, makes embarrassingly obvious the relatively few incompetent families whose chronic inability to achieve the minimum standards now set by their neighbours has earned them the title of 'problem families'. These unfortunate families may well be, however, merely the most obvious sign of the social ill-health that many think is endemic in a modern industrial society. Physical and mental ill-health and cultural and social patterns are all involved and the part played by each factor cannot clearly be seen. There is no sign of a comprehensive diagnosis, to say nothing of a cure, and perhaps to hope for one is too optimistic. All that can be attempted, at present, is to deal with breakdown as it occurs and to seek to avoid breakdown by early observation and preventive action. Not only humanity but economy makes the attempt desirable. Much physical illness and maldevelopment can, for example, be prevented by timely advice and help; the social and economic effects of illness can be mitigated; the parents who cannot manage, the aged and handicapped who are losing their ability to manage, can be supported if helped in time. It is widely held that much mental illness has its roots in social conditions generally and especially in faulty relationships within the small socially isolated family unit. The emphasis naturally lies on family welfare in a wide sense, with the mother and growing children, as the most vulnerable group, in greatest need of protection. Both clinicians and sociologists clearly have their part to play.

If a comprehensive approach is as yet impossible, it is at least desirable that fragmentary approaches should be co-ordinated. The 'problem family' attracts many social agencies and the need for a planned approach in this case is obvious and is heavily underlined in Government circulars. It is, however, only a special case of what may well happen to a lesser degree in less spectacular cases of need with equal possibilities of frustrated effort and of confusion for the family. There is a wide-spread demand for a more rational ordering of visitation of families for health and welfare purposes generally and it is often suggested that as much as possible should be done by an 'all-purpose' visitor. The practical objections to any proposal for an omnicompetent visitor are, of course, insuperable. No single worker can command the range of knowledge and ability required to observe, diagnose and provide a remedy for all medical and social problems of families in modern conditions. There may well be possibilities, however, in a limited approach. Much might be done towards reducing the number of visitors to the home and co-ordinating family welfare, if one worker with a well recognised function useful to a wide range of families at risk could act as a 'common factor' in various medical and social teams that are dealing with a part of the total social problem. Such a worker could act as a 'case finder' and rapporteur, given sufficient knowledge to recognise and describe the situation that calls for the services of other experts and to co-operate with and support their work. The Health Visitor naturally needs to be considered in this connection since she might fulfil a number of the requirements.

A wide variety of opinions about the future of Health Visiting have been expressed to us. It is fair to say that those with a medical background and those with a social science background have been in opposite camps. There is some common ground between them however. It is fairly generally agreed that the field work of Health Visitors should be among families where there are mothers with young children and that their main function should still be health education. This should be concerned with not only physical but also mental hygiene and should take account of family circumstances as a whole, so far as they can be ascertained. Equally it is agreed that health education should or could extend to such classes as the school-child, the tuberculous, the aged and chronic sick. In carrying out a health education function the Health Visitor would overlap other workers only in the sense that she was concerned with the same families. Disagreement begins with consideration of the social aspects of her work. Witnesses whose background was medical in character were advocates of the Health Visitor as a general family social worker. They thought she had special advantages because of her 'health' background, since there were health aspects to so many cases and because of her wide field of visiting for a generally acceptable purpose. Witnesses from the social science group were inclined to accept the possibility of a general family visitor (while pointing out the practical difficulties), but they doubted for a number of reasons whether the Health Visitor was suitable for the role or whether it was wise to distract her from her valuable task of health education by making her more of a social worker. Wide as it was, her field of visiting for her present purposes covered only perhaps one quarter of all families at any one time; to cover more she must give up some work. The general family visitor would, they thought, need a social worker's training not less intensive than social workers received—much longer than the Health Visitor's own public health course. Case-work functions were beyond the competence of those without proper preparation for them. They were too time-consuming to be shared with other functions and required an entirely different approach and work load from that of a routine visitor.

We shall have these views in mind in considering the field in which Health Visitors should work in future and what limitations must, of practical necessity, be put on that field. We should, however, also consider what additional functions may be added, to take the fullest advantage of a wide range of visiting. Even now the Health Visitor is in no sense an exclusive visitor. Many other workers, notably the general practitioner, have a close interest in the same subjects. As we have noted elsewhere, moreover, another Working Party has already begun to consider the role and the training of social workers in much the same field that the Health Visitor will occupy. We shall, therefore, find it necessary to consider her relationship with other workers, avoiding however rigid lines of demarcation which seem singularly inappropriate to family welfare. We shall need to review in general terms the training required leaving it to the appropriate training body, however, to work out details that may well need to be constantly reviewed to meet changing circumstances. We have noted that many think the training and experience required as a whole is unbalanced and the public health part of it too short, too formal and too cramped. We shall need to look at conditions of service generally.

Recruitment, training and field of work, are, however, interdependent. We shall bear in mind, throughout our recommendations about the Health Visitor's work, the numbers of staff of a given quality that might be attracted by reasonably good conditions of service to the profession and the kind of training that could suitably be given to them.

paras. 285–92

A FAMILY VISITOR?

A number of points stand out from our recommendations. Firstly it is obvious that the Health Visitor will have the opportunity for making contact with an extremely wide range of families. Already her work in the local health and education services may take her to perhaps two-fifths of all families and households and these will be mainly families with children, in some respects perhaps the most vulnerable group. The close association with general practitioners which we are confident will be developed will greatly add to the number of families within her field since she will be concerned also with families where there are no children. Probably in this way she may be in touch with the majority of families and households who are in need of help because there is some problem of physical or mental health. Secondly, she will be visiting for a recognised and useful purpose with the backing either of a statutory body or the family doctor. Thirdly, she will be concerned in every case with the affairs of a family and not merely with individuals. Fourthly she will inevitably be confronted with an even wider range of problems than at present, a much larger proportion of which will be "psycho-social" in character than hitherto, and will be brought into closer touch with a wider range of workers who specialise in such problems.

It would, of course, be foolish to suppose that the Health Visitor could be equally effective in all aspects of family welfare. We expect on the contrary that she will be really expert in only a few, mainly those where problems of health are dominant. It would be rash, too, to expect that all Health Visitors could adapt themselves to a wider role with equal ease. At the same time we are satisfied that the training of the Health Visitor could be so arranged that she would be better able to appreciate the problems that other workers face and the way in which they deal with them. She could thus be put into a position to observe the early signs of distress in fields in which she is not (and need not be) an expert, to consult with the appropriate worker and to help in any measures that may be arranged. Where no such advice was available she could assess what "first aid" measures she could herself safely apply. She would thus have the opportunity to share in the work of a variety of family health and welfare teams that without her might have no common membership. Her contribution would be to act as a common point of reference, a common source of information of a standard kind, a common adviser on health teaching—in a real sense, a "common factor" in family welfare. She could help to eliminate continual visiting of one family by a number of workers for purposes that are essentially the same, in particular by relieving others of the need for purely supportive visits. In many respects, therefore, it appears to us that she could satisfy the requirements for a general purpose family visitor that we outlined in Chapter IX.

paras. 314–15

2.6 Chronically Sick and Disabled Persons Act, 1970

The Chronically Sick and Disabled Persons Act was very largely the handiwork of Alfred Morris MP, who introduced it as a private member's Bill at a time when his party was in Opposition, but who had the support not only of members on both sides of the House but also of a number of voluntary organizations which had been campaigning for some years for better services and facilities for the disabled. The extent of the problem was demonstrated by figures quoted by Morris from a government survey: at least 3 million adults disabled in some degree; upwards of 1·25 million adults under the age of sixty-five disabled severely; 200,000 families with a severely disabled member but without an inside lavatory. One in five of the severely disabled, he claimed, lived alone, without the help of welfare services. For many years local health and welfare authorities had had permissive powers to provide services and assistance for these people, but Morris's Act for the first time laid on local authorities the duty of seeking out the disabled and making adequate services available to them.

Section 2 of the Act listed the facilities local authorities were called on to provide, ranging from help in adapting the home of a disabled person to meet his special needs, to making arrangements for him to have a holiday. Sections 4–8 were concerned with ensuring that all buildings open to the public, including schools, universities and colleges, were provided with means of access and toilet facilities suitable for disabled people, and Sections 9–15 with providing that disabled people should be represented on a number of government advisory bodies and local authority committees. Sections 17 and 18 dealt tentatively with the pathetic problem of the young chronic sick admitted to institutional care who were so often admitted to geriatric wards or old people's welfare homes simply because there were no other facilities for long-term care. A few voluntary organizations, such as the Cheshire Homes, had made the young chronic sick their special concern, but there was little specific provision in the public sector, and the Act attempted to give a spur to hospital and local authorities by providing that hospitals should 'use their best endeavours' to ensure 'so far as is practicable' that the young chronic sick were not cared for in geriatric wards. Local authorities were required to send returns to the Secretary of State of the numbers of young chronic sick being cared for in premises intended for the elderly. It remains to be seen how far these 'best endeavours' are successful and to what extent the saving clause 'so far as is practicable' is used as an escape hatch, but as soon as his Act was passed Alfred Morris set about belabouring local authorities slow off the mark to meet their new obligations. Birmingham, he pointed out, had provided disabled people with whistles to summon help in emergency, but Manchester had installed 400 telephones. Local authorities that were dragging their feet, he said, were dragging them at the expense of those with no feet to drag.

2.7 Report of the Committee on the Working of the Abortion Act (Lane Report)

Published: 1974

Chairman: *The Hon. Mrs Justice Lane DBE*

Members: *Miss Josephine Barnes DM, FRCP, FRCS, FRCOG; Mrs Kate Barratt JP; Professor I. R. C. Batchelor MB, ChB, FRCPE, FRCPsych., DPM, FRSE; Mrs Juliet Cheetham MA; Miss J. W. Gutteridge; R. D. Ireland QC;* A. M. Johnston QC;* Mrs Eva Learner BA, Dip. Social Studies; Miss M. E. Munro SRN, SCM; D. J. Pereira Gray MA, MB, BChir, FRCGP; Miss Diana M. Rasbach BA; E. Rosemary Rue MB, MRCP, DCH, FFCM; Professor A. C. Turnbull MD, FRCOG; D. J. Wilson FRCGP; Miss R. B. Worsley SRN, SCM, MTD, FHA; R. P. S. Hughes (secretary June 1971–March 1973); M. E. G. Fogden (secretary from March 1973); D. Rothman BSc, MB, BS, MRCOG, (medical secretary)*

*Mr Johnston resigned in October 1971 and was succeeded by Mr Ireland

Terms of Reference (1971): *To review the operation of the Abortion Act 1967 and on the basis that the conditions for legal abortions contained in paragraphs (a) and (b) of subsection (1) and in subsections (2), (3) and (4) of section 1 of the Act remain unaltered, to make recommendations.*

The Abortion Act, 1967, was the result of a private member's Bill introduced by Liberal M.P. David Steel, and the culmination of thirty years' campaigning by numerous individuals and organizations, notably by the Abortion Law Reform Association, founded in 1936, which in its early years numbered among its advisers Lord Horder, one of the most eminent medical figures of his time. Before the Act the law on abortion was in an ambiguous and unsatisfactory state. The Offences Against the Person Act of 1861 had laid down that to induce, or attempt to induce, an abortion unlawfully was a felony punishable by life imprisonment. However, the use of the word 'unlawfully' had implied the existence of a loophole, that some abortions could be lawful, and this loophole was eventually defined by Mr Justice Macnaghten in the Bourne case of 1938 in words which guided practice for the next twenty-nine years. Mr Justice Macnaghten held that certain words used in the Infant Life (Preservation) Act of 1929 indicated that abortion was not unlawful if done in good faith to save the mother's life. He went on to tell the jury that:

> If the doctor is of the opinion on reasonable grounds and with adequate knowledge that the probable consequences of the continuance of the pregnancy will be to make the woman a physical and mental wreck, the jury is quite entitled to take the view that the doctor, who, under these circumstances and in that honest belief, operates, is operating for the purpose of preserving the life of the mother.

Following this direction, Bourne, a prominent gynaecologist who aborted a girl of fourteen following her rape by two soldiers, was acquitted, and the judge's use of the term 'mental wreck' ensured that it would become common practice to refer a woman who sought an abortion to a psychiatrist for his opinion. On the other hand, doctors who took a liberal view of what the law allowed were treading a tightrope. If their good faith could be called in question, then they faced severe sentences; many of them chose not to take the risk and interpreted the law with the utmost caution. Their patients, and of course the patients of most doctors who professed the Roman Catholic faith, found themselves faced with the alternatives of allowing the pregnancy to continue or of seeking the services of a back-street abortionist. Women who took the latter course faced hazards from faulty technique and dirty instruments that in many cases led to death or disability. In latter years abortion was second only to suicide as a cause of death in women between the ages of twenty-five and forty-four.

Several attempts were made to reform the law before Mr Steel was eventually successful in securing the passage of his Bill. As passed, it confirmed the Bourne judgment that abortion was lawful if the continuance of the pregnancy would involve risk to the life of the pregnant woman, but went on to widen the grounds on which abortion could lawfully be performed to include the risk of injury to the physical or mental health of the pregnant woman or any existing children of her family. The risk did not have to be severe, only greater than the risk involved in the termination of the pregnancy (generally agreed in cases terminated before twelve weeks to be very small). Social factors ('the pregnant woman's actual or reasonably foreseeable environments') were allowed to be taken into account. The Act provided that abortions should only be carried out in National Health Service hospitals or other premises approved by the Minister, that they should be notified to the chief medical officer of the

Ministry of Health or Scottish Home and Health Department. A conscience clause was inserted for the benefit of Roman Catholic and other nurses who might object to being required to assist at abortion operations as part of their employment.

Opposition to the Act did not cease once it had become law. Abortion was still strictly only available on certain defined grounds, however these may have been widened, and in parts of the country where many doctors, and especially gynaecologists, were opposed to abortion on principle it was still difficult for women to secure the relief they sought. The opposition—the Friends of the Foetus as one writer dubbed them—missed no opportunity to claim that NHS hospitals were overwhelmed with demands for abortion and that other patients were being denied facilities in order that these might be met. The numbers of foreign women coming to Britain to take advantage of her relatively liberal laws were held to show that Britain was becoming the abortion centre of the world. Private clinics licensed by the Minister were said to be making exorbitant profits. In February 1971 the Government were sufficiently concerned to set up a committee of inquiry into the working of the Act under the chairmanship of Mrs Justice Lane. Nonetheless, in answer to a parliamentary question, Sir Keith Joseph, Secretary of State for Social Services, made it clear that 'The Enquiry will be concerned with the way the Act is working and not with the principles that underlie it.'

The committee considered a mass of evidence and commissioned some special surveys. The report was accompanied by two further volumes setting out statistical material and survey findings. Aspects considered ranged from such questions as the allegation that abortion virtually on demand was being widely practised, contrary to the intentions of Parliament, and that excessive profits were being made in the private sector, to details of surgical technique. The report rejected calls for restrictive amendments of the legislation, save on a few matters of detail. It accepted that there was inequality of access to the possibility of an abortion for women living in different parts of the country and pointed out that following the Abortion Act there was a statutory obligation on the NHS, stemming from the National Health Service Act of 1946, to provide hospital and specialist services for abortion sufficient 'to meet all reasonable requirements'. This obligation was not being met, the committee argued, in regions where lack of NHS facilities forced women to seek abortion in the private sector.

The committee considered the many suggestions that had been made for the establishment of specialist abortion units within the NHS, but felt that the disadvantages of separating abortion services from the rest of the specialty of gynaecology and obstetrics outweighed the advantages. They accepted, although reluctantly, that the obligation of the NHS to provide abortion services would mean that on occasion doctors with a conscientious objection to abortion would be discriminated against when applying for certain consultant appointments. No restriction on the right of non-resident foreign women to obtain abortion through the private sector was felt necessary for the time being, although it was recognized that abuses did exist and that if these continued legislation might be necessary.

Lane Report, 1974

SUMMARY OF CONCLUSIONS

The passing of the Act exposed many personal problems in the lives of contemporary women which had previously been hidden and the inadequacy of the services which had been instituted to alleviate these problems. By facilitating a greatly increased number of abortions the Act has relieved a vast amount of individual suffering. It has helped also to focus attention on the paramount need for preventive action, for more education in sexual life and its responsibilities, and for the widespread provision of contraceptive advice and facilities. It has served to stimulate research into all aspects of abortion and the development of safer operative techniques. These have been undeniably great benefits.

On the other hand, the passing of the Act, resulting in a greatly increased number of those seeking legal abortions, has imposed considerable strain on the N.H.S. The medical and nursing professions had scant time in which to adapt their attitudes and practice to a radically new situation and views tended initially to become polarised for and against the Act. Neither was the N.H.S. in numbers of staff and facilities equipped to meet the heavy demand for increased services. This had led to marked inequalities over the country in the provision of services. Too many women have been forced to pay for abortions when they had legitimate medical grounds for termination of pregnancy under the Act.

The real and apparent inequalities in the ease with which abortion is now obtained have been the focus of much questioning and criticism. We have no doubt that the inequalities have been too great, when one individual is compared with another, or certain hospitals or regions with others, or the N.H.S. with the private sector. It is also necessary to state that inequalities cannot be abolished altogether. The only constant in the situation is a pregnancy. There is no uniformity in the personalities and physical state of the women concerned, in the situations in which their pregnancies have arisen or in their reactions to these pregnancies. On problems which are so individual and in many respects subjective, the doctor brings to bear a clinical judgement which is also necessarily, in part at least, individual and subjective. It is in his discretion, under the Act, to decide what is best for the woman and to recommend or refuse to recommend abortion. This means inevitably that some women, whose circumstances may appear to be similar, will be treated differently. Yet we are of opinion, for reasons which we state in the body of this Report that in principle, and in the great majority of instances it is in the woman's own interest that the decision should remain a medical one.

The private sector has enabled many patients to have treatment in the privacy and with the amenities they desire, and has compensated for many deficiencies in the provision of services by the N.H.S. At the same time, it has contributed to the inequalities of which many responsible people complain. A small number of doctors, and their financial backers, have used the Act to make large sums of money; and there have been instances of gross irresponsibility in private medical practice. Some women have used the Act and the fact that they could afford private treatment to get an abortion on comparatively trivial grounds of inconvenience or embarrassment to themselves. In short, in some parts of the commercial private sector the provisions of the Act have been flouted and abortion on request has been the rule.

We are convinced that these abuses have been confined to a small minority of doctors. The great majority of the abortions which have been carried out in the N.H.S. and very many in the private sector have been, we believe, fully justified under the Act; we are fortified in this view by the evidence we have had from many witnesses that the closer one is brought into contact with the individual and her situation, the more clearly is the decision to abort seen to be justified.

For the reasons we have outlined above, and which are much more fully dealt with in the body of the Report, we are unanimous in supporting the Act and its provisions. We have no doubt that the gains facilitated by the Act have much outweighed any disadvantages for which it has been criticised. The problems which we have identified in its working, and they are admittedly considerable, are problems for which solutions should be sought by administrative and professional action, and by better education of the public. They are not, we believe, indications that the grounds set out in the Act should be amended in a restrictive way. To do so when the number of unwanted pregnancies is increasing and before comprehensive services are available to all who need them would be to increase the sum of human suffering and ill-health, and probably to drive more women to seek the squalid and dangerous help of the back-street abortionist.

The tests we have applied in coming to this conclusion will be seen to be pragmatic; but we have not been insensitive to the ethical implications of our standpoint. That the operation to abort a fetus violates the sanctity of life or extinguishes the potentiality of a life makes the decision to operate one which calls for the most serious consideration. To have to balance the life of the fetus against the health and well-being of the mother and of her existing children presents both patient and doctor with a dilemma which challenges in a most acute and often agonising form the individual consciences of both. An individual decision it must however remain: as a Committee we can only acknowledge its significance for the moral life of the individual and of society, and seek to ensure in our recommendations that such decisions are made with all the deliberation, care and earnestness they merit.

There is of course another decision for the individual conscience and that is whether or not to take any part in abortion work. No doctor or nurse is required to participate in the treatment authorised by the Act, if he or she has a conscientious objection to it on religious or ethical grounds. This is entirely proper, it is a traditional freedom which must be jealously guarded, and we have found that generally it is being very well respected. Where there is disagreement between what the individual wishes to avoid and has to do, it is far more often that he has been driven by his own feelings of loyalty and fairness to his colleagues, and by a perception of the patients' needs, into conflict with his sense of the wrongness of abortion than because he has been under any duress from seniors to take part in the work. Some of the most difficult decisions, with serious ethical implications, arise in connection with staff appointments: should priority be given to the individual's claim for religious tolerance and his right conscientiously to refuse to take part in abortion work, or to the obligation of the N.H.S. to provide a service for its patients who need abortion? We have stated the view that sometimes the needs of the many must take priority and that inevitably some who refuse this work may not obtain a particular appointment; but we came to this conclusion with great reluctance and hope that the occasions for such a decision will be rare.

Our generally tolerant attitude may disappoint those who see the Act and its workings as evidence of a serious and progressive decline in the standards of morality in sexual behaviour of this society. We understand this point of view and we sympathise with the motives of those who, disturbed by contemporary evidence of licence, press for action to curtail it. We have listened to those who wished to see the Abortion Act amended in a much more restrictive way, and we were impressed by their concern for the well-being of society. It is difficult to deny that the reaction against long-traditional social mores and in particular against what is now considered the prudishness and sexual hypocrisy of the Victorian Age, has been taken by some to unacceptable extremes of individualistic behaviour. The easing of social restraints is likely to be followed by a period of over-reaction towards licence and by the abuse of their greater freedom by a minority; and this must be lived through, for the sake of the larger advantages.

We have suggested how the services provided for abortion, both inside and outside the N.H.S., may be improved and strengthened, and how some of the abuses in the commercial private sector may be curtailed. We do not advocate for these purposes a restriction of the legal grounds for abortion: nor do we wish to give any support to those who would encourage a censorious public attitude to those who seek it. To suggest that the woman who, after anxiety, heart-searching and doubt, decides to seek an abortion, should instead summon up her will-power and accept with the best grace she can muster a situation which would often be tragic for her, is advice similar to that which has so often in the past been given to those who were suffering from nervous or mental illness—'pull yourself together'. It is advice which in the great majority of cases is crude, unfeeling and ineffectual. We do not think that the Abortion Act can be interpreted, or should be used, in a punitive way in an attempt to improve this society's morals and to diminish sexual misbehaviour. Where there has been irresponsibility or thoughtlessness, this has operated at an earlier time, when the woman has run the risk of an illegitimate or unwanted pregnancy: it is at this time that preventive action should be taken. A public educated to a more mature and responsible attitude to sexual behaviour and to contraception will be the most sure guarantee that recourse is made less often to the therapeutic abortion of unwanted pregnancies.

In the comparatively short time since the Act was passed there have been significant changes of attitude and opinion, both lay and professional. Continued social change is certain: societies throughout the world are evolving rapidly. Progress in the emancipation of women, advances in medical research and the pressures of a population explosion are only three of the factors which will ensure that further changes will occur. The conclusions formulated in this report will have therefore, we expect, only temporary relevance. We hope that they will be thought to be well-balanced, realistic in the contemporary setting, responsible and humane; and we trust that they will assist all concerned with this urgent human problem to rise co-operatively to the challenge of finding responses to it which will promote both individual happiness and social stability.

paras. 600–10

3 Social Security

Introduction

To define the Welfare State in a way that is not almost entirely arbitrary and in a way that will remain acceptable over time is so appallingly difficult that I do not propose to attempt it. The phrase is, in fact, a slogan rather than a description. The first recorded use of the term was in a book published in 1941 by Dr Temple, then Archbishop of Canterbury.

However, although the phrase appears to be so recent in its currency it is now usual to look back to the welfare legislation of the beginning of this century, and in particular to the programme of legislation embarked on by the Liberal Government that came to power in 1905, for the origins of the Welfare State. Until the introduction of old age pensions in 1908 and the passage of the National Insurance Act in 1911, only the Poor Law and private charity stood between the unfortunate and destitution. These two enactments can reasonably be held to represent the beginnings of the Welfare State and of a system of social security that was to replace the hated Poor Law.

Proposals for old age pensions and sickness insurance were put forward in a number of quarters in the 1870s and 1880s, but were opposed by the influential Charity Organisation Society, who feared the pauperization of the working classes, and by the friendly societies, who feared any diversion of the working man's savings which might be involved if the contributory principle were adopted. The friendly societies were having particular difficulties at that time because mortality rates were declining and the birth rate was also falling, so that the proportion of elderly members making heavy calls on the societies was increasing, while there were proportionately fewer young members whose contributions could adequately support the benefits that had to be paid out. At the same time, the societies possessed insufficient actuarial knowledge to make allowance for these factors, and there was fierce competition between them.

When the friendly societies were first established, old age was not seen as a time of special necessity, but by the 1880s many friendly societies were inviting bankruptcy by paying old age pensions in the guise of sickness benefit. So it is easy to understand their opposition to contributory old age pensions. It is perhaps more difficult to understand their opposition to non-contributory pensions, which might be thought likely to relieve them of a burden they were ill-fitted to support, but this was probably a reflection of their general suspicion of state intervention. Apart from the views of the friendly societies, opposition to non-contributory pensions was also widespread on grounds of cost. Charles Booth, on the other hand, argued that the provision of non-contributory pensions would reduce expenditure on poor relief.

Further thought and discussion was stimulated as news reached England that Germany had introduced old age pensions in 1889, while New Zealand followed in 1897. By the turn of the century the Labour movement had decided to back free pensions, and the friendly societies were in such desperate straits that they were compelled to come round to the same view. The COS continued their opposition, but when a Liberal Government pledged to pensions in one form or another came into power, they tried to salvage what they could from the situation by urging that stringent conditions as to character and good behaviour should be attached to the receipt of pensions.

Shortly before he became Chancellor of the Exchequer, Lloyd George wrote to his brother: 'It is time we did something that appealed straight to the people . . . it will, I think, help to stop this electoral rot. . . .' The outcome was the Old Age Pensions Act of 1908, which introduced non-contributory old age pensions of five shillings a week for the over-70s, with reduced pensions for those with incomes of over ten shillings a week. Those who were in receipt of poor relief were not eligible for pensions.

As in the case of so many pieces of social legislation, old age pensions soon started to cost very much more than those who had introduced them had bargained for. Although in 1912 there was a fall of some £600,000 (£12·5 to £11·9 million) in local expenditure on poor relief, this had to be set against a national expenditure on pensions of £11·7 million. The impact of pensions on Poor Law expenditure was necessarily limited, since many of the aged who were receiving poor relief were, by reason of infirmity, receiving indoor relief in the workhouse.

From 1908 onwards Lloyd George was the principal architect, at the political level, of the social legislation enacted by the Liberal administration, and one of the important influences on him was the knowledge he had gained of the German systems of old age pensions, social security and labour exchanges during a visit he made to that country in 1908. His greatest achievement was the National Insurance Act of 1911. This had profound importance both for the future system of social security and for the future pattern of medical practice in Britain. The fact that Beveridge worked on the unemployment insurance scheme formed a link with the next great wave of social legislation, that which followed the Second World War.

Subsequent developments in social security were influenced, even as late as the 1960s, by the need to assure people that they had a *right* to the benefits provided, that not only the Poor Law itself but the attitudes associated with it were truly dead. And yet one of the central problems that had exercised the architects of the New Poor Law remained, and remains to this day. No one dares any more to speak of the 'deserving and the undeserving poor', but it may be questioned whether any society, however advanced and however compassionate, can afford to make it more profitable to stay idle than to work.

It has been said that armies are always ready to fight the last war, never the next, and the same could be said of the architects of social security systems. The scheme of unemployment insurance devised by Churchill and Beveridge before the First World War was unable to cope with the massive unemployment of the 1920s and 1930s. Similarly the chronic inflation of the 1950s and 1960s created problems with which the post-war system of social security was ill-equipped to deal and much hardship was caused, especially to the elderly. The contributory principle solved certain problems in its day, but brought others in its train. Actuarial soundness and social justice—at least in the strongly egalitarian sense in which the term has been interpreted in recent years—seldom marched together.

The term 'social security' is used here in the narrow sense of income maintenance and supplementation, i.e. it is confined to monetary benefits of one kind or another. Thus I have used it broadly, though not precisely, in the way that Beveridge used it; not, as others have used it, as a synonym for social welfare, to include health services, the maintenance of full employment, and perhaps the provision of housing and education as well.

3.1 National Insurance Act, 1911

The National Insurance Act was originally two separate pieces of legislation, one on health insurance and the other on unemployment insurance, which were almost at the last moment combined as Parts I and II of the same Bill. The health insurance scheme was the work of David Lloyd George, then Chancellor of the Exchequer; and Winston Churchill, when President of the Board of Trade, impressed his personality and his views on the scheme of unemployment insurance. The Act marked the introduction in English social legislation of the principle of social insurance, characterized by the payment of contributions on the part of insured persons as a basis for entitlement to benefits. It is significant that William Beveridge, chief apostle of the insurance principle and author of the famous report, played a part in the preparation of Churchill's scheme of unemployment insurance. Lloyd George, at least, regarded social insurance as a temporary expedient until such time as the State was ready to assume full responsibility for the maintenance of incomes during sickness and unemployment, and there were those, such as Sidney and Beatrice Webb, who believed that that time had already come; but like many temporary expedients the insurance principle survived for more than fifty years and in 1925 a Conservative Government converted old age pensions, which had originally, in Lloyd George's 1907 scheme, been non-contributory, onto a contributory basis.

The Act was foreshadowed in Lloyd George's 1909 Budget. He made heavy increases in taxation and declared that part of the money would go to pay for sickness and unemployment insurance. In the previous year the Chancellor had visited Germany to acquaint himself with the German system of social insurance; now he sent his officials to get fuller details. His scheme, however, was by no means a copy of the German system, and in years to come it was the English model that was followed by a number of countries anxious to introduce social welfare measures.

At first the scheme did not attract much opposition, but as some of the details became known the Northcliffe Press and some of the interests that felt themselves threatened by it, or who were hostile to Lloyd George on other grounds, mounted a full-scale campaign to defeat it, or to compel the Chancellor to make important concessions. Backed by a few faithful colleagues and chosen officials, Lloyd George manœuvred his 'ambulance wagon'—his famous figure of speech for his health insurance scheme—'through the twistings and turnings and ruts of the Parliamentary road', making concessions here, disarming opposition there, sensing when proposals put up by his civil servants were politically dangerous, whatever their merits from other points of view, but keeping the essentials intact.

From the start Lloyd George intended that health insurance should be a partnership between the State and the non-profit-making friendly societies, who had pioneered this field on a voluntary basis, but the power of the commercial insurance firms compelled him to admit them into the partnership. In the event the influence of the firms' agents, calling at many thousands of homes every week, helped to win popular support for the measure. The winning slogan was 'Ninepence for Fourpence'. The working man paid fourpence a week, his employer added threepence, and the State a further twopence, and thus the benefits which the man could command were calculated on the basis of a weekly contribution of ninepence, although he only paid fourpence. Benefit consisted of a weekly sum, which varied according to age, sex and marital status, and which was paid for up to twenty-six weeks. This was followed, if necessary, by disablement benefit of five shillings a week for so long as the disablement lasted. In addition the insured person was entitled to the services of a general practitioner and to such medicines as he prescribed. The scheme also included a maternity benefit of thirty shillings, which a woman could receive either as an insured person in her own right, or by virtue of the husband's insurance.

Participation in the scheme was compulsory between the ages of sixteen and seventy for all manual workers, both men and women, and for all other workers employed under a contract of service who earned not more than £160 a year. Apart from maternity benefit, it made no provision for dependents, and thus more than half the population fell outside its scope. Nor did it provide for hospital treatment, should this be necessary. The use of friendly societies to administer the scheme had, in Treasury eyes, the advantage of keeping the administrative costs to a minimum and avoiding the necessity to develop a massive central bureaucracy. It had the consequence, however, that the benefits received for the standard contribution varied according to how well the particular society managed its finances.

One of the chief issues that had to be resolved when the Bill was drafted was whether the cost of benefits should be met from current income— the 'dividing out' principle which characterized the German scheme— or from a fund accumulated and invested over the years according to normal actuarial practice. Lloyd George at first favoured dividing out, but he was eventually persuaded by his advisers to be actuarially virtuous in order to maintain the independence of the societies, which was based on their right to manage their own funds. The initial object of the State's contribution of twopence a week was to enable the societies to calculate benefits as if all contributors came into the scheme at the age of 16, and thus paid contributions for the whole of their working lives, with the exception of such time as they were sick or unemployed. Later it was hoped that the State subvention would enable additional benefits to be paid.

Two groups who gave Lloyd George a good deal of trouble during the introduction of the health insurance scheme were the duchesses and the doctors. The revolt of the dowagers was stirred up by Northcliffe's *Daily Mail*. Lloyd George had rejected an amendment to his scheme that would have had the effect of making insurance optional for household servants. He reasoned that this would in effect exclude them from the scheme, as servants were accustomed to do as they were told and their mistresses would not want to pay contributions for them. The *Daily Mail* invited letters from its readers on the subject. Within a month the campaign reached its climax with a mass rally of mistresses and maids in the Albert Hall, London. There were speeches from a number of titled ladies. The Dowager Countess of Desart and her maid sat on the same plat-form and both spoke against the Bill. After the rally, Lady Desart started a Tax Defence Association to collect pledges from other mistresses that they would not lick stamps for their servants.

The doctors, however, were a more serious matter, as their co-operation in agreeing to treat insured persons in return for capitation fees was essential for the success of the scheme, but unlike the insurance companies they did not get all they asked for, and in some important respects Lloyd George outmanoeuvred them. As on many other occasions, the doctors were divided, and Lloyd George saw that the London leaders of the profession did not truly reflect the feelings of many general practitioners in working-class areas, for whom the terms he was offering marked an improvement on their existing incomes. On the other hand, the system followed by the friendly societies, where the doctor was under contract to the society and the patient had no choice of doctor, was universally unpopular. It was for this reason that it was agreed that local insurance committees should be set up to administer medical benefit and free choice of doctor on the part of the patient was guaranteed. The friendly societies opposed these concessions because they believed they would result in less effective control over malingering. Eventually the official British Medical Association opposition collapsed when it became evident that rank and file doctors were in fact willing to accept service under the scheme. Over the next forty years the scheme played a significant part in raising standards of practice in industrial areas by making it possible for doctors to command a living wage working among the poorer classes.

To turn to Part II of the Act, early efforts to deal with the problem of unemployment outside the provisions of the Poor Law had concentrated on providing for the unemployed work of a public nature, such as laying out parks and gardens. This system culminated in the Unemployed Workmen Act, 1905, which extended a scheme originally evolved in London to the rest of the country, and which was soon recognized to have been a failure. It was experience of this system in London that led to some of Beveridge's earlier writings on unemployment, in which he put forward the idea of a national network of labour exchanges. He took this idea with him when he became a civil servant at the Board of Trade in 1908 and had the satisfaction of seeing the Labour Exchanges Act passed in 1909. Meanwhile, he had been studying the German system of unemployment insurance and with Churchill's active interest and support he and his colleagues at the Board of Trade devised the scheme which eventually became Part II of the National Insurance Act.

The scheme was compulsory for workmen earning less than £160 a year in a group of seven trades known to be subject to short-term unemployment: building, construction; shipbuilding; mechanical engineering; ironfounding; vehicle construction; and saw-milling. The workman, his employer, and the State each contributed twopence-halfpenny a week and the unemployed workman was eligible to receive seven shillings a week for a maximum of fifteen weeks in any one year. The scheme was essentially one to deal with short-term unemployment, and was not intended to cope with long-term, cyclical unemployment of the kind that occurred between the wars. A further Act in 1920 extended the scheme to other manual and some non-manual workers—although agricultural workers were excluded—but insurance could not cope with the one million who were unemployed in 1921, and by the time the figure had risen to 3 million ten years later the 'dole'—tax-supported relief subject to a means test rather than contributions—was playing the major part. This experience taught Beveridge, among others, that unemployment insurance could not take the place of economic policies designed to promote full employment and avoid major cyclical fluctuations.

The Bill was fought fiercely in Parliament, and was forced through under closure. It came out of Parliament heavily amended, much longer than it went in. Lloyd George had, however, won his major battles, and the Act came smoothly into operation in July 1912. Separate insurance commissions were established for England, Scotland, Wales and Ireland, with a joint committee to co-ordinate their work. By 1914 2·5 million people were insured against unemployment, and nearly 14 million against interruption of earnings through sickness. In spite of the use of the friendly societies and the insurance industry to administer the sickness side of the scheme at local level, the Act imposed burdens almost without precedent on the civil service of the day. Only the Inland Revenue had experience that was in any way comparable. Sir Henry Bunbury has said: 'It was, I believe, the first time that Civil Servants had to explain novel and complex matters to the unlettered masses in plain and simple English. It is not without significance that the author of *Plain Words* began his rise to fame on the staff of the Insurance Commission. . . . There were no traditions to learn, no precedents to guide, no established routine to conform to: everything had to be created.' Some of the chief beneficiaries of the Act were the industrial insurance companies. The approved societies administered by them went from strength to strength while the friendly societies went into a slow decline from which they never recovered. There were other factors in the decline of the friendly societies. Many of them had up until that time deserved their name, and their members came together for meetings and sing-songs. As commercial entertainment became more widespread, the social life of the Lodges died out, and the admission of the companies under the 1911 Act introduced an element of competition against which the friendly societies could not maintain their position.

An interesting feature of the early working of the health insurance scheme was that although claims from men fell slightly below expectations, claims from women were well above. The scheme thus revealed for the first time the true extent of ill-health among English working-class women.

3.2 Report on Social Insurance and Allied Services

Published: 1942

By Sir William Beveridge

Terms of Reference (1941): *To undertake with special reference to the inter-relation of the schemes, a survey of the existing national schemes of social insurance and allied services, including workmen's compensation, and to make recommendations.*

Sir William Beveridge, a former civil servant turned academic, was in 1941 appointed chairman of the Inter-departmental Committee on Social Insurance and Allied Services, which was to conduct the first comprehensive survey of the British system of social insurance and provision against want. The report was published in November 1942 on the responsibility of the chairman alone, for it was realized that here was a document that dealt with broad aspects of policy and not merely with the details of administration, so that it would not have been regarded as proper for the other members of the committee, all working civil servants, to put their names publicly to it. Thus the Beveridge Report incorporated to an extent which is almost unique among such documents the vision of one man. And that one man was destined to see much of his vision turned into reality. By 1942 the thoughts of many were beginning to turn to the task of social as well as physical reconstruction that would face Britain after the war. The dearest wish of most of those who fought in the First World War was for a return to the normality which had been so rudely interrupted in August 1914, but in the Second World War it was different. The preceding decade had been one of depression and distress and no one wanted to return to that. There was a widespread desire that Britain after the war should be a better place to live in and a ready readership for what Churchill grumpily described as 'spacious plans for a new world'.

The Beveridge Report became a best-seller, and long queues formed at the Stationery Office to buy it. The armed forces read it eagerly and the

Army Bureau of Current Affairs produced a pamphlet on it. When the coalition government took fright at the possibility that it might be forced into accepting and promising to implement the Beveridge Plan in its entirety, the pamphlet was withdrawn, but so great was the outcry it had to be re-issued. In Parliament there was heavy pressure on the government to commit itself to the Beveridge recommendations.

Beveridge's survey showed 'that provision for most of the varieties of need through interruption of earnings and other causes that may arise in modern industrial communities has already been made in Britain on a scale not surpassed and hardly rivalled in any other country of the world'. He pointed out, however, that although this was generally true, some other countries were ahead of Britain in the provision of medical services, and that the other services that were provided in Britain were in certain respects defective and suffered from a serious lack of coordination. In one of the most telling passages in his report, Beveridge showed that even in the grim years before the war Britain had been wealthy enough to have abolished want if the will had been there—'want was a needless scandal due to not taking the trouble to prevent it'. Want could have been abolished by a redistribution of income stopping well short of a ruthless egalitarianism—and politically Beveridge was a Liberal, not a Socialist.

Underlying Beveridge's plan for social security were *three basic assumptions* (Beveridge's penchant for little lists like this helped to make his report easy and memorable reading). These were:

(1) children's allowances up to the age of 15 or if in full-time education up to 16;
(2) comprehensive health and rehabilitation services for the prevention and cure of disease and restoration of capacity for work, available to all members of the community;
(3) the maintenance of employment, that is to say, avoidance of mass unemployment.

Children's allowances were to take account of the relationship that had been repeatedly demonstrated between poverty and family size. The health service, Beveridge thought, would eventually pay for itself by making the nation fitter and more productive. He thus saw expenditure on health services as investment rather than consumption, a view that was not challenged until several years' experience of rising health service costs after 1948, and increasing rather than diminishing demand, forced a reappraisal and a realization that to a large extent health care was part of a high standard of living rather than a direct contribution to the nation's productive capacity. The avoidance of mass unemployment was firmly in Beveridge's mind as a prerequisite on account of the experience during the 1920s and 1930s when the unemployment insurance scheme showed itself unable to cope with a major recession. Beveridge believed that thanks to

Keynesian economics governments now had the techniques to avoid a recurrence of unemployment on such a scale.

Next Beveridge set out his *three guiding principles*. These were:

(1) Now, 'when the war is abolishing landmarks of every kind', was the time to make a fresh start.

(2) Social insurance should be treated as one part only of a comprehensive policy of social progress, attacking the *five giants* of Want, Disease, Ignorance, Squalor and Idleness. Social Insurance attacked only one of these five giants—Want.

(3) Social security must be achieved by co-operation between the State and the individual. The State should offer security, but should not, in so doing, stifle initiative, opportunity, responsibility.

There were *four conditions for the banishment of want*:

(1) that the world after the war is a world in which the nations set themselves to co-operate for production in peace;

(2) that the readjustments of British economic policy and structure that will be required by changed conditions after the war should be made so that productive employment is maintained;

(3) that a plan for social security, that is to say for income maintenance, should be adopted, free from unnecessary costs of administration and other waste of resources;

(4) that decisions as to the nature of the plan, that is to say as to the organization of social insurance and allied services, should be taken during the war.

There were *six fundamental principles of the plan for social security*:

(1) flat rate of subsistence benefit;
(2) flat rate of contribution;
(3) unification of administrative responsibility;
(4) adequacy of benefit;
(5) comprehensiveness;
(6) classification.

The Beveridge plan for social security was based on the following *twelve points*.

(1) The plan covers all citizens without upper income limit, but has regard to their different ways of life; it is a plan all-embracing in scope of persons and of needs, but is classified in application.

(2) Classification of the population into: I employees; II others gainfully employed; III housewives; IV others of working age not gainfully employed; V below working age; VI retired above working age.

(3) Children's allowances for V; retirement pensions for VI; and for all

other classes security appropriate to their circumstances. All classes covered for comprehensive medical treatment and rehabilitation and for funeral expenses.

(4) Every person in I, II and IV will pay a single security contribution by a stamp on a single insurance document each week or combination of weeks. Contributions higher for men than for women to allow for benefits to III.

(5) Subject to simple contribution conditions, I will receive unemployment and disability benefit, retirement pension, medical treatment and funeral expenses; II, all these except unemployment benefit and disability benefit during the first thirteen weeks of disability; IV, all except unemployment and disability benefit; III, maternity grant, provision for widowhood and separation and retirement pensions by virtue of husband's contributions; thirteen weeks' maternity benefit for housewives who take paid work.

(6) Unemployment and disability benefit, basic retirement pension and training benefit at subsistence rates. Maternity benefit for housewives who work at a higher rate than the single unemployment or disability rate, while their unemployment and disability benefits will be at a lower rate. Special provision for disability due to industrial accident or disease.

(7) Unemployment and disability benefits to continue at same rate as long as unemployment or disability lasts.

(8) Pensions to be paid only on retirement from work. Rate of pension increased if retirement is postponed.

(9) No permanent pensions for widows without dependent children, but temporary benefits at higher rate than unemployment benefit in early months of widowhood.

(10) For limited number of cases of need not covered by social insurance, national assistance subject to a uniform means test.

(11) Medical treatment covering all requirements to be provided by a national health service organized under the health departments for all citizens and post-medical rehabilitation for all capable of profiting by it.

(12) The setting up of a Ministry of Social Security.

A Ministry of Social Security was not set up until 1966, but the National Health Service Act was passed in 1946 and family allowances were introduced in 1945. Many of Beveridge's recommendations were incorporated in the National Insurance and National Insurance (Industrial Injuries) Acts of 1946 and in the National Assistance Act of 1948, but many of the benefits, including family allowances, were fixed at rates lower than those Beveridge had wanted, and they were further eroded by a rate of post-war inflation that he had not envisaged. The friendly societies were not brought into the State scheme in the way that Beveridge had hoped, and the actuarial principles on which Beveridge set store were disregarded when the Government decided that most old age pensioners should receive a full pension from the outset of the new scheme. Beveridge had recommended that pensions should be related to contributions so that people retiring in the early years would only have received reduced pensions. Subsequent developments in social security have almost invariably represented further departures from the principles that Beveridge laid down to govern the operation and administration of his scheme. His most lasting contribution was his vision of government's responsibility for the creation of conditions favourable to the banishment of want. This has remained a principal aim of social policy whichever party has been in power.

Beveridge Report, 1942

SIX PRINCIPLES OF SOCIAL INSURANCE

Flat Rate of Subsistence Benefit: The first fundamental principle of the social insurance scheme is provision of a flat rate of insurance benefit, irrespective of the amount of the earnings which have been interrupted by unemployment or disability or ended by retirement; exception is made only where prolonged disability has resulted from an industrial accident or disease. This principle follows from the recognition of the place and importance of voluntary insurance in social security and distinguishes the scheme proposed for Britain from the security schemes of Germany, the Soviet Union, the United States and most other countries with the exception of New Zealand. The flat rate is the same for all the principal forms of cessation of earning—unemployment, disability, retirement; for maternity and for widowhood there is a temporary benefit at a higher rate.

Flat Rate of Contribution: The second fundamental principle of the scheme is that the compulsory contribution required of each insured person or his employer is at a flat rate, irrespective of his means. All insured persons, rich or poor, will pay the same contributions for the same security; those with larger means will pay more only to the extent that as tax-payers they pay more to the National Exchequer and so to the State share of the Social Insurance Fund. This feature distinguishes the scheme proposed for Britain from the scheme recently established in New Zealand under which the contributions are graduated by income, and are in effect an income-tax assigned to a particular service. Subject moreover to one exception, the contribution will be the same irresptecive of the assumed degree of risk affecting particular individuals or forms of employment. The exception is the raising of a proportion of the special cost of benefits and pensions for industrial disability in occupations of high risk by a levy on employers proportionate to risk and pay-roll. . . .

Unification of Administrative Responsibility: The third fundamental principle is unification of administrative responsibility in the interests of efficiency and economy. For each insured person there will be a single weekly contribution, in respect of all his benefits. There will be in each locality a Security Office able to deal with claims of every kind and all sides of security. The methods of paying different kinds of cash benefit will be different and will take account of the circumstances of insured persons, providing for payment at the home or elsewhere, as is necessary. All contributions will be paid into a single Social Insurance Fund and all benefits and other insurance payments will be paid from that fund.

Adequacy of Benefit: The fourth fundamental principle is adequacy of benefit in amount and in time. The flat rate of benefit proposed is intended in itself to be sufficient without further resources to provide the minimum income needed for subsistence in all normal cases. It gives room and a basis for additional voluntary provision, but does not assume that in any case. The benefits are adequate also in time, that is to say except for contingencies of a temporary nature, they will continue indefinitely without means test, so long as the need continues, though subject to any change of conditions and treatment required by prolongation of the interruption in earning and occupation.

Comprehensiveness: The fifth fundamental principle is that social insurance should be comprehensive, in respect both of the persons covered and of their needs. It should not leave either to national assistance or to voluntary insurance any risk so general or so uniform that social insurance can be justified. For national assistance involves a means test which may discourage voluntary insurance or personal saving. And voluntary insurance can never be sure of covering the ground. For any need moreover which, like direct funeral expenses, is so general and so uniform as to be a fit subject for insurance by compulsion, social insurance is much cheaper to administer than voluntary insurance.

Classification: The sixth fundamental principle is that social insurance, while unified and comprehensive, must take account of the different ways of life of different sections of the community: of those dependent on earnings by employment under contract of service, of those earning in other ways, of those rendering vital unpaid service as housewives, of those not yet of age to earn and of those past earning. The term 'classification' is used here to denote adjustment of insurance to the differing circumstances of each of these classes and to many varieties of need and circumstance within each insurance class. But the insurance classes are not economic or social classes in the ordinary sense; the insurance scheme is one for all citizens irrespective of their means.

paras. 304–9

ABOLITION OF WANT AS A PRACTICABLE POST-WAR AIM

The aim of the Plan for Social Security is to abolish want by ensuring that every citizen willing to serve according to his powers has at all times an income sufficient to meet his responsibilities. Is this aim likely to be within our reach immediately after the present war?

The first step in considering the prospective economic resources of the community after the present war is to see what they were just before the war. The social surveys made by impartial investigators of living conditions in some of the main industrial centres of Britain between 1928 and 1937 have been used earlier in this Report to supply a diagnosis of want. They can be used also to show that the total resources of the community were sufficient to make want needless. While, in every town surveyed, substantial percentages of the families examined had less than the bare minimum for subsistence, the great bulk of them had substantially more than the minimum. In East London, in the week chosen for investigation in 1929, while one family in every nine had income below the minimum and was in want, nearly two-thirds of all the families had as least 20/- a week more than the minimum, and nearly a third had 40/- a week more than the minimum; these were actual incomes after allowing for sickness, unemployment and irregular work. In Bristol the average working-class family enjoyed a standard of living more than 100 per cent. above its minimum needs; while one Bristol family in nine in the year 1937 was in sheer physical want, two families out of every five had half as much again as they needed for subsistence. Similar contrasts were presented in every survey. Another way of putting these contrasts is to compare the surplus of those who had more than the minimum with the deficiency of those who had less. In East London, the total surplus of the working-class families above the minimum was more than thirty times the total deficiency of those below it. In York, where Mr. Rowntree in 1936 used a much higher minimum—the standard of human needs containing more than bare physical necessaries of food, clothing, fuel and housing—the three classes of the working population living above the standard had a total surplus above it at least eight times the total deficiency of the two classes living below the stand-ard. Want could have been abolished before the present war by a redistribution of income within the wage-earning classes, without touching any of the wealthier classes. This is said not to suggest that redistribution of income should be confined to the wage-earning classes; still less is it said to suggest that men should be content with avoidance of want, with subsistence incomes. It is said simply as the most convincing demonstration that abolition of want just before this war was easily within the economic resources of the community; want was a needless scandal due to not taking the trouble to prevent it.

The social surveys showed not only what was the standard of living available to the community just before the war but also that it had risen rapidly in the past thirty or forty years. The recent London and York surveys were designed to provide comparisons with earlier studies. They yielded unquestionable proof of large and general progress. When the New Survey of London Life and Labour was made in 1929, the average workman in London could buy a third more of articles of consumption in return for labour of an hour's less duration per day than he could buy forty years before at the time of Charles Booth's original survey. The standard of living available to the workpeople of York in 1936 may be put over-all at about 30 per cent. higher than it was in 1899. This improve-ment of economic conditions was reflected in improvement of physical con-ditions. In London, the crude death rate fell from 18·6 per thousand in 1900 to 11·4 in 1935 and the infant mortality rate fell from 159 to 58 per thousand. In York the infant mortality rate fell from 161 per thousand in 1899 to 55 in 1936; in the same period nearly 2 inches was added to the height of schoolchildren and nearly 5 lbs. to their weight. Growing prosperity and improving health are facts established for these towns not as general impressions but by scientific impartial investigation. What has been shown for these towns in detail applies to the country generally. The real wages of labour, what the wage-earner could buy with his earnings just before the present war, were in general about one-third higher than in 1900 for an hour less of work each day. What the wage-earner could buy, when earning had been interrupted by sickness, accident or un-employment or had been ended by old age, had increased in even larger propor-tion, though still inadequately, by development of social insurance and allied services.

The rise in the general standard of living in Britain in the thirty or forty years that ended with the present war has two morals. First, growing general prosperity and rising wages diminished want, but did not reduce want to insignificance. The moral is that new measures to spread prosperity are needed. The Plan for Social Security is designed to meet this need; to establish a national minimum above which prosperity can grow, with want abolished. Second, the period covered by the comparisons between say 1900 and 1936 includes the first world war. The moral is the encouraging one, that it is wrong to assume that the present war must bring economic progress for Britain, or for the rest of the world, to an end. After four years of open warfare and diversion of effort from useful production to the means of destruction during 1914–18, there followed an aftermath of economic conflict; international trade was given no chance to recover from the war, and Britain entered into a period of mass unemployment in her staple industries. Yet, across this waste period of destruction and disloca-tion, the permanent forces making for material progress—technical advance and the capacity of human society to adjust itself to new conditions—continued to operate; the real wealth per head in a Britain of shrunken oversea investments and lost export markets, counting in all her unemployed, was materially higher in 1938 than in 1913. The present war may be even more destructive. It is likely to complete the work of the first war in exhausting British investments overseas and to deprive Britain largely of another source of earning abroad through shipping services: in these and in other ways it will change the economic en-vironment in which the British people must live and work and may call for radical and in some ways painful readjustments. There are bound to be acute difficulties of transition; there are no easy care-free times in early prospect. But to suppose that the difficulties cannot be overcome, that power of readjust-ment has deserted the British people, that technical advance has ended or can end, that the British of the future must be permanently poor because they will have spent their fathers' savings, is defeatism without reason and against reason.

The economic argument set out above is in terms not of money, but of standards of living and of real wages. If the argument is sound, it is clear that abolition of want by re-distribution of income is within our means. The problem of how the plan should be financed in terms of money is secondary, though it is a real problem, since the fact that the whole burden, properly distributed, could be borne does not mean that it can be borne unless it is distributed wisely. Wise distribution of the burden is the object of the Social Security Budget as outlined in Part IV. There it is shown that the Plan involves for the National Exchequer an additional charge of at most £86 million in the first year of full operation. It does not seem unreasonable to hope that, even with the other calls upon the Exchequer, an additional expense of this order could be borne when actual fighting ceases. The Budget imposes a much increased burden on the Exchequer in later years to provide retirement pensions; this is an act of reasonable faith in the future of the British economic system and the proved efficiency of the British people. That, given reasonable time, this burden can be borne is hardly open to question. The exact rate at which the burden will rise is not settled finally in accepting the plan, since the length of the transition period for pensions is capable of adjustment and, if necessary, can be prolonged without serious hardship. As regards the insured person, the Budget requires of him contributions for vital security which together are materially less than he is now paying for compulsory insurance and for voluntary insurance for less important purposes, or on account of medical services for which he pays when he receives them. For the employers, the plan imposes an addition to their costs for labour which should be well repaid by the greater efficiency and content which they secure.

paras. 444–8

Want could have been abolished in Britain just before the present war. It can be abolished after the war, unless the British people are and remain very much poorer then than they were before, that is to say unless they remain less productive than they and their fathers were. There is no sense in believing, contrary to experience, that they will and must be less productive. The answer to the question whether freedom from want should be regarded as a post-war aim capable of early attainment is an affirmative—on four conditions. The four conditions are:—

(1) That the world after the war is a world in which the nations set themselves to co-operate for production in peace, rather than to plotting for mutual destruction by war, whether open or concealed;

(2) That the re-adjustments of British economic policy and structure that will be required by changed conditions after the war should be made, so that productive employment is maintained;

(3) That a Plan for Social Security, that is to say for income maintenance, should be adopted, free from unnecessary costs of administration and other waste of resources;

(4) That decisions as to the nature of the plan, that is to say as to the organisation of social insurance and allied services, should be taken during the war.

para. 450

3.3 Family Allowances Act, 1945

Children's allowances were one of the 'three basic assumptions' of the Beveridge Report. That families should be assisted in this way was not a new idea. Pitt the younger had tried to introduce children's allowances in 1796, but in more recent years the case for such allowances rested first on the assumption that it was desirable to encourage people to have more children in order to arrest the post-nineteenth century decline in the birth rate, and secondly on the recognition by social investigators from Charles Booth onwards that families in dire poverty were more often than not in this condition because of the number of children they had to support. The first argument now seems rather dated, but in the 1940s it still seemed to have some force, although there was little or no evidence that the availability of family allowances would significantly influence parents' decisions about family size.

The adoption of the term 'family allowances' and not 'children's allowances' was intended to signify that the allowances were for the benefit of the family as a whole, and not merely of the children. The original Bill proposed that they should be paid to the father, but in a free vote on an amendment proposed by Miss Eleanor Rathbone it was agreed that the allowances must be claimed by the mother though they could be paid to either the mother or the father. An allowance of five shillings a week was to be paid for every child after the first. Beveridge had recommended eight shillings a week, but the Government used the fact that free school meals and free milk were to be extended to every child as an argument for reducing the amount paid in cash to five shillings. The possibility of limiting the allowances to the poorer families had been considered, but was rejected. Instead, the allowances were made taxable so that the better-off families paid some of the money back in income tax.

The exclusion of the first child was intended to make the point that the State was not taking over the liability of parents for the support and upbringing of their children, it was only sharing this responsibility with them. An alternative would have been to give allowances in respect of all children, but at a lower rate. The rate of eight shillings suggested by Beveridge was in fact the sum he estimated was required for a child's subsistence at that time. The allowances have of course been increased several times to keep pace with inflation. In 1956, when the basic allowance was eight shillings, an extra two shillings was added for the third and each subsequent child. In October 1974 the Chancellor of the Exchequer announced that this differential would be abolished and that from April 1975 the rate would be £1·50 for the second and each subsequent child, an increase on the rates then prevailing of 60p for the second child and 50p for the others. The age limit was also raised from 16 (for full-time students and apprentices) to 18 in 1956 and to 19 in 1964.

3.4 National Insurance Act, 1946

Beveridge's vision of a unified and comprehensive scheme of social insurance was largely realized in this Act. It covered every man, woman and child in the country and provided benefits, literally, from the cradle to the grave. It was the first scheme of its kind in Britain to cover the whole population and to provide such a wide range of benefits. Previous legislation had made no provision for the insurance of (a) non-manual workers with incomes above a certain limit (£420 p.a. in 1944); (b) civil servants and others in occupational schemes which offered benefits superior to those offered in the state scheme; (c) the self-employed; (d) the non-employed. All these were now brought into the scope of national insurance.

The benefits provided under the Act were of seven kinds: (a) unemployment benefit; (b) sickness benefit; (c) maternity allowances; (d) widows' allowances; (e) guardians' allowances; (f) retirement pensions; (g) death grants. Unemployment and sickness benefit were extended to cover all occupational groups, maternity benefits were completely reorganized, the principles governing widows' allowances were drastically changed, the orphans' pensions scheme was replaced by guardians' allowances, retirement pensions replaced old age pensions—the difference is an important one—and death grants were introduced for the first time in the state scheme.

Most of Beveridge's six fundamental principles (see pp. 83-4) were supported. The scheme was characterized by flat rates of benefit and of contributions, it was comprehensive in scope and it was based on Beveridge's classification of the population into six groups: employees, the self-employed, the non-employed, married women, those below working age, and those above working age. Complete unification of administrative responsibility for social security did not come at this time, although the setting up of the Ministry of National Insurance in 1944 was a step in the right direction. The Beveridge principle most seriously compromised in the Act was that of adequacy of benefit. Because of national economic circumstances immediately after the war—it is now known that Britain was virtually bankrupt in 1940 and from that date onwards was heavily dependent on American aid—several of the benefits awarded under the Act were at a lower level than Beveridge had recommended.

The scheme was clearly presented to the nation as one based on the insurance principle, and benefits under this Act—unlike family allowances and industrial injuries benefit—were to be related to the individual's record of weekly contributions. If contributions had not been maintained for the required period of time, then there might be no entitlement, or a reduced entitlement, to benefit. On the other hand this was a purely paper operation: there was no actuarial basis for the relationship between contributions and benefits. The scheme functioned from the start almost entirely on a pay-as-you-go basis; that is, current liabilities (benefits) were met from current income (contributions and general taxation). There was no accumulation and investment of an individual's contributions to support his eventual entitlement to a retirement pension. The reasons for the emphasis on insurance were psychological and historical and it no doubt helped to gain acceptance for the scheme among members of all political parties and among the population at large. If the scheme had been intended to be actuarially sound it would not have been possible to pay out retirement pensions from the start, as was in fact done.

Unemployment benefit was made dependent on a minimum number of contributions and on the satisfaction of certain conditions designed to prevent abuse. It was only available to Class I contributors: self-employed persons were not eligible. It was limited to a year, because with experience of the 1930s in mind it was not felt that the insurance scheme could bear the burden of long-term unemployment. After twelve months, the unemployed were expected to turn to national assistance.

Sickness benefit was made payable, as under previous schemes, on production of a medical certificate signed by the claimant's doctor. Again there were provisions to prevent abuse, but sickness benefit, unlike unemployment benefit, could continue indefinitely until the person reached the age of retirement, providing only that a sufficient number of contributions had been paid before the onset of incapacity. Throughout the early years of the scheme doctors grumbled at the time they had to spend signing certificates to meet the requirements of the Act, and several changes were made in the regulations to ease the burden on them, particularly in the case of long-term illness.

The Act provided for three types of maternity benefit: (a) the maternity grant, a lump sum to meet the immediate expenses of childbirth; (b) an attendance allowance—an alternative to (c) which was abolished in 1953; and (c) maternity benefit in the form of a weekly allowance which was originally at a higher rate than sickness or unemployment benefit in order to encourage women to give up work in good time before the birth of a child and to recover fully afterwards. The difference between maternity and sickness and unemployment benefit was abolished in 1953, but the period for which maternity benefit was payable was at the same time increased from thirteen to eighteen weeks. The payment of a maternity grant was dependent on the contribution record of the woman's husband, but payment of maternity benefit was dependent on the contribution record of the woman herself. Full-time housewives were thus entitled to the maternity grant but not to maternity benefit.

The Act changed drastically the principles governing widows' pensions. Previously, widowhood as such had attracted benefit, the widow of an insured husband being entitled to ten shillings a week for life for herself, plus allowances for any children. Now, however, it was considered that a young widow without any children was perfectly capable, after a period of adjustment, of earning her own living, and she should not be entitled to any long-term pension. The Act therefore provided, for widows under 60, a relatively high allowance for the first thirteen weeks of widowhood—this was later increased to twenty-six weeks. After the period of adjustment, a widow with dependent children became entitled to a widowed mother's allowance, and a widow over 50 to a widow's pension. Otherwise she received no further benefit. It was also laid down in the Act that widows' pensions should be paid to widowed mothers who were no longer entitled to the widowed mother's allowance (because their children were off their hands) but who at that time were aged 40 or over—later this age was raised to 50. Widows' benefits were to cease on re-marriage or cohabitation and widows were initially subject to an earnings rule reducing or extinguishing their pensions if they resumed work. This rule was abolished in 1964.

Guardians' allowances were made payable to persons (not institutions or authorities) responsible for the maintenance of orphan children. They were to be paid as long as one or other of the child's parents had been insured. There were no other contribution conditions. A child's special allowance was introduced in 1957, at the suggestion of the Royal Commission on Marriage and Divorce, for the benefit of the divorced woman whose former husband has died and who has a child towards whose support he was contributing.

The substitution of retirement for old age as the ground on which pensions would be paid to the elderly was a major change linked to Beveridge's belief that the function of social insurance was to cover against interruption of earnings. Pensions should only therefore be paid when earnings ceased or dropped to a very low level. Previous pension schemes had provided for the payment of pensions automatically at pensionable age, but the 1946 Act, while setting a minimum pensionable age at 65 for men and 60 for women (on the grounds that with normal age differences this would enable the average couple to retire together), made retirement from work a requirement for the payment of a pension at that age.

Once a man reached the age of 70, or a woman 65, he would receive his pension unconditionally, but between 65 and 70 (60–65 for women) any earnings from part-time or other work above a certain fairly low level would be liable to cause a reduction in pension. Income from private insurance or an occupational pension would not affect the state pension. As with other benefits under the Act, the amounts payable have been increased from time to time. Inflation has made it necessary to review rates of benefit more frequently than the quinquennial review envisaged by Beveridge. The earnings rule, by which pensions are reduced and eventually extinguished if earnings exceed the limit laid down, was also revised in 1956 and a sliding scale was introduced to enable pensioners to earn more without losing the whole of the amount earned from their pension.

The death grants introduced under the Act were intended to help families meet the expenses of a simple funeral, and were made dependent on a certain number of contributions having been paid by the deceased person, or in the case of women and children, the husband or father. The introduction of the death grant took a good deal of business away from the industrial assurance companies, as selling policies to cover funeral expenses to the poor had been an important part of their business.

3.5 National Assistance Act, 1948

The National Assistance Act was intended to mark the end of the old Poor Law and the start of a new era. Boards of Guardians had been abolished in 1929, but their functions of administering relief to the destitute had been transferred to the public assistance committees of the major local authorities. Now the system of locally administered outdoor relief was swept away and the Assistance Board, founded in 1934 to assist those whose entitlement to unemployment benefit had run out, and given the additional task in 1941 of administering supplementary assistance to old age pensioners, was renamed the National Assistance Board and given a duty 'to assist persons in Great Britain who are without resources to meet their requirements or whose resources . . . must be supplemented in order to meet their requirements'. Financial assistance was governed by Part 2 of the Act, but under Part 3, local authorities retained other welfare functions that they had inherited from the Boards of Guardians. They were 'required to provide residential care for all persons who, by reason of age, infirmity or any other circumstance, are in need of care not otherwise available to them'.

Aneurin Bevan, Minister of Health in the post-war Labour government, believed that 'warmth and humanity of administration' could best be achieved by leaving welfare homes to be administered locally. This was all very well, but to many people legislative changes, changes in terminology, even changes in the spirit which informed legislation were less evident than the fact that the building which was now to be called a welfare home was the former public assistance institution which only a few years before had been dreaded as the workhouse. Similarly the National Assistance Board did not find it as easy as was hoped to dissociate itself from the traditions handed down from the days of 'less eligibility'.

The NAB was to retain the semi-autonomous status it had enjoyed in the 1930s, when it was thought that if it were made a part of any Ministry questions of aid to the unemployed, or even individual cases, would be caught up in party politics. Beveridge had hoped that if his scheme of social insurance were adopted the need for national assistance would eventually almost wither away. This did not happen, because national assistance benefits were not fixed at a level sufficient for subsistence, as he had recommended, but at a level which made it necessary for those without other resources to turn to the NAB for assistance. The NAB thus came to play a much larger part in the overall system of income maintenance than was envisaged when the 1948 Act was passed.

The Act forbade the payment of national assistance in supplementation of the wages of men or women in full-time work. Nor could an unemployed person be granted assistance which amounted to more than he would earn in full-time employment. This was known as the 'wages stop' and meant that in some cases the assistance paid would be less than was officially regarded as necessary for subsistence. The policy stemmed from the fact that in some occupations earnings were less than the national assistance scales, especially when family size was taken into account, and the alternative to the wages stop would have been either to supplement wages and to incur the disadvantages of such a policy, or to ensure that a man would be better off unemployed and drawing national assistance than when he was in full-time work. During the 1960s the wages stop was a prime target of such pressure groups as the Child Poverty Action Group, which pointed out that of necessity the majority of persons affected by it, and living in poverty because of it, were the child dependents of low-wage earners.

On the other hand the national assistance scales were repeatedly raised and when estimates were made of the numbers of families living 'in poverty', using these scales as a yardstick, it was sometimes forgotten that 'subsistence' in the 1960s meant a very different standard of living compared with that envisaged by Beveridge when he used the term. Poverty had become a relative concept. The use of the national assistance scales as a yardstick had the paradoxical effect that every time they were raised an increasing number of low-wage earners and wage-stopped beneficiaries appeared to be living in poverty. Campaigns about poverty were often found to be not so much about poverty in any sense of the term that Booth, Rowntree or Beveridge would have recognized, as about inequality in our society.

Eligibility for national assistance was determined by considering the applicant's resources and those of his wife and other persons dependent on him. The resources of other members of his family were not to be taken into account. Children had no liability to contribute to the maintenance of their elderly parents. In addition the NAB was required, in its assessment of a person's resources, to disregard certain assets, such as the value of a house owned and occupied by the applicant, and capital up to a certain limit. There was thus no requirement that a person should be actually destitute to receive assistance, and as time went on the rules regarding resources to be disregarded in determining entitlement to assistance were made increasingly generous.

The standard national assistance allowances did not cover rent. This was allowed for separately in the light of the general level of rents in the area. The Act also created two types of discretionary payment, an allowance to be paid weekly—in addition to the basic allowance—for special long-term needs, such as domestic help, a special diet or additional fuel, and a lump-sum exceptional needs grant for such things as major replacements of clothing, footwear and bedding.

In addition to the administration of financial assistance, the NAB was made responsible for providing reception centres to offer board and lodging to those without a settled way of life and for attempting to influence them to lead a settled life. The board could reimburse local authorities and voluntary organizations that provided such centres on its behalf. The board was also to provide re-establishment centres to help those who needed to acquire or re-acquire habits of work and to offer instruction and training when necessary.

On the day appointed for the Act to come into operation, 5 July 1948, about 100 of the 400 former public assistance institutions became chronic sick hospitals, about 200 became joint-user establishments used by both hospital authorities and welfare authorities, and the remaining 100 became welfare homes. The tricky part of this operation was to decide which of the inmates of the old institutions were 'sick' and needed nursing and medical attention, and should therefore be regarded as hospital patients, and which were merely infirm and in need of 'care and attention' only. A frail old person may not only be on the borderline between the two categories, he may change from the one category to the other week by week, or even day by day. Thus there arose a situation in which hospitals complained that their beds were 'blocked' by patients who should have been in welfare accommodation, while the staffs of old people's homes complained that they had to care for patients in need of a degree of nursing care for which they had neither the equipment nor the staff.

The economic climate of the 1950s was such that few of the new small old people's homes for 25–30 persons which Aneurin Bevan had envisaged replacing the old public assistance institutions were built at that time. The Ministry of Health encouraged conversion of existing premises rather than new building, although later it issued a circular pointing out the disadvantages of converting premises that had not been built for the purpose.

Throughout the 1950s the Ministry havered about the right size of home. Recommendations varied from homes for thirty-five residents, to sixty, to smaller homes again. The Ministry's policy also changed from single rooms for all residents to a proportion of multiple-bed rooms, and back again to a high proportion of single rooms. Gradually, however, as the economic situation improved in the 1960s an increasing number of homes were built and a number of large institutions closed.

3.6 Report of the Committee on the Economic and Financial Problems of the Provision for Old Age (Phillips Report)

Published: 1954

Chairman: *Sir Thomas Phillips GBE, KCB*

Members: *C. Bartlett; Professor A. K. Cairncross CMG; Sir Cuthbert Clegg TD, JP;* J. H. Gunlake CBE, FIA, FSS; F. J. C. Honey FIA; Sir John Imrie CBE, JP; A. McAndrews; F. A. A. Menzler CBE, BSc, FIA, FSS; J. Ross;* Dr Janet Vaughan OBE, DM, FRCP; J. Whalley and J. P. Carswell (joint secretaries)*

*Sir Cuthbert Clegg retired from the Committee in July, 1954, for health reasons, and was subsequently replaced by Mr Ross

Terms of Reference (1953): *To review the economic and financial probems involved in providing for old age, having regard to the prospective increase in the numbers of the aged, and to make recommendations.*

The Phillips report was concerned with the economic and financial problems that arose from the prospect of a steady and substantial increase in the numbers of old persons as against a working population remaining roughly constant. The primary focus of the report was on income maintenance, not only through national insurance and national assistance, but also through occupational pension schemes and other forms of private provision, but the report also touched on the need for further development of other forms of provision for the old such as local authority domiciliary welfare services, residential accommodation and specialized hospital facilities.

It was estimated that over the next twenty-five years the total and working population of Great Britain would show a moderate rate of increase, but the numbers of old people would increase much more rapidly. This increase in the numbers of elderly dependants would, however, be offset to some extent by a decrease in the number of children. However, it seemed likely that by 1979 pensions and national assistance for the elderly would cost about £1,000 million, even at the rates prevailing in 1954, compared with about £550 million in that year. The 1954 figure represented nearly 4 per cent of the national income and the 1979 figure between 5 and 6 per cent, assuming a growth rate of about 1·5 per cent per annum in the national income. There would be an increasing deficit in the national insurance fund, in the sense that if contributions were not raised or the Exchequer subsidy increased the income from current contributions would be inadequate to meet the liabilities of the fund in the form of pensions payable. A further alternative was of course that the whole basis of the national insurance scheme should be changed and the costs of pensions met out of general taxation.

However, the Phillips Committee recommended that the system under which pensions were financed largely by contributions, and under which the payment of contributions was one of the conditions for receipt of benefit, should be retained. They saw it as imposing an important social discipline in that everyone was aware that higher rates of pension must be accompanied by higher contributions. They suggested that the Exchequer should be prepared to meet any deficits which would be incurred by paying pensions at existing rates to the population including an increasing proportion of the aged, but that the cost of future increases in pension rates, as distinct from the number of pensioners, should be borne mainly by increases in the rates of contribution. They did not regard the accumulation of a capital fund as appropriate to a national scheme; the 'fund' on which the national insurance scheme must rely was that of the general resources of the community built up by all possible means including increased productivity. Nor should the principle of universality be abandoned; pensions should be payable to all who qualify, irrespective of any other provision they may have made for their old age.

In the section quoted below, the Phillips Committee argued the case for raising the pension age, in stages, to 68 for men and 63 for women, and in their discussion of occupational pension schemes they cautioned against allowing such schemes to develop on lines which would encourage early retirement. The Conservative Government rejected the committee's recommendation on pension age, stating in their election manifesto later that year: 'It is our wish to avoid any change in the present minimum pension age.'

The committee felt that pensions should continue to be conditional on retirement from work and that the rule limiting the earnings of pensioners below 70 (65 for women) should be retained, as should the system of incrementing the pensions of those who stayed at work beyond the minimum retirement age. They did not think, however, that these increments played any significant part in persuading people to postpone retirement, so there was no reason to increase them.

By implication the report rejected the Beveridge contention that pensions should be at rates sufficient for subsistence: 'A contributory scheme cannot be expected to provide a rate of pension which would enable everybody, whatever his circumstances, to live without other means. Such a pension rate would be an extravagant use of national resources.' National assistance would therefore continue to have a part to play in meeting the financial needs of many old people.

There were four reservations to the main report. Dr Janet Vaughan, the only woman member of the committee, recommended that at the same time as the minimum pension ages for men and women were raised they should be made the same for both sexes. 'If women expect the same opportunities and conditions of work as men', she wrote, 'they must also expect to make the same contribution to the productivity of the country through the length of their working life.' Mr Bartlett and Mr McAndrews in their reservation opposed the raising of the minimum pension age. Professor Cairncross argued that pensions should be paid as of right on reaching minimum pension age, without any retirement condition or rule limiting earnings, and that no additions should be made to the pensions of those who stayed at work beyond minimum retirement age. Mr Honey, one of the three actuaries on the committee, differed from his colleagues on the method of financing future increases in pensions.

Phillips Report, 1954

THE PENSION AGE
The point at which the pension age under the National Insurance Scheme is fixed is obviously a matter of major importance not only in relation to the Scheme itself, but also because it is likely to influence the age limits of other schemes and retirement practices generally. It is to be observed at the outset that what we are here considering is the minimum age at which pension becomes payable, subject to retirement, and not an age at which pension becomes automatically payable, as would be the case if there were no retirement condition. When non-contributory old age pensions payable at the age of 70 were instituted in 1908, and when contributory pensions payable at the age of 65 were introduced in 1925 (the age for women was subsequently reduced to 60), no retirement condition was imposed. This condition was first applied when the present National Insurance Scheme was introduced by the National Insurance Act, 1946; the minimum pension ages under that Act are 65 for men and 60 for women.

para. 182

In discussing the minimum age for retirement from work which would be reasonably applicable to the generality of cases, it is obviously important to seek guidance from medical evidence. The medical evidence we have had is that no definition of old age can be given which can be universally applied. The state of old age can perhaps best be described as that in which the physical and mental capacity for adult life becomes so reduced that there is a definite limitation of human activity. The point at which old age begins in this sense varies from individual to individual. To the extent that old age entails dependence on others for services previously self-supplied, old age first becomes a major contributory factor in the period from 70 to 75 years of age. This is true of both men and women. There is a regrettable lack of precise evidence as to the physical capacity of women between 60 and 65 and men between 65 and 70 to continue at their own trade, especially where this involves heavy labour in difficult conditions. But it is not unreasonable to conclude that with most men and women the age of 70 can be regarded as the point after which, in the majority of cases, the ageing process may become marked and serious in its effects. Many individuals are found who are able to continue active and regular work well over this age. There are others able and willing to work if a change to some less active employment is possible.

para. 184

The medical evidence and the numbers of people who do in fact work until ages well after the present minimum pension ages indicate that over a wide field these do not by any means represent the limit of the working life. Nor can it be doubted that with the present pension ages many people receive pensions some time before reaching old age in the physical sense. The margin of premature retirements is probably influenced by the fact that the national pension may be claimed at 65 and 60; other factors may include occupational pensions and the retirement practices of industry. Whatever the reasons, in total such retirements represent a loss of able hands to the economy.

If the minimum pension ages were raised there would be a reduction in the number of pensioners and, consequently, in the amount paid in pensions. The financial saving would be substantial but it is important not to entertain exaggerated expectations with regard to the net financial effect. During the interval before reaching the new pension ages, unemployment benefit and sickness benefit would be payable, and since the unemployment and sickness experience of this age-group would certainly be higher than the average, these benefits would more than counter-balance the contributions paid during that interval by the old people. Moreover, there would, on balance, be some reduction in total receipts from contributions, if the contributions were reassessed as presumably they would be, to take account of changes in the age limit. As an illustration of the scale of financial saving that might be expected, the following example may be given. If the minimum pension age were raised now to 68 for men and 63 for women there would be a gross annual saving in expenditure on retirement pensions rising to about £125 million by 1979–80. The net saving that would be achieved is estimated to be about £50 million, or roughly one-seventh of the deficit in that year. In addition, if more people stay in employment there would probably be some gain from increased production and increased revenue from taxes payable on earnings.

An increase in the minimum pension ages, therefore, while it would not solve the financial problem, would make a substantial contribution towards doing so. If pension ages were raised, hardship would result unless certain other measures were taken at the same time. In the first place it would not be tolerable for the invalid or the man who cannot find work—and can now take pension at 65—to be left without cover after that age because a higher pension age had been fixed in the light of a higher average limit of working capacity. Sickness and unemployment benefit would, therefore, have to be available for such people at standard rates, subject to the normal contribution conditions for those benefits. Sickness benefit is already available without limit of time, but it would be necessary to remove or adjust the limit on the payment of unemployment benefit, once the ages of 65 and 60 in the case of women, had been reached. Raising the pension ages would accentuate the problems which already exist of demarcation for the purposes of sickness and unemployment benefit where older workers who are in poor health cannot find employment. Hardship would also be caused to those at present approaching pension age if the pension ages were raised without adequate notice. Some people will already have made arrangements for retirement or there may be age limits in connection with their employment whose modification will require further consideration.

We have noted a number of indications that the desirability of encouraging and facilitating the voluntary postponement of retirement is being increasingly recognised in the public services, in the universities, and, to some extent, though as yet to a lesser extent than we should like to see, in those sections of industry and commerce which operate a fixed retiring age. The practical difficulties which still have to be overcome are fully and clearly explained in the Report of the National Advisory Committee on the Employment of Older Men and Women. It is of the greatest importance that solutions for these difficulties should be found, and applied with general acceptance, and we have no doubt that the methods suggested by the Committee for attaining this object are the right ones.

But postponement of retirement while retaining the present minimum pension ages, important though it is, is only a first step. In our opinion it will not do all that is necessary to meet the needs of the situation as it will develop in the future: in particular, under the system of increments to pension for postponing retirement, the reduction in the annual amount that would otherwise be paid in pensions will be small.

In these circumstances, and after reviewing all the evidence available to us, we have reached the conclusion that some increase in the minimum pension ages is necessary, and that positive action ought to be taken immediately to set matters in train for a future change. To avoid hardship a substantial interval of some years must be allowed before an increase in the minimum pension ages can come into force; but just because of the need for long notice before a decision can become effective an early decision is the more necessary. We are fully conscious that any such proposal is likely to meet with strenuous and sincere opposition. But financial facts must be faced. We accordingly recommend that statutory provision should be made now for raising the minimum pension ages for both men and women by one year after an interval of not less than five years. The minimum pension ages should ultimately be 68 for men and 63 for women and these levels might be reached by further increases of one year at a time at appropriate intervals. The pension payable on reaching the new minimum pension ages should be at the standard rate theretofore paid at ages 65 and 60.

We do not propose any change in the existing provision whereby retirement pension is payable at age 70 (65 for women) whether or not the claimant has retired from work; it will follow, therefore, that the period during which increments can be earned will be reduced. Concurrently with these changes the right to unemployment benefit and sickness benefit should be secured on the lines indicated in paragraph 188.

So far we have considered pension ages in the context of the existing differential of five years between men and women established by the 1940 Act. When men reached the pension age of 65 their wives were, on the average, four years younger and the change enabled the wife to qualify for pension at the same time as her husband in most cases. The 1946 Act provides for an allowance for a dependent wife of a pensioner even though she is under 60 and, therefore, one of the original justifications for the differential has disappeared. The evidence is that women live longer and it would appear that from a physiological point of view the minimum pension age of 60 for women is probably too low. There is also the view, based on sex equality, that the pension ages for the two sexes should be the same.

On the other hand we are bound to recognize that women do in practice retire sooner than men. This is no doubt due in part to the lower minimum pension age for women and there may also be reasons of health. Working women, especially single women, who have to run their homes unaided outside working hours, may wish to retire as soon as possible. The policy of employers also tends towards the earlier retirement of women than men. In our opinion, restoration of parity between pension ages for the two sexes might well be justified despite these considerations if it were likely to achieve any considerable saving, and if it were not the case that substantially the increase in the pension age would apply only to single women. An increase of pension is payable to all men pensioners for their dependent wives and this increase, which is at the same rate as the married woman's rate of pension on her husband's insurance, would still be payable in respect of married women who did not work between the ages of 60 and whatever higher age is fixed. The net savings involved would be relatively small—about £20 million—and would be at the expense of married women who had kept up their own insurance, and spinsters. On the whole, we have reached the conclusion that present conditions are not such as to justify our recommending the removal of the differential.

paras. 186–93

3.7 National Insurance Act, 1959

This Act represented a major departure from the Beveridge principle of flat-rate benefits enshrined in the National Insurance Act, 1946. It introduced retirement pensions which were related to the individual's previous earnings and based on contributions which were similarly related to earnings. The two main parties had both come to the conclusion that the basic state scheme needed supplementation and both accepted that there would have to be a provision allowing employees in occupational schemes which provided equivalent or better benefits to be contracted out of the new state scheme. In fact the growth of occupational pension schemes to supplement the basic state retirement pension had been one of the factors which had created a general opinion in favour of a departure from Beveridge principles. The occupational schemes were creating two nations, those whose pensions reflected their previous earning capacity, and those who were dependent on subsistence-level pensions from the State. The Labour Party's plan was rather more radical, and they wanted the individual to be given the privilege of choosing whether or not to contract out of the state scheme; but in 1959 the Conservatives were in power, so it was their more cautious scheme which was enacted, giving to employees the privilege of deciding whether or not to opt out of the state scheme on behalf of their workers. In any case the Registrar of Non-participating Employments would have to be satisfied that the benefits offered by the employer's scheme would be in every way as good as those offered by the state scheme, and that the employee's position would be fully protected on change of employment.

Initially, insured persons earning between £9 and £15 a week—the amounts were varied later as the value of the pound fell—were required to contribute 4·5 per cent of that part of their income which fell between £9 and £15, in addition to existing national insurance contributions, and in return they were to receive enhanced pensions. The scheme was not open to self-employed persons. The Act applied to married women equally with other employed persons, and so as far as the graduated pension scheme was concerned they lost the privileged position they enjoyed under the 1946 Act of being able to decide whether to rely on their husband's contributions for reduced benefits or to pay full contributions themselves and receive full benefit.

The Government estimated that 2·5 million employees would be contracted out of the scheme; in the event nearly twice this number were contracted out by the end of 1966. About half of them were in the public service or in nationalized industries. The Act probably encouraged the further growth of private occupational pension schemes, since the benefits offered under the state scheme were very modest and it was not difficult to better them. This was partly because the earnings-related contributions were used not only to finance the enhanced pensions (on a pay-as-you-go basis—see introduction to National Insurance Act, 1946), but to rescue the finances of the flat-rate pension scheme, which was then heavily in deficit and going in deeper each year. This could of course have been achieved from general taxation, but the scheme would then have lost any pretence of being an insurance scheme, and although the reality had long been lost the time was not felt ripe to drop the pretence.

This Act was followed in 1966 by a further Act extending the principle of earnings-related benefits to unemployment, sickness and industrial injuries benefits. Again, benefits were related to the middle range of earnings so that no account was taken in determining benefits or assessing contributions of earnings above a certain level (currently £30 a week) and the very low paid do not participate. Contributions were levied at the rate of 0·5 per cent of the relevant earnings.

The 1966 Act also merged the tribunals set up to settle disputes relating to benefits under the National Insurance Act, 1946, and the National Insurance (Industrial Injuries) Act, 1946.

3.8 Ministry of Social Security Act, 1966

This Act represented a further step towards the realization of Beveridge's recommendation that administrative responsibility for social security should be concentrated in one government department. The earlier merger of the Ministry of Pensions and the Ministry of National Insurance was taken a step further when the Ministry of Social Security succeeded the Ministry of Pensions and National Insurance and absorbed the National Assistance Board, which now became known as the Supplementary Benefits Commission. The government's reasons for the change were said to be: (1) to ensure the coordination of policy for all social security benefits; (2) to ensure that people who claim contributory benefits also get any non-contributory benefits to which they are entitled; (3) to make possible the development of a comprehensive service for the public so that inquiries across the whole range of social security can be dealt with at one point of contact; and (4) to end the sharp distinction between contributory and non-contributory benefits in the hope that people would be less reluctant to apply for non-contributory benefits when they were entitled to them.

This last point was also behind the change in terminology from 'national assistance' to 'supplementary benefits'. Supplementary benefits were to be 'claimed', not, like national assistance, 'applied for'; when awarded to persons over retirement age, supplementary benefits were to be known as supplementary pensions, and when awarded below retirement age as supplementary allowances. At the same time as these changes in terminology were introduced, the rates of benefit were increased and certain of the procedures and regulations governing assistance were made more flexible and sensitive in application. Retirement pensions and supplementary pensions were made payable on the same book in a further attempt to avoid any embarrassment to an old person who claimed supplementary benefit.

These measures had their effect, and by the following year the number of applications for supplementary pensions was more than a third higher than the previous applications from retirement pensioners for national assistance.

3.9 Family Income Supplement Act, 1970

With this Act the wheel turned full circle and the Speenhamland system of supplementation of wages below a certain level was reintroduced on the English scene. The Act was preceded by a campaign by the Child Poverty Action Group which had obliged the incoming Conservative Government to pledge itself to assist families with children living in relative poverty in spite of the fact that the head of the family was in full-time work. At first it had been thought that the Government's answer to this problem would be to increase family allowances but to recover the increase from the better-off families through income tax, thus leaving it to benefit only the lower-paid. On closer examination this was not found to be a practicable solution, given the existing tax structure. For one thing, the increased allowances would be 'clawed back'—the image reflects the English view of the tax collector as a predator—from families they were intended to help. For another, the administrative costs of paying out large sums of money and then taking most of it back would be considerable.

The Family Income Supplement was therefore designed to enable cash payments to be made to families where the income of the head of the family fell below a certain level. The payment would make up half the deficit, subject to a maximum payment initially fixed at £3 a week and successively increased to £4 and to £5 as the stated income level for a family with one child rose from £15 to £18 and then to £20. The Act applied to families with a head in full-time work and the supplement could be claimed on production of five weekly pay-slips. It would then be paid for six months without further review. In addition to the cash supplement, families receiving FIS were also automatically eligible for free school meals and exempted from health charges. The administration of FIS and the interpretation of regulations was placed in the hands of the Supplementary Benefits Commission.

FIS probably provided bigger benefits for poor families than any feasible increase in family allowances would have done, and it also provided these in respect of the first or only child in a family. On the other hand it brought with it all the disadvantages of supplementing low wages in such a way that increased effort on the part of the wage earner brought him little reward. He would lose in state benefits most of what he gained in increased earnings.

The other problem which the Act encountered was a reluctance on the part of those eligible to claim the supplement. In the first year only about half the families thought to be entitled to FIS put in their claims. The Government had estimated that 134,000 couples and 54,000 single persons with children would be eligible and about 85 per cent of these would claim, and an intensive publicity campaign accompanied the Act's coming into operation in the summer of 1971. It is uncertain to what extent this campaign failed in its object of making families aware of their entitlement to claim FIS, but it seems likely that many of those who could have claimed did not do so because of the persistent dislike among the English working classes of means-tested benefits.

3.10 National Insurance (Old Persons and Widows Pensions and Attendance Allowance) Act, 1970

This modest but useful Act fulfilled a Conservative election pledge to grant pensions, as of right, to the over-80s who were already over pensionable age in 1948 when the National Insurance Act, 1946, came into operation, and who were not entitled to pensions under earlier schemes. The previous Labour Government had refused pensions to this group on the grounds that it was important to uphold the principle that pensions were granted in return for contributions, and had pointed out that in the absence of a contributory pension these old people were entitled to claim non-contributory pensions from the Supplementary Benefits Commission. This many of them were reluctant to do, in spite of the attempts which had been made to remove the stigma that had previously attached to national assistance. It was estimated that about 100,000 people would be eligible for the new pension, but in the event 120,000 old people claimed it. Many of these had no doubt previously received a supplementary pension and the new pension merely replaced this, but it is likely that the Act relieved a number who were living in dire poverty. On the other hand, the pension was a small one. Taking into account an increase granted in the following year, it amounted to £3·85 compared with the normal single person's retirement pension of £6.

The 1970 Act also enabled widows between 40 and 50 years of age without dependent children to receive a widow's pension and introduced an attendance allowance of £4·80 a week to be paid when a severely physically or mentally disabled person being cared for in his own home required frequent attention throughout the day and prolonged or repeated attention during the night, or continual supervision to prevent his being a danger to himself or others. An Attendance Allowance Board was set up to determine eligibility. Within three weeks of the Act coming into operation on 6 December 1971, nearly 100,000 claims had been lodged, almost twice as many as the number of people previously estimated to be eligible.

4 Provision and Organization of Health Services

Introduction

This section spans a period of more than fifty years, from the Dawson Report of 1920 to the National Health Service Reorganisation Act of 1973, and the National Health Service Act of 1946 falls almost exactly in the middle. Looking back over this period, the most recent reorganization can be seen as an attempt to remedy some of the features of the 1946 Act which were seen at the time, or very soon afterwards, to be unfortunate, but which then appeared to be inescapable in the light of contemporary political pressures and realities. The 1946 Act in its turn aspired to provide the free and comprehensive health service which had been envisaged by Dawson in 1920. Subsequent reports and drafts tried to give this vision an acceptable form, and it soon became clear that the doctors, the local authorities and the voluntary hospitals were the main interest groups to be taken into account. The election of a Labour Government in 1945 brought in overtones of political ideology which on the whole had been absent from previous discussions. It is doubtful if any but a Labour Government would have nationalized the voluntary hospitals.

The cost of the new service exceeded all expectations, but the Guillebaud Committee in 1956 issued a reassuring report which said that although the cost might be more than the nation had bargained for, it was at least not going up so steeply as had been feared. It was, however, 1962 before governments felt able to devote much attention to the future development of the service and to launch a capital building programme. In the same year, the medical profession itself produced a report, the Porritt Report, which voiced the discontent which many had been feeling with the tripartite structure of the service and suggested unification under area health boards. Discussion of the structure of the service gathered momentum after the publication of Kenneth Robinson's Green Paper in 1968, when it became clear that the Government intended to embark upon legislation.

Like the Act of 1946, the Act of 1973 embodied numerous compromises. Sadly, perhaps, the implementation of the Seebohm Report in the Local

Authority Social Services Act of 1970 (see pp. 448–60), and the reluctance of the doctors to have the health service run by local authorities, meant that health and social services would continue to be administered by two separate sets of authorities. There were many ready to predict that another fifteen years would see a further reorganization designed to bring the two together.

Again like the Act of 1946, the 1973 Act was influenced by ideology; not this time the ideology of a political party, but a managerial ideology which sought to ensure efficiency in the management of the new service by an insistence on the close definition of roles, responsibilities and lines of authority. The 'Grey Book' setting out the management arrangements for the reorganized health service was drawn up by a study group advised by Professor Elliott Jaques of the Brunel School of Social Science and by McKinsey and Company, the international management consultants. Much of the new terminology that the service had to learn to describe managerial relationships and processes derived from Professor Jacques's work on organizational analysis. The McKinsey influence was shown in such matters as the decision that administrators of health districts should not be accountable to their area counterparts, but directly to the area health authority, and that area officers should thus function in a 'staff' rather than a 'line' capacity.

Thus both the concepts and the language used in the management of the health service became rather more sophisticated and precise than had previously been the case. The new approach had its critics, however, who were ready to argue that it would prove insufficiently flexible and responsive to change, and that it was likely to aggravate all the problems inherent in very large, centrally controlled organizations. The Department of Health talked about 'maximum delegation downwards matched by maximum accountability upwards', but many health service administrators saw in the flood of 'guidance' circulars that issued from the Department immediately before and after the appointed day a clear intention to tighten central control and limit local discretion. Time alone will show whether the new structure and the new philosophy of management bring about improved efficiency and a more effective service to the people, or whether the critics are right.

4.1 Report on the Future Provision of Medical and Allied Services (Dawson Report)

An Interim Report to the Minister of Health by the Consultative Council on Medical and Allied Services

Published: 1920

Chairman: *The Rt Hon. Lord Dawson of Penn GCVO, KCMG, CB, MD, FRCP*

Members: *C. J. Bond CMG, FRCS (vice-chairman); N. G. Bennett MB, BCh, LDS Eng.; R. A. Bolam OBE, MD, MRCP; Victor Bonney FRCS; H. G. Dain MB, MRCS; A. Fulton MB; Sir William S. Glyn-Jones; T. A. Goodfellow CBE, MD, MRCS; T. Eustace Hill OBE, MB, BSc; F. G. Hopkins DSc, FRS; Miss M. H. F. Ivens M.B, MS; Miss Janet E. Lane-Claypon MD, DSc; A. Linnell MRCS; J. A. Macdonald LLD, MD; E. W. Morris CBE; John Robertson CMG, OBE, MD,; T. W. Shore MD, MRCS; Sir William A. Tilden DSc, FRS*

Terms of Reference (1919): *To consider and make recommendations as to the scheme or schemes requisite for the systematised provision of such forms of medical and allied services as should, in the opinion of the Council, be available for the inhabitants of a given area.*

Fifty years after publication of the Dawson Report many of its arguments and proposals still seem relevant. It is certainly entitled to be regarded as one of the founding documents of the National Health Service. A. G. L. Ives declared that although for many years its recommendations failed to be implemented in Britain it 'became a guiding star in many parts of the world', and Sir Arthur MacNalty described it as 'the parent of all regional schemes of health services'. In the long term it has been an immensely influential document; in the short term it was quietly shelved within a few months of publication.

The report was produced in the period immediately after World War I when it did not seem unrealistic to propose sweeping remedies for social ills, to ignore history and to argue from first principles. After all, the Lloyd George Government was pledged to create a land fit for heroes. Sir Bertrand Dawson—he became Lord Dawson of Penn in April 1920; the report was published in May—had shown the visionary quality of his thinking in a striking lecture on the future of the medical profession given in July 1918, and the creation of a Ministry of Health, with a doctor, Dr Addison, as Minister, in 1919 gave a further stimulus and opportunity for radical thinking on matters of health care. The Labour Party had already produced a report entitled *The Organization of the Preventive and Curative Medical Services and Hospital and Laboratory Systems under a Ministry of Health.* This urged the integration of curative and preventive services, the creation of a free national health service staffed mainly by full-time salaried doctors, and a nation-wide network of health centres. In its election manifesto, the Liberal Party declared that 'all services relating to the care and treatment of the sick and infirm should not be administered as part of the Poor Law but should be made a part of the general health services of the country.' When Dr Addison took up his post as Minister one of his first acts was the creation of the Consultative Council on Medical and Allied Services.

However, although the report was given a good press when it appeared—it was even initially welcomed by the BMA—the Government was by then facing both economic and political problems that made it less than sympathetic to radical reforms demanding the expenditure of large sums of public money. The report was an interim one, but no further meetings of the Consultative Council were called although a small group of members, including Dawson, continued to meet from time to time as an advisory body to the Ministry. Britain had to wait until after another World War for its National Health Service, and even then this did not bring with it the total integration of preventive and curative, first line and second line, medical services which the Dawson Report envisaged. Even the comprehensive survey of existing hospitals which it recommended should take place 'at an early date' was not undertaken until the Nuffield surveys of World War II laid the basis for regional planning under the NHS.

The origin of the term 'health centre', which features so largely in the report, is difficult to trace, but it was the Dawson Report that gave it wide, indeed international, currency. The concept was incorporated in a limited form in the National Health Service Act, but few centres were actually brought into operation until the late 1960s. The pioneer health centre was the Peckham experiment between the wars, and like the primary health centres described in the Dawson Report it placed great emphasis on recreational and 'keep fit' facilities, but health centres under the NHS have played down this kind of provision. Changing times, standards of living and nutrition, and the growth of alternative recreational facilities have made the stress which Dawson placed on 'physical culture' (paras. 134–44) outmoded, but it was very characteristic of its time.

The earliest true NHS health centre was the William Budd Centre, opened at Bristol in 1952, and providing facilities for local authority clinics and other health activities and for eleven general practitioners, supported by a staff of secretaries and nurses. Some later centres have included provision for x-ray and laboratory investigation and for consultant clinics, and some have been closely associated with or based at a hospital, thus moving closer to the Dawson pattern.

The text of the Dawson Report was illustrated with plans and elevations of three hypothetical primary health centres, varying in size and the facilities provided. There was also a diagram showing the distribution of services over an area, and a map showing details of a scheme that had actually been agreed by local and hospital authorities in Gloucestershire and was very much on Dawson lines.

Dawson Report, 1920

Preventive and curative medicine cannot be separated on any sound principle, and in any scheme of medical services must be brought together in close co-ordination. They must likewise be both brought within the sphere of the general practitioner, whose duties should embrace the work of communal as well as individual medicine. It appears that the present trend of the public health service towards the inclusion of certain special branches of curative work is tending to deprive both the medical student and the practitioner of the experience they need in these directions.

Any scheme of services must be available for all classes of the community, under conditions to be hereafter determined. In using the word 'available,' we do not mean that the services are to be free; we exclude for the moment the question how they are to be paid for. Any scheme must further be such that it can grow and expand, and be adapted to varying local conditions. It must be capable of comprising all those medical services necessary to the health of the people.

paras. 6–7

THE PRIMARY HEALTH CENTRE

The domiciliary services of a given district would be based on a *Primary Health Centre*—an institution equipped for services of curative and preventive medicine to be conducted by the general practitioners of that district, in conjunction with an efficient nursing service and with the aid of visiting consultants and specialists. Primary Health Centres would vary in their size and complexity according to local needs, and as to their situation in town or country, but they would for the most part be staffed by the general practitioners of their district, the patients retaining the services of their own doctors.

para. 101

Accommodation.—There would be wards of varying sizes, and for varying purposes, including provision for midwifery. The increasing employment of open-air treatment of illness would be provided for. Clinics would be equipped where doctors could see their patients and consult with each other.

Further accommodation might include the following:—

Operating room, with the necessary equipment;
Radiography rooms;
Laboratory for simple investigations;
Dispensary;
Baths, including simple hydro-therapy;
Equipment needed for Massage Electricity, Physical Culture;
A Public Mortuary;
A Common Room which would serve as a meeting-place for the general practitioners of the district, and to store Clinical Records on an agreed and standardised basis.

Only some of these facilities would be found in smaller Centres, and the more fully-equipped Centres would render aid to those less well equipped.

Communal Services.—There would be accommodation for communal services such as those for pre-natal care, child welfare, medical inspection and treatment of school children, physical culture, examination of suspected cases of tuberculosis and occupational diseases, &c. These services should, where possible, be aggregated at the Primary Centre.

So far as midwives were not available in particular districts under other arrangements, their services could be provided from the Centre, and at the Centre residential accommodation could be found not only for nurses and midwives working there, but also for those engaged in rendering similar services in the neighbourhood.

paras. 37–40

. . . In many instances, existing buildings such as Poor Law infirmaries transferred to the Health Authority, or cottage hospitals, could be adapted for the purpose, at any rate as a beginning. On the other hand it would be important to guard against making expensive alterations to buildings which, from their positions or structures, could only be makeshifts. Health Centres and hospitals require adequate ground, so as to provide not only for future expansion, but also for open-air clinics, convalescent treatment, physical culture, and such like services. Many War Memorial Hospital schemes are likely to be defective because their promoters ignore these considerations and fail to realise that a modern hospital should be part of a more comprehensive organisation.

The Personnel.—The general practitioner would attend at the Primary Centre such of his patients as required hospital treatment, irrespective of their status, though under varying conditions of service. Consultants and specialists from the staff of the Secondary Health Centre, to which the Primary Centre was attached, would attend under the conditions of the service at fixed intervals, and, under circumstances of emergency, on special summons. These or other consultants could attend patients other than those provided for at the Centre, if the patient paid for their services.

paras. 46–7

The Primary Centre would be the home of the health organisation and of the intellectual life of the doctors of that unit. Those doctors, instead of being isolated as now from each other, would be brought together and in contact with consultants and specialists; there would develop an intellectual traffic and a camaraderie to the great advantage of the service. No doubt discussions and post-graduate instruction would in time be organised and 'study leave' to teaching hospitals could easily and advantageously be arranged.

para. 50

The custom whereby each general practitioner has his consulting rooms at his own house should, under ordinary circumstances, continue, but where, as in certain congested areas it is impossible for a doctor to provide adequate accommodation at his own expense, it should be possible, if the public interest demanded it, for the Health Authority to provide such accommodation at the Primary Health Centre, or elsewhere, on such terms as are reasonable, and after previous consultation with a Local Medical Advisory Council. Where local conditions, and medical opinion, favoured the plan, collective surgeries might with advantage be tried, either attached to a Primary Health Centre, or set up elsewhere.

Work in preventive medicine by the general practitioner would be carried out both in the homes of his patients and in the Primary Health Centre, and the Health Authority should be enabled to make specific payments for such work.

We think that in any scheme of improved medical services the duty of the general practitioner to advise how to prevent disease and to improve the conditions of life among his patients should be an important element in his work.

paras. 21–3

Whole-time and Part-time Services.—The alternative of a whole-time salaried service for all doctors has received our careful consideration, and we are of opinion that by its adoption the public would be serious losers.

No doubt laboratory workers and medical administrators who do not come in personal contact with the sick can, with advantage, be paid entirely by salary.

The clinical worker, however, requires knowledge not only of the disease but of the patient; his work is more individual, and if he is to win the confidence so vital to the treatment of illness, there must be a basis not only of sound knowledge but of personal harmony. The voluntary character of the association between doctor and patient stimulates in the former the desire to excel both in skill and helpfulness. It is a true instinct which demands 'free choice of doctor,' and there should be every effort, wherever possible, to make this choice a reality. In no calling is there such a gap between perfunctory routine and the best endeavour, and the latter, in our opinion, would not be obtained under a whole-time State salaried service, which would tend, by its machinery, to discourage initiative, to diminish the sense of responsibility, and to encourage mediocrity.

para. 52

THE SECONDARY HEALTH CENTRE

A group of Primary Health Centres should in turn be based on a *Secondary Health Centre*. Here cases of difficulty, or cases requiring special treatment, would be referred from Primary Centres, whether the latter were situated in the town itself or in the country round. The equipment of the Secondary Centres would be more extensive, and the medical personnel more specialised. Patients entering a Secondary Health Centre would pass from the hands of their own doctors under the care of the medical staff of that centre. Whereas a Primary Health Centre would be mainly staffed by general practitioners, a Secondary Health Centre would be mainly staffed by consultants and specialists. It would be a consultant service in function and would be carried out by specialists or by general practitioners acting in a consulting capacity.

para. 11

The services of the Secondary Health Centres would be mainly of a consultative type. The Centres would receive cases referred to them by the Primary Centres, either on account of difficulties of diagnosis or because in their diagnosis or treatment a highly specialised equipment was needful. On the other hand, Primary Centres would ease the work of the Secondary Centres by treating less complex cases which are now sent to the larger hospitals, and by receiving patients from the Secondary Centres when the acute stage of their illness had passed. Although in some places, *e.g.*, in smaller towns, it would be necessary to have primary services also performed in Secondary Health Centres, these should not be allowed to interfere with the consulting functions of the Secondary Centre.

para. 54

A Secondary Health Centre should be completely equipped, since on the excellence of its service and organisation the efficiency of the Primary Health Centres and domiciliary services based upon it would, to a large extent, depend.

Such equipment would include:—

General Services.—Medical, Surgical.
Special Services.—Obstetric, Gynæcological, Ophthalmological, Throat and Ear, Dermatological, Orthopædic, Genito-urinary, Dental and Industrial Hygiene.
Laboratories.—Pathology in all its branches.
Other Services.—Pharmacy, Radiology, Electrotherapy, Hydrotherapy, Radiant Heat, Physical Culture, Massage, Nursing.

In existing circumstances some of these services might have to be in separated, though closely co-ordinated, institutions.

All these services would be in consultant relationship, and in some instances in administrative relationship with the Primary Centres. For instance, the organisation of the Nursing Service should be based on a Secondary Health Centre. Only in this way could the varying needs of the different districts be met, a high standard of nursing maintained, and that change of work secured which is so necessary to retain a nurse's efficiency.

The Curative Services of Secondary Health Centres would have as their nucleus existing hospitals, for to and from these latter flow the currents of medical work, and they are part of the life of their districts.

In the comprehensive organisation contemplated, the functions of existing hospitals would be considerably extended, and the present buildings would not be large enough for such purposes, and would need to be either supplemented or enlarged.

In those areas in which there are modern and well-equipped Poor Law Infirmaries the necessary accommodation might be partly provided by the transfer of these institutions from the Guardians to the Health Authority. . . .

paras. 56–9

PAYMENT FOR TREATMENT AT HEALTH CENTRES

Certain members of the Council are of the opinion that curative services at Health Centres should be provided by the Health Authority free of charge to the individual patient. The majority of the members, however, consider that this course would impose a heavy burden on public funds. Preventive services must of necessity be publicly provided: their relation to the individual is less obvious and personal. On the other hand, illness is a direct personal concern, and experience has shown that the patient, when able, is willing to contribute in some form or other to the cost of its treatment. It could, as a rule, only be a contribution to the cost, for it has already been pointed out that efficient treatment will often be beyond the means of most citizens to provide in its entirety.

We recommend that standard charges should be made in the public wards and for other curative services, though it is possible this standard charge might vary in different parts of the country.

We contemplate that such charges would more often be met by some method of insurance, though private patients recommended by their doctors would have the right to avail themselves of these services by direct payment.

paras. 71–2

DOMICILIARY NURSING

Domiciliary nursing is an essential part of a health service.

This need, so strongly felt, has led to a variety of earnest efforts to meet it by various voluntary nursing associations. These associations are mainly supported by voluntary subscriptions, by fees, and by contributions from public authorities and societies. Concentration of effort is aimed at by the affiliation of district associations to County Nursing Associations, some of which in their turn are affiliated to Queen Victoria's Jubilee Institute for Nurses. These associations, however, cannot fully meet the need.

In our opinion nursing should be available for all illnesses and all persons when the doctor deems it necessary. The services of nursing for a district should be based on the corresponding Primary and Secondary Health Centres (*see* paragraphs 40 and 58 below).

The responsibility for the provision of a nursing service would rest with the Health Authority, which would no doubt avail itself, where possible, of the excellent existing organisations.

paras. 29–31

TEACHING HOSPITALS

Secondary Health Centres should in turn be brought into relation with a *Teaching Hospital* having a Medical School. This is desirable, first in the interest of the individual patient, that in difficult cases he may have the advantages of the highest skill available, and secondly in the interest of the medical men attached to the Primary and Secondary Centres, that they may have the opportunity to follow the later stages of an illness in which they have been concerned at the beginning, to make themselves acquainted with the treatment adopted, and to appreciate the needs of a patient after his return to his home.

In those towns where Teaching Hospitals exist, Secondary Health Centres would sometimes be merged in them.

Supplementary Services.—Certain supplementary services would be a necessary part of the scheme. They would be in relation to both Primary and Secondary Health Centres, would often serve a wide area, and would require special staffs. They would comprise provision for patients suffering from such conditions as tuberculosis, mental diseases, epilepsy, certain infectious diseases, and for those in need of orthopædic treatment.

paras. 13–14

In those parts of the country where it is geograpihcally possible, it is desirable that every Secondary Health Centre should be brought into relationship with a Teaching Hospital. The academic influence, and the spirit of inquiry and progress associated with a Teaching Hospital, would permeate the system of secondary and primary health services within the allotted sphere of influence of such a medical school.

para. 75

THE VOLUNTARY HOSPITALS

That the hospitals have fallen on evil days is known to all. The reason is two-fold. One is that the prices of all the commodities a hospital has to buy—its coal, food, linen, &c., as well as the salaries and wages it has to pay, have increased. The other reason is that the investigation and treatment of disease are becoming increasingly complex. So that not only are the old items of expenditure more costly, but there is hardly a year but some new method of diagnosis or treatment makes it necessary to incur fresh expenditure, and capital expenditure in a hospital differs from capital expenditure in business, in that when a business house grows, it grows in earning capacity, but when a hospital grows it grows in spending capacity. And therefore almost without exception every hospital in the country is facing increasing difficulty in carrying on its work.

para. 82

We hope that the scheme we have suggested will help these institutions, since these institutions are an essential part of the scheme. They should receive grants in aid for work carried out, and we hope that those of them which are suitably equipped may receive grants in aid for carrying on research, and that those with schools attached may also be assisted in their most important work of medical education.

para. 84

ADMINISTRATION

We have set forth in outline a scheme of services, proceeding from the simple to the complex. In it, all the services, curative and preventive, would be brought together in close coordination under a single Health Authority for each area.

Wherever possible, the buildings needed to accommodate the services of all types should be grouped in such juxtaposition as to form one institution styled a 'Health Centre.' . . .

para. 92

It is vital to the success of any scheme of Health Service that there should be unity of idea and purpose, and complete and reciprocal communication between the associated Teaching Hospitals, Secondary Health Centres, Primary Health Centres, and the Domiciliary Services, whether the Centres are situated in town or country.

Existing methods of Health Administration, involving as they do considerable diversity of responsibility, would not secure this essential condition, and there will be need for a new type of Health Authority to bring about unity of local control for all health services, curative and preventive.

As regards the nature of this new Health Authority, there are some who favour a Statutory Committee of an existing Local Authority, whereas there are others who favour the establishment of an *ad hoc* independent body for the purpose of administering health services alone. The question which of these courses is preferable is one upon which we would rather defer any final expression of opinion.

paras. 93–4

The Composition of the Health Authority.—The representatives elected by popular vote should hold a majority on the Health Authority. We suggest that they should constitute three-fifths of the membership, and that the remaining two-fifths be made up of persons whose special knowledge would be of value in health questions, a majority of whom should be medical representatives nominated by the Local Medical Advisory Council.

By such an arrangement, the elected representatives would hold the majority of votes, and the nominated members would contribute to the skilled knowledge necessary for successful deliberation.

Methods should be provided whereby the Health Authority could obtain the advice and ascertain the collective opinions of those engaged in allied services, such as pharmacists, nurses, or midwives.

Local Medical Advisory Council.—In any areas in which there is established a Health Authority, we advise the setting up of a Local Medical Advisory Council, consisting of, say, ten to twenty members, the number varying according to the needs of the area. This Council should be elected periodically by and from all the registered practitioners resident in the area by means of the postal vote or otherwise, and the Health Authority might be made responsible for conducting the election. The Principal Medical Officer and the two Chief Assistant Medical Officers (as defined below) should be ex-officio members of this Advisory Council.

paras. 98–9

Medical Officers of the Health Authority.—The Principal Medical Officer of the new Health Authority would be the administrative head of the medical service, whether under a readjustment of the existing authorities or under an *ad hoc* authority, and would have duties and responsibilities more extensive than those attaching to the existing Medical Officer of Health.

Under the Principal Medical Officer, we recommend that there should be two

Chief Assistant Medical Officers, of whom one would be specially concerned with the administration of the curative services, and the other would be occupied more especially with preventive services. Under these again would be Assistant Medical Officers, the number varying with the size and needs of the area concerned. On the staff of the Principal Medical Officer would be the professional heads of the various services in the area, *e.g.*, the Principal Dental Officer, the Principal Matron, &c.

paras. 103–4

4.2 A General Medical Service for the Nation

Published: 1938

A General Medical Service for the Nation was a revised version of the *Proposals for a General Medical Service for the Nation* published by the British Medical Association in 1929. The earlier document had brought together a number of proposals previously made by the BMA for the extension of the national health insurance scheme to cover dependents and others not previously eligible for benefit, and to provide for maternity and consultant services. The service would revolve around the family doctor, who would have links with every hospital in his area and would be responsible for co-ordinating services to his patients.

The revised document, nine years later, took account of further developments in medical opinion and of the publication in 1937 of the Report of the Voluntary Hospitals Commission (Sankey Report), which had called for machinery to co-ordinate the work of the voluntary hospitals and to give financial assistance to the less wealthy of them. The revision was carried out by Dr Charles (later Lord) Hill, then deputy secretary, later secretary, of the BMA, and ultimately a Minister (not of health) in a Conservative Government, and chairman of the Independent Television Authority. Dr Hill, who achieved popular fame during the war years as the 'Radio Doctor' who dispensed homely advice on aperients and healthy living, and who led the BMA in its post-war confrontation with Aneurin Bevan, continued in his redraft to place the emphasis firmly on the general practitioner. The main basic principles of the scheme were said to be four in number:

(1) That the system of medical service should be directed to the achievement of positive health and the prevention of disease no less than to the relief of sickness.
(2) That there should be provided for every individual the services of a general practitioner or family doctor of his own choice.

(3) That consultants and specialists, laboratory services, and all necessary auxiliary services, together with institutional provision when required, should be available for the individual patient, normally through the agency of the family doctor.

(4) That the several parts of the complete medical service should be closely co-ordinated and developed by the application of a planned national health policy.

The principle that access to institutional and specialist services should normally be through the general practitioner was to be applied to hospital outpatients departments as well as to inpatient beds. The BMA waxed eloquent on the subject of 'abuse' of hospital outpatient departments by patients who needed only the type of service which could be provided by a general practitioner, but who preferred to go to a voluntary hospital and receive treatment free rather than attend their family doctor and pay him his fee. The outpatient department, it was argued, should be complementary to, and not a substitute for, general practice. However, if national health insurance were extended to all those with incomes below £250 a year, the temptation to 'abuse' the hospital outpatients department would be lessened and the convention that—except in emergency—hospital doctors only saw patients who had been referred by general practitioners would be generally accepted.

The BMA decided it would not be practicable to include hospital services in the benefits of an extended national health insurance scheme, but envisaged the continuation of the two main types of hospital, voluntary and local authority, dependent on separate sources of finance. There should, however, be regional co-ordinating machinery on the lines suggested in the 1937 Report of the Voluntary Hospitals Commission (the Sankey Report). Unlike the Sankey Report, the BMA document was unequivocal about the payment of hospital medical staffs. The Sankey Commission thought that in some hospitals, particularly teaching hospitals, doctors derived such substantial benefits from their appointment to the staff that there was no need to pay them, but the BMA argued that doctors should be paid whenever the institution itself received payment, whether from the patient, from a contributory scheme, or from an insurance fund.

The extension of national health insurance benefits to consultant services meant that some criteria would have to be laid down to define which doctors were entitled to consultant status. Under the National Health Service it became the case that consultant status was defined by appointment to a consultant post with a hospital authority, but the situation was by no means as clear as this in 1938. Doctors practised as consultants without necessarily holding a hospital appointment—although such an appointment, especially with a voluntary hospital, was obviously an advantage to them—and some doctors practised both as family doctors and as consultants. The BMA suggested that before becoming eligible for inclusion on the list of consultants and specialists a doctor should satisfy a representative committee of doctors that:

(a) he has held hospital or other appointments affording special opportunities for acquiring special skill and experience of the kind required for the performance of the service rendered, and has had actual recent practice in performing the service rendered or services of a similar character; or

(b) he has had special academic or postgraduate study of a subject which comprises the service rendered, and has had actual recent practice as aforesaid; or

(c) That he is generally recognized by other practitioners in the area as having special proficiency and experience in a subject which comprises the service rendered.

The document laid down principles which should govern dealings between general practitioners and consultants, principles again designed to protect the position of the family doctor as the pivot round which the whole service revolved.

A General Medical Service for the Nation, 1938

THE NATION'S HOSPITALS

As a result of the interplay of many factors—social, scientific, and legislative—the hospital situation in this country has become exceedingly complicated. The voluntary hospital, which at one time was primarily the place in which the poor could obtain the treatment they needed, is to-day serving a class which constitutes four-fifths of the community. Formerly it provided a complete medical service for the poor: now it offers a specialized service to the great majority of the population, comprising not only the poor but those who can and do pay, in part or in whole, for the service they receive. Although the income from charitable sources is still considerable, the payments to voluntary hospitals by or on behalf of patients treated, made directly or by contributory schemes or local authorities, have in recent years risen greatly, and in 1935 they constituted nearly 40 per cent. of the total income in London and nearly 60 per cent. in the provinces. No fewer than ten million persons are covered by existing contributory schemes.

Until 1930 the voluntary hospital was the main agency providing an institutional service of a specialist character. As a result of the Local Government Act, 1929, it has now been joined in this field by county and county borough councils. Under the Poor Law there had in 100 years grown up a system of institutional provision which had a bed capacity approximately twice that of the voluntary hospital. This provision, however, was available not to the community generally, but only to those who could satisfy the criterion of destitution; in fact, it was used largely for the chronic sick. The Local Government Act of 1929 transferred these institutions to the administrative control of county councils and county borough councils, giving them at the same time power to remove these institutions from their Poor Law associations. In the large towns local authorities have not been slow to exercise these powers, while in the counties there are signs of greater activity in this direction. There has thus appeared a new and powerful agency in the sphere of hospital activity.

The local authorities which have used their powers are, in many cases, planning and rebuilding, re-equipping, and restaffing many of these transferred hospitals in an endeavour to bring them up to, or even beyond, the standard of the voluntary hospital. The hospitals thus transferred and administered under Public Health Acts (in Scotland under the Local Government (Scotland) Act, 1929) will be open not only to the poor but *to all the inhabitants of the area.* Under Section 16 of the Local Government Act local authorities are required, subject to the patient's capacity to pay, to charge the whole or part of the cost of maintenance and treatment; in Scotland, under Section 28 of the Local Government (Scotland) Act, 1929, local authorities are empowered to make this charge. Local authorities in both countries are, however, empowered to accept payment from contributory scheme funds in lieu of direct payment by the patient.

Hospital provision should be included in a comprehensive national medical service. Practical considerations have led the Association to share the opinion expressed by the Royal Commission on National Health Insurance of 1926, and by the Departmental Committee on Scottish Health Services, 1936, that the inclusion of hospital provision in an insurance service is not possible. Among these considerations are the coexistence of two hospital systems as yet not fully correlated; the special characters, historical, administrative, and scientific, of the voluntary hospital system; the inadequacy of hospital accommodation; and the existence of a large contributory scheme movement at present making payments to hospitals in respect of ten million people. It is, however, of first importance that the hospitals of the country, both voluntary and municipal, should work as one service, that voluntary and statutory authorities should devise efficient machinery for co-operation with each other and with non-institutional health services, and that the available hospital accommodation should be adequate. Some of the problems of hospital co-operation, accommodation, staffing, and administration are dealt with in Sections IV (*b*) and V of this report.

paras. 41–4

For many years the Association has envisaged the evolution of a hospital system on a regional basis. In each region all the hospitals would be grouped around a central or base hospital, which would be one of the larger voluntary or council hospitals, either associated with a medical school or possessing outstanding advantages in regard to staff and equipment for undertaking the more specialized methods of treatment. Around such a base hospital or hospitals would be grouped all other hospitals in the area. These, which would include both special and cottage hospitals, would provide such services as were within their competence, patients being passed on where necessary to the central or base hospital.

The services of such a region or area would be developed as an integrated whole, and a patient would be directed to one or other of the institutions according to the conditions from which he suffers and not because of individual prejudice or preference. It is probable that such a development would render necessary the absorption of some hospitals, particularly special hospitals, and the establishment of others in order that the regional institutional service may be economical and efficient as well as complete.

Machinery for Co-operation and Consultation. Such an ideal will remain unattainable until more authoritative and comprehensive machinery of co-operation and consultation has been created. All too often voluntary hospitals have grown up in isolation without contact or co-operation with neighbouring institutions of the same kind. In order to remedy this situation the Voluntary Hospitals Commission recommended in 1937 the division of the country into hospital regions and the establishment of a regional council in each region, representative of the voluntary hospitals of the area, and a central council, representative of the voluntary hospitals of the country. The Commission suggests that while the central council would secure that no overlapping occurred between regional areas, the regional councils would, through a regional office, be responsible for the distribution of patients, the keeping of patients' records, the arrangement for the transfer of patients to and from hospitals, and the control of ambulance and other auxiliary services. It is hoped, further, that the organization of joint purchasing schemes, the giving of advice on new buildings and extensions, and the establishment of local funds on the lines of the King Edward's Fund for London would be amongst its duties. Such regional organizations linked by a central body would effect a substantial improvement in the present situation.

Although the Commission made the suggestion that representatives of local authorities should be invited to serve on regional councils, it is not to be expected that the adoption of the Commission's proposals on the subject would of itself result in the establishment of the necessary machinery for the other and extremely important form of co-operation, that between the local authority and the voluntary hospital authorities in its area. Between these agencies something more than the co-operation imposed by Section 13 of the Local Government Act, 1929, is required. A local authority can discharge its legal obligations under this section by consulting the voluntary hospital committee on the restricted subject of accommodation, and a voluntary hospital can be established or extended regardless of the statutory provision of the area. In some areas, where Section 13 committees have been set up, the consultation has been either rigid, limited and official, or completely absent. Co-operation is vital, but it would be unwise to rely merely on legal obligations.

What is wanted is the degree of consultation referred to by the Minister of Health in 1930:

'It is the confident hope and expectation of the Minister that as procedure under Section 13 becomes established and regular, it may lead to wider arrangements for the fullest consultation between the local authority and the medical profession, not merely in regard to institutional accommodation and its use, but also in regard to those numerous developments in the health provision of the people which are implicit in the new organization laid down by the Act.'

In those consultations all interests should be considered, including those of the general practitioner. In some areas local authorities will prefer to make substantial contributions to voluntary hospitals for the performance of certain work.

In others they will prefer to make their provision direct. But in every case the needs of the area should be studied. No spirit of wasteful competition should appear between agencies concerned with one purpose—the provision of the necessary hospital accommodation for the area.

In some areas there are signs of a close and continuous co-operation. In others the fact that the boundaries of the natural hospital area are not coterminous with those of the local authority has militated against the establishment of an effective machinery of co-operation. While the rearrangement of local government boundaries to meet the situation is, for a number of reasons, hardly practicable, the creation of larger units of public health administration, by the removal of such functions from local authorities below a certain size, would make it possible to treat hospital services as well as the related medical services on a wider basis as regional problems. This subject is dealt with more fully in the section devoted to Administration. . . . Until some such steps are taken, the problem of co-ordination between the two hospital agencies will prove difficult to solve.

Contributory schemes have aided to a remarkable extent the finances of voluntary hospitals, and it is possible to make arrangements whereby contributors are admitted to local authority as well as to voluntary hospitals, and payments from contributory schemes accepted by local authorities in lieu of direct assessment. Bearing in mind that the local authority must charge (and in Scotland may charge), it is clear that this provision not only makes financial co-operation between the local authority, the voluntary hospital, and the contributory scheme desirable, but emphasizes the need for separating contributory schemes from particular voluntary hospitals, and giving them reference to groups of hospitals over a wide area.

paras. 57–64

PAYMENT OF HOSPITAL STAFFS

Consideration of the change in clientele and of the change in the law leads inevitably to certain conclusions. The strictly charitable basis of the voluntary hospital now exists only to the extent that some of the poor are still treated gratuitously; the majority of persons obtaining treatment are those who can pay, desire to pay, and do in fact pay, directly or indirectly, towards their maintenance and treatment. Although the medical profession will gladly give, as always, its services gratuitously to those who cannot afford to pay for them, it is inequitable to require it to give its services without remuneration in voluntary hospitals which treat persons able to pay and which, in practice, collect payments from a large number of their patients. The field of private practice has inevitably contracted, with the result that consultants, and in particular the younger consultants, are finding it increasingly difficult to secure and maintain a standard of living which represents a reasonable reward for their services and which enables them to maintain the highest possible standard of professional efficiency. In the view of the Association there should be remuneration of the medical staff in respect of all medical services in hospital for which payment is made, directly or indirectly, by contributory scheme, by local authority, by employer, by patient, or by massed contribution. In an area where the powers conferred under the Local Government Act are being properly utilized, the voluntary hospital and the county or county borough authority are serving the same section of the community, and the principle of remuneration for services rendered should be adopted in both kinds of hospital.

para. 69

4.3 White Paper on a National Health Service, 1944

The 1942 Beveridge Report (p. 79) laid down as one of the basic assumptions underlying post-war plans for social security that there should be 'comprehensive health and rehabilitation services for the prevention and cure of disease and restoration of capacity for work, available to all members of the community'. The 1911 health insurance scheme had paved the way for the idea of a national health service, and between the wars rising costs of medical care—which in turn stemmed from the introduction of more complex and expensive techniques of treatment and investigation —rendered imperative a new approach to the financing of health care. Several reports from 1920 onwards recommended measures to co-ordinate more effectively the fragmented hospital and general practitioner services and to bolster up the (at times) rather shaky finances of the voluntary hospitals.

The Dawson Report (p. 111) was followed by the 1926 Report of the Royal Commission on National Health Insurance, which discussed the financing of medical services. In 1937 the Report of the Voluntary Hospitals Commission, the Sankey Report, put forward a plan to co-ordinate the activities of the voluntary hospitals through regional councils. The BMA's *A General Medical Service for the Nation* (p. 121), published the following year, was succeeded in 1942 by the Interim Report of the Medical Planning Commission, an influential body set up by the BMA in collaboration with the Royal College of Physicians, the Royal College of Surgeons, and other medical bodies. This report envisaged the extension of national health insurance to cover the whole 90 per cent of the population whom it was estimated could not afford private medical care, and to provide specialist as well as general medical services. Hospitals would, however, continue to charge fees according to the patient's means. Voluntary and local authority hospitals would again be co-ordinated by regional councils with a representative membership, and the regional councils would in turn be co-ordinated by provincial councils answerable to a government department, or perhaps a public corporation, headed by a Minister.

The ground was therefore well prepared for Beveridge's proposal, although he did not go into detail as to what form the service was to take. The principle of a national health service was accepted, along with the other chief recommendations of the report, by the Coalition Government of the day, and discussions started with the voluntary hospitals, the local authority interests, and the doctors. The Minister of Health at that time was Ernest Brown, who before the Beveridge Report was published had announced the Government's decision to set up machinery after the war to continue the co-operation between local authority and voluntary hospitals which characterized the wartime Emergency Medical Service and which had disclosed to the horrified eyes of teaching hospital consult-ants the poor standards of equipment and practice that prevailed in many local authority hospitals. Brown now put before representatives of the BMA a plan in which the health service would be administered by local govern-ment, although the voluntary hospitals would retain a substantial degree of independence, and general practitioners would be salaried officials. This plan was not well received by the BMA, who described it as 'an unfruitful basis for discussion', and at the end of 1943 Brown was replaced as Minister by H. U. Willink.

Willink found himself confronted by a BMA which had laid down that it would only co-operate in the setting up of a national health service if the 'character, terms and conditions of the medical service' were determined by negotiation and agreement with the medical profession and if the posi-tion of private practice were protected. By February 1944 he and his advisers had prepared a White Paper which embodied a number of concessions to the doctors. This was in fact the first published account of the Govern-ment's intentions. The Brown Plan was never published. The White Paper recorded the Government's acceptance of the Beveridge recom-mendation that access to medical services should be determined by need and not by ability to pay—'the real need being to bring the country's full resources to bear upon reducing ill health and promoting good health in all its citizens'. As in the Brown Plan, local government had an important part to play, but general practitioners were to be given the choice of salaried service or payment by capitation fees, unless they worked in health centres provided by local authorities, in which case they would be salaried. The terms of doctors' contracts would be negotiated by the Ministry of Health with the medical profession, and a Central Medical Board would be set up to administer the contracts and to try to improve the distribution of doctors over the country as a whole. Under this plan doctors would not have been deprived of the right to sell their practices.

County and county borough councils would be responsible for primary and preventive health services and joint authorities would be set up to administer hospital and specialist services and to draw up plans for the future development of health services as a whole. The joint authorities would control the municipal hospitals directly and make contractual arrangements with the voluntary hospitals for the use of their facilities. The Minister of Health, who would carry the ultimate responsibility to Parliament, would have a Central Health Services Council to advise him. There would also be a Local Health Services Council to advise the joint authority. The service would be financed by National Insurance contributions, local rates and general taxation. Both municipal and voluntary hospitals would receive financial aid from the Government, and the Government would pay both part-time and full-time specialists for their services.

When the White Paper was debated in the House of Commons the Minister set out the four basic principles of the plan as:

(1) the provision of a comprehensive service, available to all;
(2) freedom for both doctors and patients to take part in the service or not as they wished;
(3) democratic control through Parliament and the elected local authorities;
(4) machinery to ensure that the views of the professions were taken into account in the development of the service.

The White Paper was notable for the extent to which it used existing machinery whilst at the same time giving considerable weight to the views of the medical profession. In spite of this, the plan was not well received by the doctors. Most of them were gravely suspicious of any hint of salaried service. Many doctors favoured the White Paper's proposals for health centres, but the official BMA reaction was one of caution. There was strong opposition to the administration of the health service by local authorities. At both local and national level doctors were anxious for a system of administration that would keep the service 'out of politics'. At national level they favoured a public corporation largely controlled by professionals rather than the normal government department staffed by civil servants.

In the postal poll organized by the BMA, general practitioners came out strongly against the scheme outlined in the White Paper, but the consultants and specialists showed themselves to be more receptive, thus revealing the major split in the profession of which Aneurin Bevan was later to take such skilful advantage. It was also significant that the younger doctors tended to favour the scheme more than their senior colleagues. Many doctors expressed fears for the future of private practice alongside a National Health Service, even though the White Paper was careful to reserve the rights of both general practitioners and specialists to engage in private sector medicine. The poll highlighted the poor view taken by most doctors of local authority administration and their profound suspicion that the new health service would be bureaucratic and authoritarian in tone. They did not always distinguish between clinical freedom to treat their patients as they thought best and the personal freedom to maximize their incomes and arrange their work to their own convenience which had traditionally characterized medical practice.

In many ways the proposals of the White Paper were little more advanced than those put forward by the medical profession itself in the Interim Report of the Medical Planning Commission. It therefore seems possible that the opposition of the profession to the White Paper stemmed largely from the threat to private practice presented by the difference between the 90 per cent coverage envisaged by the Commission and the comprehensive service proposed by the Government. The Government may not have excluded private practice, but how long could private practice last if a comprehensive medical service was to be available to all, without payment at the time of use? The BMA also feared for the future of the voluntary hospitals, seeing the joint authorities and government financial aid as the thin edge of the wedge which would eventually undermine their independence and cause their traditional sources of finance to dry up. There may have been a consciousness, too, that at last a national health service was really about to happen and that the coming months would see the Government and the doctors engaged in hard bargaining over the terms on which doctors would enter the service. The BMA would be in a stronger position if it did not appear too eager to accept the Government's proposals at the start.

The reception accorded to the White Paper among the public at large was much more favourable. They were less concerned with questions of how the service was to be administered and how doctors were to be paid; to the public the main thing was that the service would be freely available to all. The British Hospital Association, the representative body of the voluntary hospitals, echoed the doctors' fears for the future of the voluntary hospitals if the White Paper were accepted, while the different local authority associations spoke with different voices; the two most powerful—the County Councils Association and the Association of Municipal Corporations—insisting that the joint authorities should be limited to planning and have no executive functions. Smaller authorities objected to the concentration of health functions in the hands of the larger councils and the new joint authorities.

Discussions continued throughout 1944 and by early 1945 Willink had evolved a further set of proposals and was ready to start drafting a Bill. He had abandoned the Central Medical Board and instead proposed to set up local committees to administer general practitioners' contracts. Hospital planning groups, consisting of representatives of both voluntary and municipal hospitals, would be created to prepare plans for submission to regional planning authorities based on the teaching hospitals. These regional authorities would also receive proposals for the non-hospital services from area planning authorities which were to replace the joint authorities of the White Paper. Local authorities would continue to administer their own hospitals, as would the governing bodies of the voluntary hospitals.

Willink's Bill never saw the light of day because in the summer of 1945 a general election took place, a Labour Government came to power, and Willink was replaced as Minister by Aneurin Bevan, to whom it was to fall to bring into being a National Health Service clearly deriving from many of the earlier proposals but with certain important features that would probably not have been introduced by any but a Labour Government.

White Paper on a National Health Service, 1944

LOCAL ORGANISATION

Suggestions have been made for a completely new kind of local or 'regional' authority—sometimes proposed as a vocational or technical body (like the special kind of central organisation already mentioned). In so far as those suggestions would conflict with the principle of public responsibility, they need not be considered here. Both the principles applied to central organisation—that of democratic responsibility and that of full professional guidance—must be equally applied to local organisation.

The present local government system amply embodies the former of these principles—that of democratic responsibility—and the existing local authorities are already responsible for many kinds of personal health service which will need to be incorporated in the new and wider service in future. It is certainly no part of the Government's intention to supersede and to waste these good existing resources, or needlessly to interfere with the well-tested machinery of local government as it is already known; nor would the record and experience of the existing local authorities in the personal health services justify such a course. On the contrary the Government propose to take as the basis of the local administration of the new service the county and county borough councils. But there are some requirements of the new service which the county and county borough councils cannot fulfil if they continue to act separately, each for its independent area; and changes will be necessary. In particular, for the future hospital service, it will be essential to obtain larger local areas than at present, both for planning and administration. The special needs of this service can be considered first. . . .

The essential needs of a reorganised hospital service, based on a new public duty to provide it in all its branches, are these—

(*a*) The organising area needs to cover a population and financial resources sufficient for an adequate service to be secured on an efficient and economical basis.

(*b*) The area needs to be normally of a kind where town and country requirements can be regarded as blended parts of a single problem, and catered for accordingly.

(c) The area needs to be so defined as to allow of most of the varied hospital and specialist services being organised within its boundaries (leaving for inter-area arrangement only a few specialised services).

In the majority of the areas of existing authorities none of the three conditions would be met.

It is therefore necessary to decide what the form of authority for these larger hospital areas should be. On this, various alternatives are examined in Appendix C to this Paper. The course most convenient—and indeed, in the Government's view, the only course possible at the present time—will be to create the larger area authorities by combining for this purpose the existing county and county borough councils, in joint boards operating over areas to be settled by the Minister after consultation with local interests at the outset of the scheme. There will be some exceptional cases (the county of London is the most obvious) where no combination is necessary at all; in such cases an existing authority will fulfil both its own functions and those of the new form of authority—but this will be unusual. Where the new form of joint authority is referred to in the rest of this Paper it should be taken as including any individual council which, in such exceptional circumstances may be acting in the two capacities.

While both planning and administration will usually need to be based on larger areas, this does not mean that a standard-sized area need be, or can be, prescribed for the hospital services. Local conditions—distribution of population, natural trends to various main centres of treatment, geography, transport and accessibility—must determine the size and shape of the optimum area. Sometimes simple combination of a county with the county boroughs within its boundary (i.e. the geographical county as a unit) will be sufficient; sometimes the linking of two or three small counties will be needed, sometimes other variations. . . .

As will be seen, when the hospital services are fully considered in chapter IV, the function of the new joint authorities will be to secure a complete hospital and consultant service of all kinds for each of the new and larger areas—partly by their own direct provision and partly by arrangement with voluntary hospitals, and all on the basis of an area hospital plan which they will formulate in consultation with the hospitals and others concerned, and which will require the Minister's final settlement and approval. The existing powers and duties of the present local authorities in regard to hospital services—including tuberculosis, infectious diseases and mental health—will pass to the joint authorities, together with the existing hospitals and other institutions concerned.

Outside the hospital and consultant services—that is, in the kinds of service appropriately given in local clinics and similar premises, or by domiciliary visiting (like midwifery or home-nursing)—the case for centralising all administration in the one authority over the larger area is not the same, and it is the Government's view that there should be as little upsetting of the existing organisation for these services as is compatible with achieving a unified health service for all. It will not be enough, however, simply to leave all these separate services exactly as they are now. What is essential is that, although still locally conducted with all the advantages of local knowledge and enthusiasm, they should be regarded in future as the related parts of a wider whole and should fit in with all the other branches of a comprehensive service in their planning and their distribution. For this purpose it must be the single responsibility of some authority to plan the whole, although not necessarily to provide the parts, and the obvious authority to do this—from the point of view both of its area of operation and of its constitution—will be the new joint authority.

The new joint authority will therefore be charged to examine the general needs of the area from the point of view of the health service as a whole—not only in the hospital services for which it will itself be responsible but also in these more local services. It will have the duty of producing, in consultation with the local authorities and others concerned, an area arrangement or plan for a related service of all kinds—and this will need the approval of the Minister. But, within the general framework of the approved plan, the provision and administration of most of the local services—including some new kinds of service—will normally rest with the individual county and county borough councils, and the joint authority will be concerned only to watch that the general area arrangement proves to be the right one when put into actual operation, that in fact it works out as intended, and that any subsequent additions to it, or amendments of it, which seems to be required are put in hand and submitted to the Minister. . . .

An important task, therefore, of the new joint authorities will be to unify and to co-ordinate the service. They will be the instrument through which, with the Minister, a rational and effective plan for all branches of the health service in their respective areas is secured. It will be their responsibility to see that their proposals provide for all that the inhabitants of their areas will require, to submit the proposals to the Minister as an area plan for final settlement, and subsequently to keep the plan up to date as requirements develop and to bring before the Minister any necessary changes if the plan is found not to be working out in the manner designed. They will not themselves provide and operate all the services for which the approved area plan provides; nor is there any need for them to do so. They will usually administer themselves only those branches of the service which demand direct administration over the larger area as a whole, and not those which can suitably be administered (when once a unified plan is settled) on a more localised basis. In short, the existing major local authorities will combine to secure, with the Minister, a unified general plan of the whole service for their grouped areas; they will then combine to carry out those parts of this plan which demand a single administration over all their areas together; but they will be charged individually to carry out those parts which can be separately and locally administered.

pp. 14–19

FINANCIAL ARRANGEMENTS WITH THE VOLUNTARY HOSPITALS

As already emphasised, it is the aim of the Government to enable the voluntary hospitals to take their important part in the service without loss of identity or autonomy. But it is essential to this conception that the hospitals should still look substantially to their own financial resources, to personal benefactions and the continuing support of those who believe in the voluntary hospital movement. So long, and so long only, can they retain their individuality. If once the situation were to arise in which the whole cost of the voluntary hospitals' part in the public service (a service designed for the whole population) was repaid from public money, or indeed in which it was recognised that public funds were to be used to guarantee those hospitals' financial security, the end of the voluntary movement would be near at hand.

On this footing, the financial relation between the joint authority and the individual voluntary hospital must be that of an agreement to pay a specified sum in return for services rendered or to be rendered, and this should not be assessed as a total reimbursement of costs incurred. Whether the sum will be calculated in terms of beds or occupied beds, or otherwise, is for the moment immaterial. In order to avoid a large number of individual bargains, and the risk of competitive bargaining leading to undesirable results, it will be convenient for standard payments, in respect of different kinds of hospital service which involve different levels of expense, to be settled centrally. These payments will be made by the joint authorities and will fall on local rates, assisted by exchequer grant.

In addition, both the municipal and the voluntary hospitals will receive a direct grant from central funds which will include the share, attributable to hospital services, of any sum allocated towards the cost of the comprehensive health service from the contributions of the public to any scheme of social insurance. So far as this sum represented contributions by potential patients of hospitals it could fairly be said that the Government would have collected money which might otherwise have been paid to the hospitals direct, and that the proposed grant would thus restore the balance. This grant could be based on the number of beds provided by each hospital, but in the case of voluntary hospitals it would be feasible, if so desired, to regard the aggregate of their share of the payments as a central pool from which payments to individual hospitals could be varied according to the needs and resources of each.

In either case it will be the Minister's responsibility to see that the conditions of the grant are fulfilled. If the idea of a variable grant to the voluntary hospitals is adopted, the Minister will be prepared to be guided in questions of relative need by some suitable body representing the hospitals, though the final responsibility and decision must remain with him.

Particular regard will need to be given, in connection with the area plans, to the position of hospitals used for the clinical teaching of medical students, and the question of financial assistance in respect of teaching work will be reviewed when the report is available of the Committee on Medical Schools now sitting under the chairmanship of Sir William Goodenough.

pp. 23–4

4.4 National Health Service Act, 1946

The National Health Service Act came into operation on 5 July 1948, two years after its passage through Parliament. These two years were taken up not only with administrative preparations for setting up the new health service authorities, but with prolonged and at times bitter wrangling between the medical profession and the Minister of Health, ex-miner Aneurin Bevan. It was a remarkable case of history repeating itself, with many echoes of the disputes, nearly forty years earlier, between the doctors and another Welshman, David Lloyd George, on the subject of National Health Insurance.

When Labour came to power in 1945, Bevan did not immediately enter into discussions with the doctors, but kept his own counsel for several months. When he was ready to discuss his proposals, he refused to be placed in the position of negotiating with outside bodies and interests. It was improper, he held, for a Minister to enter into understandings with outside bodies which would tie his hands in Parliament. He would consult, but not negotiate.

The British Medical Association did not care much for this approach, but real trouble with the doctors did not come until the Bill had passed through Parliament with the large majorities that the new Government was then able to command; it did not come in fact until the early months of 1948. After several months of discussion with Bevan on features of the Act which the doctors regarded as unsatisfactory, and on the terms on which they would be asked to enter the Service, a representative meeting of the BMA resolved, in January 1948, that the Act was 'so grossly at variance with the essential principles of our profession that it should be rejected absolutely by all practitioners'. Bitter leading articles in the *British Medical Journal*, the official voice of the BMA, whipped up feeling against the Act and against Bevan as its author.

The doctors' chief worry was how they would be paid. This was not specified in the Act but was to be determined by regulation. Bevan had declared against a salaried service, although there were many in his party who would have preferred it, but there were hints in some of his earlier speeches that he might be thinking of introducing it later on, when the shouting had died down. His suggestion of a basic practice allowance to help young doctors in their early years in general practice was seen as the thin end of the wedge.

Consultants and specialists were happy for the most part to receive a salary for work that most of them had previously done without payment. The problem was the general practitioners, many of whom also objected to the proposal to abolish the sale of practices. It was intended to set aside £66 million to compensate them for the loss of this right, but Dr Dain, chairman of the BMA Council, said that the amount, which was based on 1938 values plus a 16 per cent allowance for subsequent inflation, was too low.

Again, the doctors were troubled by the threat to private practice represented by the nationalization of the voluntary hospitals. Some 200 nursing homes where doctors treated their private patients were to be 'disclaimed' under the Act and left to operate outside the National Health Service, but it was feared that they might subsequently be nationalized, leaving doctors with only 'grace and favour' beds provided by the state hospitals for the use of private patients.

On many points Bevan offered ample assurances, but he was firm on the abolition of the right to sell practices. His object was to secure more flexibility in the distribution of doctors over the country in order to correct excessive inequalities. A committee consisting mainly of doctors, the Medical Practices Committee, was to be created with the power to deny doctors permission to set up in practice in areas considered to be already over-doctored.

A basic factor was that the doctors, and the BMA leadership in particular, did not trust Labour and they did not trust Bevan personally. The secretary of the BMA at the time was Dr Charles (later Lord) Hill, who was to become a few years later a prominent Conservative politician (see also p. 121). The attacks on Bevan took such a personal turn that it was little wonder he eventually lost patience and told the House of Commons that 'the whole thing begins to look more like a squalid political conspiracy than the representations of an honoured and learned profession'. He had in fact compromised heavily to satisfy the doctors. He had compromised both Labour policy and his own personal views. He would probably have preferred to abolish private practice. The health service should represent, he said, 'access, when ill, to the best that medical skill can provide'. He rejected the idea of an income limit for the health service because it would lead to 'a two-standard health service'. This would mean that 'Even if the service given is the same in both categories, there will always be the suspicion in the mind of the patient that it is not so. . . .'

The creation of regional hospital boards, hospital management committees and boards of governors to run the hospital service, and of the executive

councils to administer the contracts of general practitioners, were concessions to the doctors' dislike of working for local authorities. But just as
Bevan stood firm on the sale of practices, his strong views did not allow
him to compromise on the nationalization of the voluntary hospitals.
He not only wanted to bring them into a unified system, he disliked their
dependence on charitable appeals: 'I have always felt a shudder of repulsion
when I see nurses and sisters who ought to be at their work, and students
who ought to be at their work, going about the streets collecting money
for the hospitals'.

And so, only six months before the Act was due to come into operation,
discussions with the BMA broke down. Deadlock lasted until April when
Bevan, adopting a more conciliatory tone than he had used in the past,
repeated his earlier assurances and furthermore agreed to introduce an
amending Act (the National Health Service (Amendment) Act, 1949)
specifically prohibiting the introduction of a full-time salaried medical
service. The BMA polled its members with, this time, an inconclusive
result. In earlier polls there had been heavy majorities for non-coopera-
tion, but now it was clear that many doctors would be willing to accept
service under the Act. A stormy Special Representative Assembly of the
BMA in May brought the split in the profession into the open and eventually
resolved to accept the Act and the Minister's assurances. Within three months
of the appointed day, 86 per cent of general practitioners had accepted
service under the Act, and eventually the total rose to about 98 per cent.

While Bevan had been wrangling with the BMA, he had been wining and
dining with the Royal Colleges which were the stronghold of the consultant
branch of the profession. A number of consultants were, of course,
opposed to certain features of the Act, and in particular to the nationalization of the voluntary hospitals, and none was more vocal in opposition to
Bevan and all his works than Lord Horder, the most eminent doctor of his
day, who predicted that the Act would set back the progress of British
medicine 100 years. But the consultants had had the experience of the
Emergency Medical Service to teach them that government intervention
and government money did not necessarily mean interference with clinical
and personal freedom, and they were also being offered payment for the
hospital work which they had previously done without payment
in order to establish a reputation which would attract private patients to
their consulting rooms. They were therefore prepared to receive the Minister
with open minds and, at times, to try to moderate the fury of the BMA.
It is perhaps significant that for many years after the inception of the service
the consultants appeared relatively happy with their lot, while the general
practitioners were in a state of simmering discontent which was not
finally resolved until the late 1960s.

The National Health Service Act made no new resources available for
health care, for many years it built no new hospitals, and the training of

doctors and nurses went on much as before, without any positive intervention by the Government. The Act did, however, impose a new administrative framework and introduced a new system of financing health care. It removed any immediate financial barrier between the patient and the care or treatment he required, but it offered no guarantee, in spite of the fulsome speeches of politicians, that every demand for treatment or care would be promptly met. One immediate consequence of the Act was that by far the greater part of the costs of health care was to be met by and was therefore under the control of the Exchequer. It has, therefore been argued that the British people spent less on health care after 1948 than they might have chosen to spend if the total amount had continued to be the aggregate of many thousands of decisions by individuals, by local authorities, by voluntary hospitals, and perhaps by private health insurance schemes.

Certainly the cost of the health service came as a shock to a Government that had had to cope since 1945 with one economic crisis after another. Britain had finished the war bankrupt and in debt to America. Labour celebrated peace by embarking on a major programme of social legislation, much of which represented the fulfilment of pledges given to the people during the war by the Coalition Government. Apart from the introduction of the NHS, 5 July 1948 was also the appointed day for the National Assistance Act, 1948, the National Insurance Act, 1946, and the National Insurance (Industrial Injuries) Act, 1946. It had been hoped that the National Health Service at least would represent not pure consumption, an absolute drain on the nation's resources, but an investment which would be realized in the increased productive efficiency which would flow from a fitter population.

Before this theory could be fairly tested, however, Ministers were horrified by the spectacle of thousands of gallons of medicines cascading down the throats of the British people, and of a rush for free dentures that showed all too clearly how cost had operated as a barrier before the appointed day. Financial ceilings and certain charges had to be imposed (Bevan resigned over this) and the Guillebaud Committee (p. 142) was set up to examine the situation.

If the Act did not entirely solve the problems of financing health care, there is also a good deal of evidence that it left other problems unsolved too. The pre-war system had been fragmented, with local authority hospitals and voluntary hospitals, general practitioners for some, and local authority clinics and hospital outpatient departments for others. The post-war system was also fragmented, and lack of co-ordination between the hospital, general practitioner and local authority services was to remain a problem for the next twenty-five years and was to be the prime reason offered to the public for the next major upheaval, the health service reorganization of 1974.

The inequalities in the provision of health services, whether of hospital beds or of general practitioners, between one part of the country and another, that were so noticeable when Aneurin Bevan surveyed the scene in 1946, were still very much in evidence in 1966, so the passage of the Act did not solve that problem either. In fact the achievements of the health service, as distinct from the developments in health care and in medical science which would probably have taken place in any case, are difficult to identify and measure. The Act was a product of its time, of the party that was in power and of the man who was Minister at that time. It was also the product of the preceding discussions of the Beveridge Report itself, of the Brown Plan, the 1944 White Paper and the Willink Plan. It now seems curiously dated, with its naive belief that a new administrative structure would usher in an era of vastly better provision for the health of the people, and Bevan's simplistic view of the relations between himself as Minister and the medical profession—'My job is to give you all the facilities, resources, apparatus and help I can, and then to leave you alone as professional men and women to use your skill and judgement without hindrance.' One has the impression that the medical profession clung to this model of the relationship long after the Ministry of Health had realized that in assuming responsibility for a National Health Service it had assumed responsibility for decisions about priorities and developments for which this model made no provision.

Part I of the Act conferred on the Minister of Health the duty 'to promote the establishment in England and Wales of a comprehensive health service' and provided for the setting up of a Central Health Services Council to advise the Minister.

Part II vested in the Minister the vast majority of both municipal and voluntary hospitals and provided for the setting up of regional hospital boards, hospital management committees and boards of governors.

Part III designated county and county borough councils as local health authorities for the purpose of administering a range of public health and domiciliary health services and, curiously, ambulance services. The duty of every local authority to provide health centres was given a prominent place in this part of the Act, but this duty was allowed to go very largely by default for the first twenty years of the Service. It was quickly discovered that not only would it be rather expensive to build large numbers of health centres, but that the doctors were not prepared to work in them (see also pp. 259–60).

Part IV dealt with the administration of general medical and dental services, pharmaceutical services and supplementary ophthalmic services. Executive councils were to be set up for each local health authority's area to discharge the limited range of functions which were compatible with the position of general practitioners, dentists, pharmacists and opticians as independent contractors. This part contained provision for doctors to be compensated for the loss of the right to sell their practices.

Part V included special provisions relating to mental health services, including the transfer to the Minister of Health of the former functions of the Board of Control (see p. 370). Part VI consisted of a number of miscellaneous financial and administrative clauses.

As soon as the parliamentary schedule permitted Bevan, fulfilled his pledge to the doctors, and the National Health Service (Amendment) Act 1949 was passed. This had the effect of ensuring that any decision to introduce full-time salaried service for general medical and dental practitioners would require further legislation, as would any decision to require that all hospital consultants would be employed full-time.

National Health Service Act, 1946

OBJECTIVES

1.—(1) It shall be the duty of the Minister of Health (hereafter in this Act referred to as 'the Minister') to promote the establishment in England and Wales of a comprehensive health service designed to secure improvement in the physical and mental health of the people of England and Wales and the prevention, diagnosis and treatment of illness, and for that purpose to provide or secure the effective provision of services in accordance with the following provisions of this Act.

(2) The services so provided shall be free of charge, except where any provision of this Act expressly provides for the making and recovery of charges.

S.1

2.—(1) As from the appointed day, it shall be the duty of the Minister to provide throughout England and Wales, to such extent as he considers necessary to meet all reasonable requirements, accommodation and services of the following descriptions, that is to say:—

    (*a*) hospital accommodation;
    (*b*) medical, nursing and other services required at or for the purposes of hospitals;
    (*c*) the services of specialists, whether at a hospital, a health centre provided under Part III of this Act or a clinic or, if necessary on medical grounds, at the home of the patient;

and any accommodation and services provided under this section are in this Act referred to as 'hospital and specialist services'.

(2) Regulations may provide for the making and recovery by the Minister of such charges as may be prescribed—

    (*a*) in respect of the supply, as part of the hospital and specialist services, of any appliance which is, at the request of the person supplied, of a more expensive type than the prescribed type, or in respect of the replacement or repair of any such appliance; or (*b*) in respect of the replacement or repair of any appliance supplied as part of the services aforesaid, if it is determined in the prescribed manner that the replacement or repair is necessitated by lack of care on the part of the person supplied.

S.3 (1)–(2)

4.5 Report of the Committee of Enquiry into the Cost of the National Health Service (Guillebaud Report)

Published: 1956

Chairman: *C. W. Guillebaud CBE*

Members: *Dr J. W. Cook FRS; Miss B. A. Godwin OBE; Sir John Maud KCB; Sir Geoffrey Vickers VC*

Terms of Reference (1953): *To review the present and prospective cost of the National Health Service; to suggest means, whether by modifications in organization or otherwise, of ensuring the most effective control and efficient use of such Exchequer funds as may be made available; to advise how, in view of the burdens on the Exchequer, a rising charge upon it can be avoided while providing for the maintenance of an adequate Service; and to make recommendations.*

In an appendix to the Beveridge Report the government actuary had hazarded the guess—it could have been little more than a guess—that a national health service for Great Britain might cost about £170 million a year. Other government estimates before 1948 were around £180 million (gross cost), with a net cost to the Exchequer, after allowing for contributions from local authorities, the national insurance fund, certain limited charges to users of the service (e.g. amenity bed charges) and other sources, of about 68 per cent of this. However, in its first full year the National Health Service cost more than twice what had been estimated, £402 million, with £305 million of this falling on the Exchequer. The ophthalmic service, which had been expected to cost less than £1 million, cost £22 million; the dental service had not been expected to spend £10 million, but succeeded in swallowing up £43 million. No one had realized that there would be such a rush for free spectacles and dentures, but at least demand for these items was finite and levelled off as the backlog was dealt with, in contrast to the demand for and the cost of drugs and other services. It was not surprising that the early estimates should have been wide of the mark, for they were based on data that were often sketchy and confused, as for example the costs of the voluntary hospital system, and had to incorporate predictions about the behaviour of people in circumstances where there were few precedents to offer guidance. Nonetheless the extent of the miscalculation came as a shock to the Government which had introduced the scheme, and was immediately seized upon by the Conservative Opposition.

Stringent economy measures followed and the Minister of Health, Aneurin Bevan, besought the medical profession not to prescribe expensive drugs where cheap ones would do, and not to prescribe unnecessarily. The following year drug costs and the costs of the service as a whole increased further. In the spring of 1951 the Labour Government introduced charges for spectacles and dentures, and Aneurin Bevan resigned in protest. Later that year a general election brought the Conservatives to power and additional charges were imposed, including a prescription charge and a charge of £1 for a course of dental treatment. To all these charges there were certain exemptions and in cases of harship there was provision for help to be given by the National Assistance authorities, but the object of the charges was not only to bring additional money to the Exchequer but also to check 'abuse', which many of those seeking a scapegoat for the rising costs of the service claimed to be widespread.

However, the Conservatives were no more successful in controlling rising costs than Labour had been. Among the many attempts made to explain the situation was a book by Dr Ffrangcon Roberts, *The Cost of Health*, in which he argued that the demand for health services was potentially infinite—an attack on the position which had been held by many, including Beveridge, before 1948, and which considered that a national health service would produce a healthier population and an eventual reduction in the reservoir of disease requiring treatment.

So although it was recognized that inflation played a part in the continuing increase in the cost of the service, it was not thought to be a very large part—inflation had not become so recognizably a feature of the British way of life at that time—and apart from Dr Roberts' thesis, most emphasis in public discussion was placed on abuse, bureaucracy and waste. Until the Guillebaud Committee reported it did not seem to occur to anyone that, apart from the initial understandable miscalculation, the rising cost of the service was almost entirely an illusion brought about by the fall in the value of money.

The Guillebaud Committee were appointed in 1953 with wide terms of reference and membership which deliberately excluded anyone directly involved in the National Health Service. The Government assured a suspicious Labour Opposition that the inquiry would be completely impartial and was not intended, as Aneurin Bevan had suggested, to be an instrument to 'mutilate the National Health Service'. The committee took evidence from more than 100 organizations and groups but in addition commissioned a study of health service costs by the National Institute for Economic and Social Research. This study was carried out by Brian Abel-Smith and Richard Titmuss and was later published separately by the NIESR, but its conclusions formed the basis of Part I of the Guillebaud Report, dealing with 'Present and Prospective Cost of the National Health Service in England and Wales'.

Abel-Smith and Titmuss showed that once the cost figures were corrected for the fall in the value of money between 1949–50 and 1953-4, the rise in net cost in 'real' terms was only £11 million over the four years, compared with the nominal rise of £59 million, Moreover, not only had the value of money fallen but the national income had increased quite considerably, and expressed as a proportion of gross national product the current net cost of the service fell from 3·75 per cent in 1949–50 to 3·25 per cent in 1953–4. They also pointed out that the population had increased by nearly 2 per cent during the four years under review, and that the cost of the National Health Service per head of population was therefore, at constant prices, almost exactly the same in 1953-4 as in 1949–50.

Other facts which emerged from the study were that the hospitals were claiming an increasing, and the executive council services a declining, share of total health service resources, and that capital investment in the service had declined from 0·8 to 0·5 per cent of national fixed capital formation over the four years, in spite of the fact that 45 per cent of all hospitals had originally been erected before 1891 and many were seriously in need of replacement.

The Guillebaud Committee found that:

the Service's record of performance since the Appointed Day has been one of real achievement. The rising cost of the Service in real terms during the years 1948–54 was kept within narrow bounds; while many of the services provided were substantially expanded and improved during the period. Any charge that there has been widespread extravagance in the National Health Service, whether in respect of the spending of money or the use of manpower, is not borne out by our evidence.

Parts II–V of the report dealt in turn with the general structure of the National Health Service; the hospital and specialist services; the family practitioner services; and the local health authority services; Part VI with Whitley Council machinery; and Part VII with various general topics, including a proposal for the setting up of a research and statistics department within the Ministry of Health.

The committee concluded that no major change was required in the general administrative structure of the NHS and that unification of the three branches—the hospital service, local authority services and executive council services—was not at that time practicable. Nor was it feasible to remove the service from direct parliamentary control by the setting up of a national board or corporation to run it.

It was acknowledged that it was not possible to define for all time what constituted an 'adequate service' and that the aim had to be simply to provide the best service possible within the limits of the available resources, but the committee warned that the idea that the service could be self-limiting in the way that Beveridge had envisaged was an illusion.

In the recommendations on the hospital service the committee suggested that some of the ministry controls on capital expenditure and staff establishments should be eased and that some of the larger hospital groups should be split. Simplification of the committee structure at group level and a ceiling of 25 per cent on medical membership of hospital authorities were also recommended. The existing system of hospital cost accounts was regarded as unsatisfactory and the Guillebaud Committee gave their blessing to the introduction of a system of departmental costing which had recently been recommended by a ministry working party.

In reviewing the executive council and local health authority services the Guillebaud Committee declared against major changes, in favour of closer co-operation between these branches and the hospital service, and thought that those who had criticized the NHS for spending too much on disease and too little on prevention had tended to overstate their case. The report did however express concern on the subject of the maternity services, which were 'in a state of some confusion, which must impair their usefulness, and which should not be allowed to continue', and called for the setting up of a separate committee to review the organization of the maternity services at an early date—this in due course led to the appointment of the Cranbrook Committee, which reported in 1959.

The Whitley Council machinery which had been set up to negotiate salaries and conditions of service of staff in the NHS was criticized in Part VI for the rigidity and inflexibility of the terms in which agreements were drawn up, and for under-representation of the actual employing authorities—the hospital management committees and regional hospital boards—on the staff sides, compared with the central government health departments.

The report was signed by all members of the committee but in the case of Miss Godwin and Sir John Maud this was subject to reservations that were printed with the report. Miss Godwin wanted the teaching hospitals of England and Wales to be taken under the wing of the regional hospital boards, like their counterparts in Scotland, instead of having boards of governors directly responsible to the Ministry; she wanted most of the existing charges which had been introduced since 1948 abolished; and she wanted provision for paying patients' travelling expenses other than through the National Assistance Board. Sir John Maud in his reservation reviewed the arguments for unifying the service and whilst agreeing that at that time radical reorganization was inadvisable thought the ultimate aim should be unification under local government, even though this might only be possible after a reorganization of local government itself which would have as one of its principal objects making local government administratively and financially able to accept responsibility for the National Health Service. Many years later, as Lord Redcliffe-Maud, Sir John had the opportunity to chair a Royal Commission on Local Government which recommended just such a reorganization.

Guillebaud Report, 1956

THE STRUCTURE OF THE NATIONAL HEALTH SERVICE

We believe that the structure of the National Health Service laid down in the Acts of 1946 and 1947 was framed broadly on sound lines, having regard to the historical pattern of the medical and social services of this country. It is very true that it suffers from many defects as a result of the division of functions between different authorities, and that there is a lack of co-ordination between the different parts of the Service. But the framers of the Acts of 1946 and 1947 had not the advantage of a clean slate; they had to take account of the basic realities of the situation as it had evolved. It is also true that even now, after only seven years of operation, the Service works much better in practice than it looks on paper. That it should be possible to say this is a remarkable tribute to the sense of responsibility and devoted efforts of the vast majority of all those engaged in the Service, and also to their determination to make the system work.

We are strongly of opinion that it would be altogether premature at the present time to propose any fundamental change in the structure of the National Health Service. It is still a very young service and it is only beginning to grapple with the deeper and wider problems which confront it. We repeat what we said earlier—that what is most needed at the present time is the prospect of a period of stability over the next few years, in order that all the various authorities and representative bodies can think and plan ahead with the knowledge that they will be building on firm foundations.

The present National Health Service is both too recent in origin and also bears too much the imprint of the historical circumstances from which it sprang, for any one to be able to do more than make a guess at the lines along which it may be expected to evolve. Those who have spent the greater part of their working lives under quite different conditions—for example consultants serving voluntary hospitals in an honorary capacity; Medical Officers of Health; members of local authorities in charge of municipal hospitals—these and many others have not always found it easy to adapt themselves to the new order of things. Some of the strains and stresses of the National Health Service are attributable to the difficulty experienced by many, who had grown up under the old system, when called upon to operate a service administered on different lines. Longer experience of the working of the Service and the gradual emergence of a new generation may make comparatively simple many things which now appear difficult or impracticable.

What is essential is the recognition that the hospitals, the general practitioners and the local authorities have each an indispensable task to fulfil in their respective spheres. They are however each severally only a part of a single National Health Service; and the efficiency of the Service depends not merely on the quality and quantity of the work that each of these branches performs within its own sphere, but on the degree to which they co-operate with one another to accomplish the ends for which the Service as a whole exists.

We conclude therefore that no sufficiently strong case has been made out for transferring either the hospital service or the Executive Council services to the local health authorities, nor for transferring the Executive Council services to the Regional Hospital Boards.

In our view, a more important cleavage than the division of the National Health Service into three parts is that between the hospital service and the services provided by the local authorities under Part III of the National Assistance Act, and we come back to this point in Part V of our Report when dealing with the services relating to the care of the aged.

paras. 147–51

THE TEACHING HOSPITALS

We do not feel that a convincing case has been made out for transferring the teaching hospitals to the Regional Hospital Boards.

It seems to us that one of the dangers of a national hospital system lies in over-standardisation and uniformity. There is a distinct advantage therefore in preserving the separate status of the teaching hospitals outside the Regional Hospital Board framework. In the past, the great advances in medical techniques and knowledge have come from the teaching centres, and these benefits have accrued thereafter to the non-teaching hospitals. In our view, it would be a short-sighted policy now to subordinate these institutions upon which so much depends for the future development of the service, to the Regional Hospital Boards. The medical and nursing standards of the whole service are set by the teaching hospitals who send out trained staff to work in the regional hospitals. It is entirely fitting therefore that the standards of the teaching hospitals themselves should be maintained at the highest possible level.

If the teaching hospitals continue to maintain the standards and the reputation to which they are in our view entitled, it is inevitable that they will attract medical and nursing staff more readily than the non-teaching hospitals, whatever administrative system is adopted. This is a fundamental characteristic of the teaching hospital and is not the result of their separate administration under Boards of Governors. So far as the nurses are concerned, we have been told that some might refuse to take up employment in the service if an appointment could not be secured with a teaching hospital, while it does not follow that nurses deliberately diverted from teaching hospitals would necessarily accept posts elsewhere.

The special role of the teaching hospitals, however, does not imply that the

Boards of Governors should work in isolation from the other authorities providing services under the National Health Service Acts. Nor should they resent the same careful examination of their annual expenditures as that carried out with other hospital authorities, to ensure that good value is received for money spent, and that savings are effected both in money and manpower wherever possible.

From the evidence we have heard, it is clear that some Boards of Governors and Regional Hospital Boards have solved the problem of co-operation satisfactorily and are planning their services and working together in very close harmony. Relations in other areas are not so harmonious, and where this is the case, there is evident need to ensure that the services of teaching and non-teaching hospitals are developed together to their mutual advantage. This is not a question of machinery, but of the will to co-operate, and we consider it a matter of very great importance that all Boards of Governors and Regional Hospital Boards should do their utmost whether through the use of Joint Committees or other means, to effect a smooth administration of the hospital service as a whole.

The introduction of a more satisfactory system of hospital costing should make it possible to throw more light on the relatively high running costs of the teaching hospitals in England and Wales—particularly the London teaching hospitals. So far as the actual control of expenditure is concerned, however, we do not believe that the Regional Hospital Boards would be any better placed than the Ministry to make the annual allocations of money to the teaching hospitals and to examine their annual running costs. The Ministry is in a position to weigh the needs of one teaching hospital against other teaching hospitals in the service, while many Regional Boards would be judging the disparate needs of one teaching hospital against a large number of non-teaching hospitals in their Regions. In our view therefore it is appropriate that the Ministry should continue to carry out this function in preference to the Regional Boards. When a more satisfactory system of hospital costing is in operation, it will give Boards of Governors, in conjunction with the Ministry, a better opportunity for examining their detailed running costs in order to ascertain the precise reasons for their excess over the corresponding costs of other hospitals in the service and for seeing whether the excess is entirely justified. It has been put to us that in the past some Boards of Governors have not taken this matter as seriously as they might—perhaps because the existing Costing Returns have been regarded as inadequate for the purpose of carrying out any realistic comparison of costs. There can be no doubt that the relatively high costs of the teaching hospitals are a source of irritation to, and criticism by, many Regional Boards and Management Committees, and the onus lies on the Boards of Governors to prove that the whole of their expenditure is in fact fully justified.

In short, while we support the separate administration of teaching hospitals through the Boards of Governors, we would stress that their separate status brings with it a heavy responsibility both for the fullest co-operation with other organisations in the Health Service and for the most efficient and economical management within the teaching hospitals themselves. If the teaching hospitals are to justify their special position, they must demonstrate, as a number of them already do, both their willingness to co-operate with the Regional Hospital

Boards in fulfilling their obligations to the Regions in which they are placed and also their determination to keep expenditure within reasonable bounds.

paras. 183–8

REGIONAL HOSPITAL BOARDS

We should make it clear at the outset that we consider two levels of management —i.e., the regional and group levels—to be essential for the efficient administration of a service which deals with more than 3,000 hospitals in England and Wales and some 400 in Scotland. We do not agree therefore with those who have recommended that:—

(*a*) the Regional Boards should be abolished, or
(*b*) that the number of Regional Boards should be increased (e.g., to 40 in England and Wales), and the Hospital Management Committees (and Boards of Management in Scotland) eliminated altogether.

If there were say 40 Regional Boards in England and Wales, it seems to us that their areas would be too small for efficient planning and yet much too large for the efficient management of hospitals. The service undoubtedly requires both regional authorities covering areas large enough for purposes of planning and general supervision, and also group management authorities with responsibility for the day-to-day running of the service.

A further advantage which we can see in the existence of a system of Regional Hospital Boards is the scope which it affords for some measure of variation in the way in which problems of the hospital service are treated in the different Regions. While it is essential that matters of major policy should be determined centrally, it is desirable, in the interest of avoiding excessive uniformity and standardisation that the individual Regional Boards should have adequate freedom both to experiment and to adopt measures which have regard to their own special conditions and requirements...

We are of the opinion that the primary need now is to give more emphasis, in England and Wales, to the Regional Boards' responsibility for the general oversight and supervision of the service (in addition to their planning functions), though without in any way detracting from the Hospital Management Committees' direct responsibility for day-to-day management. We agree therefore with the trend which appears to us to have been taking place in the distribution of powers and functions since 1951.

It should be clearly recognised throughout the service in England and Wales that Hospital Management Committees are responsible to their Regional Boards for the efficient administration of their services, and that the Boards in their turn are responsible to the Minister. We understand that this is the system which prevails in Scotland where it has been established both in principle and in practice since the inception of the National Health Service; and we believe that it represents the proper relationship which should exist between these different levels of management and trust. As the Regional Hospital Boards have the task of allocating regional funds between the Management Committees, they must have the knowledge to enable them to make the right allocations, and to satisfy themselves that Management Committees are exercising their functions in a responsible and efficient manner, and that there is no unnecessary expenditure of public funds. We derived from our evidence the strong impression that some Regional Hospital Boards feel that they lack the authority for fulfilling this role, not through any insufficiency of formal powers, but because their responsibility for supervision has lacked both the necessary support from above and the necessary acceptance from below. To some extent this is inevitable in a new service. The acceptance of authority (by which we do not mean dictation) is only one aspect of a relationship which takes time to grow and which, when developed, links the different levels of management in a nexus of mutual dependence. To create this relationship is a major duty of all concerned at every level.

We consider that it is neither necessary nor desirable to define in detail the powers and functions of each level of management. We are confident that Boards and Committees can be relied on to find their own means of striking a balance; and if, exceptionally, they should be unable to reach agreement on any matter, the issue can be referred to the Health Departments for settlement. This is the normal administrative practice in any chain of command; each level of management must learn to "carry along with it" the authorities for whom it is responsible; and in a unified service each level must equally recognise its duty to act responsibly as members of the larger organisation.

We conclude that Regional Hospital Boards should be told, and Hospital Management Committees should accept, that the Regional Boards are responsible for exercising a general oversight and supervision over the administration of the hospital service in their Regions. It is a corollary of this recommendation that the Ministry should leave the task of supervising the Hospital Management Committees to the Regional Boards and should not itself undertake this task over the head of the Boards.

paras. 207, 211–12

LOCAL HEALTH AND WELFARE SERVICES

We appreciate that, strictly, our terms of reference do not relate to the welfare services, but there are points where the welfare services are so closely related to the Health Service—particularly in relation to the care of the aged—that we cannot deal properly with our remit without paying some regard to their provision. We have noted with interest that a number of authorities have taken steps with satisfactory results to combine the administration of their local health and welfare services under one committee (the health committee) of the council. In the majority of areas however, these services are still administered by two separate committees of the county council or county borough council—i.e., the health committee and the welfare committee.

In view of the very close relationship which exists between the domiciliary services provided under the National Health Service Acts and the National Assistance Act, and bearing in mind the close connection between the services for the aged under the National Health Service and the provision of residential accommodation for old people under the National Assistance Act, we recommend that all authorities who have not yet done so should review the working of their health and welfare services to see whether their efficiency might be improved, and the interests of patients better served, by combining their administration under one committee of the council, or under a joint sub-committee.

para. 606

4.6 A Hospital Plan for England and Wales

Published: 1962

The *Hospital Plan* was published by the Ministry of Health while Enoch Powell was Minister, and marked the resumption of major hospital construction in Britain after a gap of more than twenty years due to the war and its aftermath. In 1948 the National Health Service inherited from the local authorities and voluntary bodies in England and Wales some 2,800 hospitals with slightly more than 500,000 beds; nearly half these hospitals had been built before 1891 and one in five before 1861. The outbreak of war in 1939 had led not only to a virtual standstill in hospital construction but also to twenty years' neglect in the maintenance of these very old buildings. The physical fabric of the National Health Service was therefore in very poor shape.

The Plan was based on a comprehensive review, region by region, of the country's hospitals and the relationship of existing provision to the needs of the population. Estimates were made of the appropriate number of acute, geriatric, maternity, mental and mental subnormality beds per thousand population; these estimates broke new ground and were based on such limited research studies as were available along with the experience of those regions that had perforce had to manage with a relatively low proportion of beds to population. For acute beds the new norm was 3·3/1,000 (against the existing national figure of 3·9/1,000—a figure which concealed substantial inter-regional variations); maternity beds 0·58/1,000 (0·45/1,000); geriatric beds 1·4/1,000 (1·5/1,000); mental illness beds 1·8/1,000 (3·3/1,000); mental subnormality beds 1·3/1,000 (1·3/1,000).

The Plan thus implied a reduction in the total number of beds as new, larger hospitals replaced numbers of older, smaller establishments, and as hospital beds came to be more effectively used. The costs of keeping patients in hospital were rising fast and in some parts of the country, notably the Oxford region, it had been demonstrated that the average length of stay in hospital could be markedly reduced without, as far as could be seen, any ill effects on the patients' recovery. In addition it was hoped that for many geriatric and mentally ill patients the emphasis would change from care in the hospital to care in the community. An exception to this general trend was maternity care, for it was expected that as time went by more women would expect to have their babies in hospital, so more beds would be required. The existing figure for mental subnormality beds was accepted simply because there was so little information on which to base an estimate of true requirements.

The cornerstone of the *Hospital Plan* was the idea of the district general hospital, a hospital of 600–800 beds serving a population of 100,000–150,000 and providing treatment and diagnostic facilities for both in-patients and out-patients in all the commoner specialties. The Plan did, however, concede (as the later Bonham-Carter Report, q.v., p. 160, did not) that separate provision would have to be made for long-stay geriatric and psychiatric care, and for the mentally subnormal.

Not surprisingly, the proposals to close many small hospitals as new district general hospitals were built aroused substantial local opposition, particularly in such areas as the Welsh valleys where communications were difficult and a good deal of local sentiment attached to the local hospital. Problems arose too with the cost of the new hospitals, which proved to be rather more expensive to build than had been envisaged. Again there had been no experience on which to base realistic estimates for the last twenty years. The plan announced that standards and cost limits were to be laid down which would govern all subsequent hospital building and that the possibility of standardizing building components was being explored.

The most controversial aspect of the Plan was probably the proposal to reduce the number of mental illness beds over a period of fifteen years from 3·3/1,000 population to 1·8/1,000. This reflected the belief that there were many long-stay patients in mental hospitals who could be discharged into the community if an active programme of rehabilitation were pursued, and that with modern methods of treatment fewer patients would become chronically ill and require long-term care. It was, however, extremely disturbing to the staff of the mental hospitals to be told that beds were likely to close on such a massive scale and for a year or two morale in the mental hospitals was at a very low ebb. It only started to recover when it was realized that—as indeed the Plan had pointed out—more intensive methods of treatment required more staff to care for a smaller number of patients.

The Plan set out in detail for each hospital region the new hospitals and major hospital buildings that were thought to be required, with approximate starting dates, and lists of hospitals likely to be closed by about 1975. There were several subsequent revisions of the Plan in order to keep it abreast of changing requirements and resources, but the basic principles remained unchanged, although the Bonham-Carter Report (q.v., p. 160) in 1969 pronounced in favour of larger and more comprehensive hospital complexes to serve populations upwards of 200,000.

A Hospital Plan for England and Wales, 1962

THE DISTRICT GENERAL HOSPITAL

In recent years there has been a trend towards greater interdependence of the various branches of medicine and also an increasing realisation of the need to bring together a wide range of the facilities required for diagnosis and treatment. Hence the concept of the district general hospital (described in more detail in the Ministry of Health's Building Note No. 3) which provides treatment and diagnostic facilities both for in-patients and out-patients and includes a maternity unit, a short-stay psychiatric unit, a geriatric unit and facilities for the isolation of infectious diseases. Provision is made for all other ordinary specialties, but there are a small number of specialties, such as radiotherapy, neurosurgery, plastic surgery and thoracic surgery which need a larger catchment area and would be provided only at certain hospitals. The size of hospital this concept implies would normally be of 600–800 beds serving a population of 100,000–150,000. Some district general hospitals particularly where more specialties are provided, might be larger. Others would be smaller, though they would rarely be of less than about 300 beds. Each would be located in or near the centre or one of the centres of population of the area which it serves. The district general hospital offers the most practicable method of placing the full range of hospital facilities at the disposal of patients and this consideration far outweighs the disadvantage of longer travel for some patients and their visitors.

Changes which have been developing in hospital practice will require increased facilities for out-patient treatment to be provided in the district general hospital. The out-patient departments are likely to include operating theatres for out-patients only and more day wards where patients undergoing investigations or operations may recover from them without occupying beds as in-patients. There will often be a need for the establishment of peripheral clinics or diagnostic centres where consultation can be undertaken locally without the full resources of the general hospital. Some existing small hospitals may be suitable for this purpose.

The accident services are the subject of more than one study proceeding at the present time, but it is clear that the need will be for the development of an accident and emergency service organised on a regional basis and providing continuous cover by expert medical staff. The pattern of district general hospitals fits this conception: most, but not necessarily all, of them will contain fully developed accident and emergency departments, each of which will be linked with appropriate centres providing regional specialist services.

A maternity unit will be a normal part of the district general hospital where full and continuous consultant cover will be at hand for all beds, including those which should be available to general practitioners for the care of their own patients undergoing normal confinements. There will sometimes be justification on geographical grounds for providing maternity units at peripheral towns where the population to be served is sufficient to support a viable unit. Thus the retention of a local maternity unit of 15 to 25 beds serving a population of 35–50,000 might be regarded as justified if the nearest district general hospital was 15 to 20 miles away. In all circumstances however, potentially abnormal deliveries should take place in the district general hospital.

Each district general hospital will include an active geriatric unit. It is through this unit that elderly people likely to require prolonged treatment will usually be first admitted. Others will be transferred to it from acute wards. Normally, some beds for long stay also will be at the district general hospital; but limitations on the size of the main hospital or its distance from smaller towns which it serves will often justify long-stay annexes on separate sites or geriatric provision at small hospitals.

The district general hospitals will provide (apart from psychiatry and regional specialties) the great majority of the beds which are needed, and as they are developed a large number of the existing small hospitals will cease to be needed. This is implicit in the new pattern and indeed is part and parcel of the improvement of the service for hospital patients. But many small hospitals will still be needed. Some will be retained as maternity units (para. 23), though any additional provision will nearly always be at the district general hospital. Others will provide long-stay geriatric units (para. 24). Others again, where a local population is remote or inaccessible, or where isolated towns receive an exceptional seasonal influx of visitors, will continue to admit medical emergencies which do not require specialist facilities. Finally, though this is not indicated in detail in the plan, many small hospitals where no beds, or at least no acute beds, need eventually be retained will be suitable for providing out-patient services (para. 21).

It is now generally accepted that short-stay patients should be treated in units nearer to their homes than is generally possible with large isolated mental hospitals and that it will usually be desirable to have these units attached to general hospitals. The plan therefore provides for a considerable increase in the number of short-stay units of this kind. To ensure adequate treatment they need to be of a certain size, which will range from 30 beds up to 60 or more depending on the population to be served. As the majority of patients in such a unit will not require nursing in bed, their treatment and rehabilitation proceed more favourably if they can go in and out of the hospital during the day and so participate in the various activities of the general community. To facilitate this, the accommodation should preferably be on the lower floors or in a separate building in the grounds of the general hospital. Patients who need longer periods of treatment must have a more specialised regime and facilities; but units for their treatment also must not be too large, and should not be in isolated positions. In this new pattern there will be no place for many of the existing mental hospitals. Some can probably continue if reduced in size and improved, but a large number will in course of time be abandoned.

Beds for subnormal and severely subnormal patients do not need to be at the district general hospital. Subnormal patients should be cared for separately from the severely subnormal and in comparatively small units, preferably of not more than 200 beds, which are best located in areas where after training the patients can be employed and so eventually may return to the community. Severely subnormal patients should be cared for in separate hospitals except that severely subnormal children who suffer from physical handicap can be looked after in a separate ward of the paediatric unit at a district general hospital.

paras. 20–5, 27–8

COMMUNITY SERVICES

While the local authority services affect the number of hospital beds required for all types of illness and infirmity, physical and mental, acute and chronic, they have a special bearing on hospital provision for the elderly, for maternity and for mental disorder.

The ratio of 10 geriatric beds per 1,000 population over the age of 65, or 1·4 per 1,000 total population (para. 16), assumes that the standard of services for the elderly outside hospital will be brought generally up to the level of the best current practice. Even this level is capable of being raised further, and some areas fall well below it. The services for the elderly include not only health visitors, social workers, home nurses and home helps, but also residential accommodation provided under Part III of the National Assistance Act for those in need of care and attention. The total number of people in residential accommodation provided by a local authority either directly or by arrangement with a voluntary organisation increased from 79,877 (of whom 69,340 were aged) at the end of 1958 to 82,017 (71,412 aged) at the end of 1959, and 84,556 (73,881 aged) at the end of 1960. The 73,881 aged persons at the latter date represented 13·54 per 1,000 population over the age of 65. In addition the increase in housing accommodation for old people, ranging from separate, specially designed dwellings to group schemes with a warden and communal services, has also made it possible for more to be cared for outside hospital.

The increase forecast in hospital confinements (para. 15) does not imply that a domiciliary midwifery service is less important than in the past. It is true that a decrease is assumed in the proportion of confinements that will take place at home. But there is some tendency to reduce the length of stay in hospital in selected cases, and should this tendency spread it may be associated with a still lower proportion of home confinements. These trends must materially affect the volume and nature of the work of local authority midwives. The type of work required following early discharge from hospital is very suitable for midwives with family responsibilities who give part-time service. The employment of more part-time midwives may well prove an important aid to the domiciliary service in meeting its future tasks.

The ratio of 1·8 hospital beds per 1,000 population adopted as the probable limit of requirements for the mentally ill by 1975 (para. 17) takes no account of any contribution from expanded community mental health services. These services are still very much in their infancy. Thus only four residential hostels specially designed for the mentally ill have so far been provided by local authorities. But many more are planned: over 150 are included in their programmes for the next few years. Concurrently, there should be a notable increase in the amount of home care, as more trained social workers are recruited for work with the mentally ill, especially with the stimulus of the national training council for which provision is made in the Health Visitors and Social Workers Training Bill now before Parliament. All this expansion of local authority services cannot fail to have a considerable effect on the hospital provision that will need to be made for the mentally ill in the future.

In setting the ratio of hospital beds for the subnormal and severely subnormal, paragraph 18 assumes that there will be a further expansion of the community services. These services, which can avoid or postpone the need for hospital admission, and enable more patients to be discharged, have grown considerably during the past few years. For example, the following table shows the rise each year between the end of 1955 and the end of 1960 in the numbers of the sub-normal receiving training in training centres:—

			1955	1956	1957	1958	1959	1960
Juniors	..	..	8,055	8,665	9,108	9,804	10,566	11,614
Adults	..	..	4,317	4,761	5,243	6,009	6,987	8,182

This training was given in 468 centres at the end of 1960. Twenty more centres have since been opened and about 350 are planned by local authorities over the next few years. Expansion may be expected also in other community services for the subnormal, including residential hostels and facilities for sheltered employment.

paras. 38–42

4.7 Health and Welfare: the Development of Community Care

Plans for the Health and Welfare Services of the Local Authorities in England and Wales.

Published: 1963

When *A Hospital Plan for England and Wales* was published in 1962 it was expressly intended to be 'complementary to the expected development of the services for prevention and for care in the community'. All local health and welfare authorities were therefore invited at the beginning of 1962 to prepare plans for the development of their services over the ten years from 1962–3 to 1971–2. No attempt was made to indicate common standards to which plans should conform, nor was any attempt made to get the plans of individual authorities modified to bring them into conformity with any standards or norms before they were published in *Health and Welfare: the Development of Community Care*.

Authorities were asked to prepare summaries showing, for each year up to 1966–7, and for the five-year period from 1967–8 to 1971–2, the staff they would require to give effect to their plans, the buildings they hoped to erect, and the estimated capital and revenue expenditure involved. The responses showed that local authorities contemplated an overall increase in staff from the 85,000 employed in local health and welfare services in 1963 to 119,000 by 1972, an increase of 39 per cent in nine years. (Over the previous five years the estimated increase had been 20 per cent.) The plans submitted envisaged capital expenditure of about £150 million in the first half of the decade and £70 million in the second half, estimates which led the Ministry of Health to suggest that perhaps local authorities had greatly overestimated the likely rate of progress in the earlier years and underestimated it for the later years. The rate of estimated increase in revenue expenditure—47 per cent in nine years—was approximately the same as during the preceding five years, but again the rate of growth likely appeared to have been overestimated in the earlier years and underestimated in the later years—possibly reflecting the similar distortion of the capital investment plan.

The Ministry's introductory comments drew attention to the change of emphasis from the provision of particular services to the meeting of particular needs, and the text (comprising the first fifty pages of the blue book, the remaining 320 pages being devoted to the local authority plans set out in the form of statistical tables) was organized in chapters based on the needs of four broad groups of people: mothers and young children; the elderly; the mentally disordered; and the physically handicapped. These were followed by chapters on some other groups in need of community care; the ambulance service; and voluntary effort.

Apart from the predictably wide variations between authorities there were some interesting general tendencies to overestimate or underestimate for particular groups of staff or forms of investment. Many local authorities appeared not to realize how steadily domiciliary confinements were declining in number, and the figure of 6,509 midwives (0·13 per 1,000 population) which local authority plans envisaged for 1972 seemed likely to be substantially higher than would be required. In fact by 30 September 1971 local authorities were employing only 4,081 midwives (full-time equivalents). Conversely, the widening scope of the health visitor—originally largely concerned with mothers and very young children, but by 1962 undertaking rapidly increasing responsibilities with other groups in the population, especially the elderly—did not seem to be taken fully into account in the estimate that 7,607 health visitors would be required by 1972. The Ministry thought the figure should be nearer 8,600, or 0·17 rather than 0·15 per 1,000 population, but by 30 September 1971 local authorities had only the equivalent of 6,035 full-time health visitors. The Ministry were also uneasy about the envisaged rate of development of residential homes for the elderly and of residential accommodation for the mentally handicapped, and suggested that if local authorities thought 0·46 places per 1,000 population was the right ratio for training centres for mentally subnormal children then they ought to plan for rather more than the 0·55 places per 1,000 population envisaged for adults. The estimates of need for social workers were also on the low side and the Ministry thought that, as training facilities increased as a result of the recommendations of the Younghusband Report, local authorities might find it possible to build up their social work staffs rather more rapidly, perhaps to 0·11 per 1,000 population instead of the 0·10 per 1,000 envisaged in the plans.

Significantly, health centres hardly figured at all in local authority plans at this point in time. Proposals for four new centres, in addition to the seventeen which had already been set up, were at an advanced stage, and local authorities planned to provide a further twenty-six within the next decade, bringing the total for the country as a whole to forty-seven. The Ministry saw nothing to criticize here, but commented on health centres: 'The circumstances which now justify their provision do not arise frequently: there must be a local need for new premises, coinciding with a keen desire on the part of both local health authority and general practitioners to develop this particular form of co-operation.' This 'keen desire' was obviously not very prevalent at the time, but by the end of the 1960s the situation had changed completely. In the Annual Report of the Ministry of Health for 1966 an upsurge in demand for health centres was noted and by 1970 there were nearly 100 open and 200 more in the pipeline, far outstripping the 1963 predictions.

Several subsequent revisions of the health and welfare plan, based on local authorities' revised forecasts, were published.

4.8 Report on the Committee on the Functions of the District General Hospital (Bonham-Carter Report)

Published: 1969

Chairman: *Sir Desmond Bonham-Carter KB, TD*

Members: *A. A. Driver MD, DPH; J. R. Edge MD, MRCP; C. M. Fletcher CBE, MD, FRCP;* A. B. Gilmour MB, BS, LMSSA;† W. J. B. Groves FHA; Miss C. H. Hall SRN; D. H. Irvine MD, DObst RCOG;‡ H. H. Langston MB, BS, FRCS; Professor T. McKeown PhD., DPhil, MD; A. J. Oldham MD, DPM; Dame Muriel Powell DBE, SRN, SCM, RNT; J. J. A. Reid TD, MD, MSc, MRCP, MRCPE, DPH; Professor C. Scott Russell MD, FRCS, FRCOG; J. A. Shepherd VRD, MD, FRCS, FRCS (E); L. Slater MA, JP; Professor A. G. Watkins CBE, MD, FRCP; S. R. F. Whittaker DL, MA, MD, FRCP; J. A. W. McDonald* (*secretary*)

*Resigned December 1967 †*Resigned July 1967* ‡*Appointed August 1967*

Terms of Reference: *To consider the concept of the district general hospital promulgated in 1961–2, in the light of developments since that time; and to redefine the functions which the district general hospital should perform in the health service of the future.*

The Bonham-Carter Report represented the first official review of the concept of the district general hospital embodied in *A Hospital Plan for England and Wales* (q.v., p. 151) some eight years earlier. The setting up of the committee followed a meeting of the Central Health Services Council which was addressed by Professor T. McKeown, professor of social medicine, University of Birmingham, and Dr J. O. F. Davies, then senior administrative medical officer, Oxford Regional Hospital Board. Professor McKeown had for some years been arguing the case for what he termed the 'balanced hospital community'. His arguments are set out at length in his book *Medicine and Modern Society* (Allen & Unwin, 1965). He became a member of the Bonham-Carter Committee and his stamp is set firmly upon the report which urges the integration of hospital psychiatric and geriatric services on the same site and under the same administration as the acute medical and surgical facilities. McKeown had all along argued that any other solution was to condemn psychiatric and geriatric patients to second class facilities and second class care.

This, together with certain arguments about minimum levels of consult-ant staffing, and about the organization of supporting services, led the Bonham-Carter Committee to recommend much larger district general hospitals than had formerly been envisaged. The *Hospital Plan* had spoken of hospitals of 600–800 beds each serving a population of 100,000–150,000. Bonham-Carter revised the population figure to upwards of 200,000; in the larger cities and conurbations 300,000 was the figure suggested. This meant hospitals of 1,000–1,750 beds.

The report accepted the necessity to retain some small hospitals in peripheral areas from which it was difficult to reach the district general hospital but described a more limited role for these hospitals than had been set out in the *Hospital Plan*. They should undertake only work that could suitably be undertaken on the basis of day-to-day staffing by general practitioners, with only such help from the specialists of the district general hospital as could be given at a distance or on occasional visits.

In a foreword by the Central Health Services Council it was pointed out that the report was to be seen not simply as a report about district general hospitals, but as one about the part that district general hospitals should play within the National Health Service as a whole; the committee's recommendations on the organization of the hospital service assumed a corresponding development of the community services, both in quality and in quantity.

Of course, by the time the report was published a good deal of hospital building was under way as a result of the earlier *Plan*. In Great Britain the planning and construction of a major new hospital is a lengthy business —ten years is not uncommon. No immediate impact on the pattern of hospital construction was therefore to be expected in any case, but in the event the report was accorded a lukewarm reception by the Government and was at least temporarily shelved pending the outcome of discussions that were going on at that time about the future organization of the health service as a whole.

An indication that the Government was prepared to go part, but not all, of the way suggested by the Bonham-Carter Committee was given by the Secretary of State, Sir Keith Joseph, in a speech early in 1972. 'One found-ation of the new National Health Service', he said, 'will be on the hospital side, the district general hospitals, each providing comprehensive services for populations up to about 250,000 people. There will be something like

230 of them. Perhaps three-quarters of them will have more than 600 beds and the 1,000-bed hospital will not be uncommon.'

But Sir Keith went on to say that he had been taking a fresh look at the place of the local hospital in the scheme of things.

I am a healthy sceptic of over-centralization and there *will* be local hospitals. The Government sees the need for what we are now calling community hospitals—for patients who need hospital care but do not need all the expensive facilities of a district general hospital. In these local hospitals they can be looked after nearer their homes and friends, benefiting from the goodwill and service, whether voluntary or paid, that can be focused on a small hospital serving its local community.

4.9 Domiciliary Midwifery and Maternity Bed Needs (Peel Report)

Report of a Sub-committee of the Standing Maternity and Midwifery Advisory Committee of the Central Health Services Council

Published: 1970

Chairman: *Sir John Peel KCVO, FRCS, PRCOG*

Members: *H. G. E. Arthure CBE, MD, FRCS, FRCOG; T. R. Bryant OBE, MB, BCh, JP; Miss W. Frost SRN, SCM, HV Cert, QN; Mrs J. M. Goodman SRN, SCM, MTD, QN; Professor T. N. A. Jeffcoate MD, FRCS (Edin.), PRCOG; J. Leiper MBE, TD, MB, ChB, DPH; Professor S. Shone OBE, MD, FRCP; Dr Margaret M. Bates and R. L. Gordon (joint secretaries)*

Terms of Reference (1967): *To consider the future of the domiciliary midwifery service and the question of bed needs for maternity patients and to make recommendations.*

The Cranbrook Committee,when it reviewed the maternity services in the late 1950s, did not see any overwhelming need to unify the administration of hospital and domiciliary maternity services, and their report set a target for hospital deliveries of 70 per cent of all births. Given correct selection for hospital or home confinement the committee felt that the remaining 30 per cent of mothers could safely and appropriately be delivered in their own homes. Subsequent experience, however, showed that this correct selection was not easily achieved. The Perinatal Mortality Survey demonstrated that women were being booked for delivery at home who might reasonably be expected to experience complications in labour, and as a result they were having to be transferred to hospital at a late stage, with enhanced risk to both mother and child. Professional judgment was not always at fault; often it was the high-risk mother, for example the woman who had had three or more children, who was the most difficult to persuade to accept hospital delivery before complications developed.

Between 1959 and 1968 the national trend was towards the delivery of an increasing proportion of women in hospital. By 1965 the Cranbrook target of 70 per cent had been reached and in 1968 the national figure (which concealed important regional variations) was over 80 per cent. As a consequence it was becoming difficult to maintain, or justify economically, a satisfactory domiciliary midwifery service. Local authority midwives were underemployed, and were dissatisfied because the trend to hospital confinement deprived them of the opportunity to use their professional skills; in many parts of the country high hospital confinement rates were being achieved by cutting the length of stay and discharging mothers and babies to the care of the domiciliary midwife shortly after delivery. This meant that the domiciliary midwife was deprived of the satisfaction of presiding over labour, and was only permitted to function as a maternity nurse. Cranbrook accepted the traditional ten-day stay as the norm, but many women were now being discharged after forty-eight hours.

In some areas arrangements had been made to enable the domiciliary midwives to come into hospital to deliver patients whose antenatal care they had supervised, and for whom the general practitioner retained medical responsibility until he felt the necessity of calling in a consultant. Increasingly, too, midwives were attached to general practitioners and cared for the practice patients rather than for patients who lived in a defined geographical area, and together general practitioners and their attached midwives were gradually taking over from local authority medical officers the staffing of maternity and child health clinics.

All these developments suggested the necessity for a new review of the maternity services and the committee that was set up could hardly have been more high-powered, with both the incoming and the outgoing presidents of the Royal College of Obstetricians and Gynaecologists, and the president of the Royal College of Midwives among its members. It spoke out firmly for 100 per cent hospital deliveries and put forward interim proposals to give, in effect, a unified maternity service pending the full unification of the three branches of the health service as a whole. Medical and midwifery care should be provided, the report said, by consultants, general practitioners and midwives working as teams, and general practitioner obstetric beds should be provided in combined consultant and general practitioner units in district general hospitals, sharing the same staff and facilities. Those isolated general practitioner units which it was felt necessary to retain for the time being should be linked as closely as possible with the consultant units.

The interim arrangements for the unification of the service proposed that local authorities should take advantage of the provisions of the Health Services and Public Health Act, 1968, to make arrangements with hospitals to provide a domiciliary maternity service (insofar as such a service was still required—there would probably always be a small number of women who resolutely declined hospital delivery). This would enable all midwives to be employed by the hospitals, and to be deployed flexibly so as to make the best use of their skills. The report included a large number of statistical tables providing a mine of information about recent trends in maternity services, and some useful appendices, including two dealing with the calculation of bed needs to serve defined populations and the calculation of numbers of delivery beds required on various assumptions regarding organization and obstetric technique.

4.10 White Paper on National Health Service Reorganisation: England

Published: 1972

The first indication that major reconstruction of the National Health Service was seriously in prospect was the publication in 1968 of the Labour Government's Green Paper on the Administrative Structure of the Medical and Related Services in England and Wales. A 'Green Paper' is intended to embody tentative proposals which the Government would like the public, and in particular interested parties, to discuss and comment on before decisions are taken. It thus represents an earlier stage in the evolution of policy than a White Paper, which is normally a fairly firm statement of the Government's views and intentions. In this case, widespread debate followed the publication of the Green Paper and it became clear that although there was general acceptance of the fundamental point that the three parts of the health service—the hospitals, local health authority services, and the executive council services—should be unified, this general agreement did not extend to many of the detailed proposals, such as the sharp reduction in the numbers of committees and boards and in the numbers of people required to give voluntary service on these committees and boards.

When the 1968 Green Paper was published, Kenneth Robinson was Minister of Health, but when later that year the government departments concerned with the social services were reorganized and Richard Crossman became Secretary of State for Social Services, he announced that he would prepare revised proposals taking into account many of the comments and criticisms that had been made. In 1970 Crossman published a second Green Paper, in which he announced three firm decisions by the Government as a result of the earlier discussions and of the Report of the Royal Commission on Local Government, which had been published in the summer of 1969.

The three firm decisions were: (a) that the National Health Service would not be administered by local government but by area health authorities directly responsible to the Secretary of State; (b) that the boundary between the health service and the personal social services provided by local authorities should be determined by the skills of the providers rather than the needs of the users, i.e. health authorities would be responsible for services where the primary skill needed was that of the health professions, while local authorities would be responsible for services where the primary skill was social care or support; (c) the geographical boundaries of the health service areas should match those of the new local authorities; there would thus be ninety areas or thereabouts, compared with the 40–50 proposed in Green Paper I. Green Paper II also restored the regional tier which had been omitted in Green Paper I.

When the Conservatives came to power in late 1970 Crossman was succeeded as Secretary of State for Social Services by Sir Keith Joseph, who brought a touch of briskness to the continuing discussions on reorganization. 'We are perhaps in danger', he wrote in his foreword to the Consultative Document which his Department published in 1971, 'of a surfeit of plans and prospectuses: there must be early decisions, so that enthusiasm for reform does not wither away.' The Consultative Document endorsed the principle of administrative unification of the existing tripartite structure and the principle that the new area health authorities should have the same geographical boundaries as the new local authorities which were to be created in 1974. 1 April 1974 was fixed as the date for the establishment of both sets of authorities.

Sir Keith pointed out that the essence of the new Government's proposals—and their basic difference from earlier proposals—was the emphasis placed on effective management. 'The importance of good management in making the best use of resources can hardly be overstated.' So the regional tier was firmly established as part of a classical chain-of-command structure, passing orders to the area boards and receiving from them accounts of how they had discharged their delegated responsibilities.

Following the two Green Papers and the Consultative Document, the 1972 White Paper set out the Government's intentions at a time when the necessary legislation for the reorganization of the health service must have been at an advanced stage of drafting. It was based firmly on the Consultative Document and contained few significant new proposals. The health service was to be unified administratively under regional and area health authorities. There was to be no question of the community health services swallowing up the hospitals or, a more common suspicion, *vice versa*. The NHS administering bodies were to be entirely new bodies covering the whole field of health care, domiciliary and institutional. Their membership and administrative structure would be such that they would not be dominated by people whose main interests lay in one or other service. They would be responsible for balancing needs and selecting priorities so as to provide the right combination of services for the benefit of the public. They would be answerable to the Department of Health and Social Security and would operate under the scrutiny of community health councils established at district level to represent the views of the consumer.

The services to be brought together under the new bodies were the hospital and specialist services administered by regional hospital boards, hospital management committees and boards of governors, the family practitioner services administered by the executive councils, the personal health services administered by local authorities through their health committees, and the school health service. The personal social services would continue to be provided by local authorities, which would also continue to have responsibilities for environmental health, e.g. measures for preventing the spread of communicable disease (other than routine immunization, some epidemiological investigation, and treatment); powers relating to food safety and hygiene, port health, and diseases of animals insofar as they affect human health; and the enforcement of requirements about environmental conditions at places of work. In discharging these environmental health responsibilities, local authorities would look to the health authorities for the advice and assistance of their medical staff, although the statutory responsibility would rest on the local authorities and not on the health authorities. The occupational health services provided through the Department of Employment were also left outside the scope of the new health authorities.

The regional health authorities would be based on the fourteen planning regions already established for the hospital service. The area health authorities would share the boundaries of the new non-metropolitan counties and metropolitan districts. Thus there would be seventy-two area health authorities outside London. The White Paper devoted a separate chapter to the special problems of London, and proposed that while health areas would be formed out of single London boroughs or groups of boroughs, the health districts would not always follow the borough boundaries. The special arrangements for London also included keeping in existence boards of governors for the postgraduate hospitals after 1 April 1974, until such time as these hospitals became sufficiently closely associated with other hospitals and services in the vicinity to make it feasible for them to be administered by the new health authorities. These arrangements reflected a good deal of controversy which had been taking place, largely behind closed doors, about the future of both undergraduate and postgraduate teaching hospitals and medical schools in the London area.

The teaching hospitals generally scored an important success in the White Paper, which replaced the Consultative Document's notion of 'teaching districts', subordinate to area health authorities but with some special privileges, with the concept of the 'teaching area' managed by an area health authority whose members would include some chosen from the membership of existing boards of governors and university hospital management committees and which would be known as an AHA(T).

The AHA(T)s would, however, be accountable to the regional health authority in the same way as other AHAs.

In the chapter referring to the membership of regional and area health authorities the controversial phrase 'management ability', which had been used in the Consultative Document, was dropped. Instead, the work of the members would call for 'general ability and personality . . . an unbiased, questioning yet constructive approach and good judgment', so as to give 'guidance and direction on policies to their chief officers . . . to set high standards and provide vigorous leadership'. Authorities would be relatively small, with normally about fifteen members. Like members of hospital authorities before them, members of the new health authorities would be unpaid, but there would be provision in the legislation for the chairmen to be paid on a part-time basis so that no financial barrier should prevent those with other commitments from giving adequate time to this 'heavy and time-consuming job'.

The regional authorities would be responsible for strategic planning, for co-ordinating, supervising and checking the performance of the AHAs, and for certain executive functions that needed to be undertaken from a regional base, notably the design and construction of new buildings; the provision of a blood transfusion service; and in some parts of the country of the ambulance service; sponsorship of some research projects; certain supplies functions; and the provision of the more specialized management services. The White Paper tentatively (a review was promised after the first five years) perpetuated one of the anomalies of the existing service that the medical profession had been keen to retain. Although all other staff at operational level in the service were to be employed by area health authorities, medical and dental consultants and senior registrars were, as in the past, to be employed by the regional authority. This promised to give them the same quasi-independence in relation to area health authorities as they had previously enjoyed in relation to hospital management committees. Presumably too there would continue to be no objection to a doctor's serving as a member of an authority for which he provided medical services, on the grounds that he was not technically employed by that authority, but by the next tier up. This irritated the other professions who had not been allowed to serve on the authority which employed them, although in the event some concessions were made on this point.

An exception to the rule that senior medical staff would be employed by the regional authority was made for AHA(T)s. They would employ their own, as boards of governors had previously done.

The area health authority would be responsible for the provision and operation of comprehensive health services to meet the needs of the population, but the day-to-day running of services would be based on districts—there would be a number of one-district authorities, but some would have two, three, four or even five districts. The districts would be officer-run and there would be no formal authority constituted at district level. As proposed in the Consultative Document, each area authority would be obliged to set up a Family Practitioner Committee to administer the contracts of family doctors, dentists, pharmacists and opticians, in succession to the former executive councils. Planning of the family practitioner services would, however, be the responsibility of the AHA.

The two main appendices to the White Paper set out the proposed functions of the health service commissioner, and summarized the management study which had been carried out by the working group of civil servants, NHS officers and management consultants following the publication of the Consultative Document. The task of the working group had been to develop proposals for the internal management arrangements of the new authorities within the broad organizational principles laid down in the Consultative Document—principles such as 'clear delegation downwards, matched by accountability upwards', and the provision of a 'fully integrated service'. The full study was subsequently published as *Management Arrangements for the Reorganised National Health Service*, and quickly became known as the 'Grey Book', a title which reflected both the colour of its covers and the quality of its prose.

At district level a district management team was envisaged, consisting of two elected medical representatives, one from the specialists, one from the general practitioners; a community physician; a nursing officer; a finance officer; and an administrator. Considerable scepticism was created by the statement that 'The team would be a consensus group, that is, all decisions it makes would have to be unanimous.' Within the districts, teams drawn from all the professions concerned would provide services for 'patient groups' with identifiable needs, e.g. geriatric patients, the mentally handicapped etc. Senior area staff would again come together as a team to co-ordinate their activities. Corporate management would be the pattern from district to regional level, and at no level was there to be a single executive head. Each level would monitor, i.e. continually check, the work of the level below.

One of the significant changes in management practice proposed in the White Paper itself was the introduction of more flexibility in the financing of the service. Authorities would have freedom, within limits, to use funds allocated for capital expenditure to meet revenue expenditure and *vice versa*. They would also be enabled to carry unspent revenue allocations over from one year to the next. Previously this had not been allowed and as a result a great deal of panic spending generally occurred towards the end of the financial year to avoid unspent balances having to be returned to the Treasury. The White Paper did not explain why these two changes, which had previously been claimed to be out of the question because of the requirements of parliamentary accountability, had now become possible.

The penultimate chapter of the White Paper dealt with 'Preparing for

1974' and referred to the setting up of joint liaison committees to enable existing NHS authorities to prepare the way for the setting up of 'shadow authorities' as soon as possible after the passage of the necessary legislation. A National Health Service Staff Commission was also to be created to make arrangements for the appointment of officers and the transfer of staff to the new authorities.

National Health Service Reorganisation: England, 1972

WHY REORGANIZE?

For two years I have been responsible for the National Health Service—and for the personal social services.

Throughout this time my respect for the achievements of the National Health Service has steadily grown. Whatever its defects we would be utterly wrong to take for granted the massive performance of this remarkable network of services and the ease of mind that it has brought to all the people of this country. I am sure that they feel a deep sense of gratitude to all those involved: to the members of the governing authorities; to the men and women who make their careers in the service, whether in direct contact with patients or in supporting services; and to the voluntary workers.

But at the same time I have come to recognise, as many others have, that while this good work will continue, nothing like its full potential can be realised without changes in the administrative organisation of the service.

Hence this White Paper. It is about administration, not about treatment and care. But the purpose behind the changes proposed is a better, more sensitive, service to the public. Administration is not of course an end in itself. But both the patients and those who provide treatment and care will gain if the administration embodies both a clear duty to improve the service and the facilities for doing so.

Let me illustrate this. Everyone is aware of gaps in our health services. Even for acute illness, where we provide at least as good a service for our whole population as any country in the world, there are some respects in which we achieve less than we could. On the non-acute side the services for the elderly, for the disabled, and for the mentally ill and the mentally handicapped have failed to attract the attention and indeed the resources which they need—and all the more credit to the staff who have toiled so tirelessly for their patients despite the difficulties.

It is well understood now, moreover, that the domiciliary and community services are under-developed—that there is a need for far more home helps, home nurses, hostels and day centres and other services that support people outside hospital. Often what there is could achieve more if it were better co-ordinated with other services in and out of hospital. It is well understood too that there must be more emphasis on prevention—or at the least on early detection and treatment.

For the imbalances and the gaps Governments must take their share of the responsibility. Resources were and still are stretched. The acute services had a legitimate priority. But the shortcomings were not rational. They did not result from a calculation as to the best way to deploy scarce resources. They just happened.

Why did they just happen? Because it has never been the responsibility—nor has it been within the power—of any single named authority to provide for the population of a given area of a comprehensible size the best health service that the money and skills available can provide. There has been no identified authority whose task it has been, in co-operation with those responsible for complementary services, to balance needs and priorities rationally and to plan and provide the right combination of services for the benefit of the public.

It is to enable such an authority to operate in each area, with the best professional advice, that the Government proposes to reorganise the administration of the National Health Service as explained in this White Paper.

The National Health Service is one of the largest civilian organisations in the world. Its staff is growing rapidly. It contains an ever-growing multitude of skills that depend on and interact with each other. It serves an ever-growing range of health needs with ever more complex treatments and techniques. And though the Government has made substantial additions to a programme of expenditure which was already planned to grow at an above-average rate, there is never enough money—and never likely to be—for everything that ideally requires to be done. Nor, despite the great increases since 1948, are there ever enough skilled men and women.

Real needs must therefore be identified, and decisions must be taken and periodically reviewed, as to the order of priorities among them. Plans must be worked out to meet these needs and management and drive must be continually applied to put the plans into action, assess their effectiveness and modify them as needs change or as ways are found to make the plans more effective.

Effective for what?—to improve the service for the benefit of all. The plans must therefore be effective in providing what patients need: primarily, treatment and care in hospital; support at home; diagnosis and treatment in surgery, health centre or out-patient clinic; or day care.

Furthermore they must include arrangements whereby the public can express their wishes and preferences, and know that notice will be taken of them. That is why I attach great importance to the establishment of strong community health councils, and to improved methods for enquiring into complaints, including the appointment of a health ombudsman.

The health services depend crucially on the humane planning and provision of the personal social services, and therefore on effective and understanding collaboration with local government. No doubt arguments will continue about the theoretical advantages of making both health and social services the responsibility of a single agency. But the formidable practical difficulties, which have been fully argued elsewhere, rule this out as a realistic solution, and require us to concentrate instead on ensuring that the two parallel authorities—one local, one health—with their separate statutory responsibilities shall work together in partnership for the health and social care of the population. This White Paper demonstrates the Government's concern to see that arrangements are evolved under which a more coherent and smoothly interlocking range of services will develop for all the needs of the population.

The doctor and other professional workers will gain too. The organisational changes will not affect the professional relationship between individual patients and individual professional workers on which the complex of health services is so largely built. The professional workers will retain their clinical freedom—governed as it is by the bounds of professional knowledge and ethics and by the resources that are available—to do as they think best for their patients. This freedom is cherished by the professions and accepted by the Government. It is a safeguard for patients today and an insurance for future improvements.

But the organisational changes will also bring positive gains to the professional worker. He—or she—will have the opportunity of organising his or her own work better and of playing a much greater part than hitherto in the management decisions that are taken in each area. At the same time the more systematic and comprehensive analysis of needs and priorities that will lie behind the planning and operations of each area will help professional workers to ensure that their skills bring the greatest possible benefit to their patients.

We are issuing a White Paper, and promoting legislation about the administration of the National Health Service, solely in order to improve the health care of the public. Administrative reorganisation within a unified health service that is closely linked with parallel local government services will provide a sure foundation for better services for all.

Foreword by the Secretary of State, Sir Keith Joseph

In the final analysis, health care depends on the effective delivery at the right time and place of the skills and devotion of those providing the services required. We are indeed fortunate in this country in the quality of the staff of our health teams, and we have good reason to be proud of the achievement of the National Health Service.

Nevertheless, no one would claim that it is perfect. The proposed reorganisation offers the chance to establish a framework within which a more integrated and improved service can be offered to the public. The purpose of this White Paper and of the Bill that will follow is to provide a better health service for all.

How in fact will the public benefit from reorganisation? A more informed judgment of priorities will concentrate more of the available resources where they are most needed. There will be better co-ordinated provision for their health and social needs. Professional skills will be grouped into teams to meet the needs of particular categories of patients—the old, the handicapped, the acutely ill, mothers and children, the mentally sick. Strong community health councils will ensure that the public's views are known and that the service is run with full regard to them. Improved arrangements will be made for enquiring into complaints, and an ombudsman for the health service will be appointed.

Reorganisation will be of equal benefit in helping those who provide or manage health services to improve the quality of care given to the public. The health professions will have the support of a well organised NHS for the exercise of their professional skills and will be freed from some of the frustrations which the lack of this in the past has caused. Furthermore, they will make an important contribution to the management of the service: the governing authorities will include members of the main health professions and will reach their decisions on the basis of advice from strong professional advisory committees and from their chief professional officers. Those of the professions who are independent contractors will be strongly represented on special committees for administering their contractual relationship with the service.

The staff of the NHS, including the professional staff, will in a unified service have wider scope and opportunities than is now the case. They will be fully consulted about the changes, and care will be taken, by the establishment of a Staff Commission and in other ways, to safeguard their interests when the changes are being made.

The members of the new health authorities, and their administrative staff, will be able to develop comprehensive services without running into the artificial administrative barriers which now divide the sectors of what should be a single service. The administrator will have full scope for personal initiative within clearly allocated responsibilities. This will give him the satisfaction of being able to do a worthwhile job well, of securing value for money and providing a framework and the necessary support for an efficient and sensitive health service.

This White Paper proposes a framework which will co-ordinate the many and varied skills of all those who work in the National Health Service and will focus them on the needs of the individual citizen of this country. Its purpose is to enable an improved health service for all to be provided.

paras. 202–8

COMMUNITY HEALTH COUNCILS

In planning and running their services, the health authorities must be in a position to know the views taken of them by the communities for whom the services are provided. They must also take full account of those views in the decisions they make. A lively and continuing interaction between management and the users of services is of direct benefit to both parties. It helps to make sure that the public has a full say in what is done in its name, and it helps the managing authorities by making them better informed on priorities, needs and deficiencies in service.

The expression of local public opinion can be catered for in one of two ways. It can be done indirectly by including in the membership of the health authorities local people serving in a representative capacity. Or it can be done more directly, through bodies specially set up for this purpose, with direct links to the authorities. The Government prefer the second course. It allows each of the interests—management and the community—to concentrate on its own special function, avoids a confusion between the direction of services and representation of those receiving them, encourages a constructive interplay of ideas and makes possible the expression of a wider cross-section of local opinion than is feasible where the authority itself contains members serving as representatives.

Bodies to represent the views of the consumer—the community health councils—will therefore be established. There will be one for each of the areas' health districts. It is at the district, rather than at the (often large) area, where there is real local interest. Special arrangements will be made where the people living within a health district look for a large part of their services to a neighbouring district (which might be administered by a different area health authority).

Each council will be made up of people with particular interest in the health services. Half its members will be appointed by the local government district council(s), and the rest by the AHA, mainly on the nomination of voluntary bodies concerned locally with the NHS and some after consultation with other organisations. No upper or lower limit of membership will be set, but a total of between 20 and 30 members would normally be about right for ensuring a proper spread of local interests within an effective and coherent working unit. Councils will appoint their chairmen from among their own members.

The council's basic job will be to represent to the AHA the interests of the public in the health service in its district. It will be for each council to decide how best to go about this, but they will be expected to influence area policy by contributing their own ideas on how services should be operated and developed. To help them do this effectively, councils will have powers to secure information, will have the right to visit hospitals and other institutions, and will have access to the area authority and in particular to its senior officers administering district services. Some council members may want to take a special interest in particular institutions or services or parts of their district, especially where the districts are large.

Councils will be well placed to bring to the notice of the AHA and its district staff potential causes of local complaint, especially those of a general nature, but their function will be distinct from that of the AHA's complaints machinery and of the Health Service Commissioner. . . . There will be well understood procedures for the investigation of individual complaints in the reorganised service but a community health council might well wish, on request, to provide information about these procedures, to advise complainants how to lodge a complaint and to provide a 'patient's friend' where one is needed. The volume and type of individual complaints about a service or institution will be of legitimate concern to councils as a measurement of public satisfaction.

For their part, the AHA will be expected to consult the councils on its plans for health service developments, and particularly on proposals for important variations in services affecting the public. New services, closures of hospitals or departments of hospitals or their change of use, are examples. The full AHA will meet representatives of all its community health councils at least once a year; that meeting would of course be additional to the regular, less formal meetings which will take place between the authority's members and officers and council representatives. The councils will publish annual reports and may publish other reports; the AHA will be required to publish replies recording action taken on issues raised in them.

The AHA will meet the council's reasonable expenditure, including expenses incurred by their members, and will provide accommodation for meetings and secretarial staff.

paras. 105–12

4.11 National Health Service Reorganisation Act, 1973

The Act closely followed the lines of the White Paper, and its main purposes were set out in the explanatory memorandum as:

(a) to unify the local administration of the National Health Service under new health authorities covering the whole field of health care;

(b) to provide means in each area of representing the interests of the community;

(c) to ensure that the views of the health professions are given full weight in the planning and management of services;

(d) to continue the National Health Service responsibility for providing facilities in support of the medical and dental teaching functions of universities;

(e) to provide for collaboration between the National Health Service and the services for which local authorities are responsible, and between the National Health Service and voluntary organizations;

(f) to provide for the establishment of Health Service Commissioners for England and for Wales to investigate complaints against Health Service Authorities.

Part I placed upon the Secretary of State the duty to reorganize the NHS in accordance with the provisions of the Act and transferred to him functions previously exercised by local health and education authorities. The education functions transferred to him were of course those relating to school health services. Subsequent clauses outlined the new structure of regional and area health authorities, area health authorities (teaching), family practitioner committees, local professional advisory committees, and community health councils. Clause 10 required health authorities and the new local authorities to co-operate with one another and to establish area joint consultative committees.

Part II provided for the abolition of the existing health authorities, with the exception of the boards of governors of certain London postgraduate teaching hospitals which were to be kept in existence for the time being, until the future of these hospitals could be sorted out. These were hospitals that provided a national rather than a local or even a regional service, and they had fought hard to avoid absorption. Clauses 16–17 dealt with the transfer of property, rights and liabilities from local health authorities and executive councils; Clauses 18–19 with the transfer of staff and the protection of their interests. Clause 20 provided for the setting up of Staff Commissions for England and for Wales. These bodies had already been set up in the form of advisory committees and had done a good deal of work by the time the Act was passed, but they only took on their full status and powers after the Act. Clauses 21–30 dealt with the transfer and administration of existing hospital endowments.

Part III authorized the appointment of Health Service Commissioners for England and for Wales to investigate complaints against NHS authorities that were not dealt with by those authorities to the satisfaction of the complainant. The commissioners were precluded from investigating matters of clinical judgment and matters in which the aggrieved person had a remedy through a statutory tribunal or action at law.

Part IV contained a number of miscellaneous provisions, including one to bring the special hospitals, such as Broadmoor, Rampton and Moss Side, currently administered directly by the DHSS, within the National Health Service and to make it possible for the administration of these hospitals to be transferred to a subordinate health authority if at any time this was considered to be desirable.

There were five schedules to the Act, the most significant being the first, which specified the membership and manner of appointment of the new health authorities, and which empowered the Secretary of State to pay chairmen—with the exception of chairmen of family practitioner committees—a salary agreed with the Minister for the Civil Service.

The National Health Service Reorganisation Bill started its career in the House of Lords and was there subjected to a number of minor amendments, of which perhaps the most interesting was the prohibition of charges for family planning advice and the supply of contraceptives. Clause 4, which laid on the Secretary of State the duty of providing a family planning service, originally laid down that 'regulations may provide for the making and recovery, in respect of treatment given and articles supplied in pursuance of the arrangements, of charges prescribed by or determined under the regulations'. The Lords altered this to 'such arrangements shall provide that no charge shall be made for any such medical examination or treatment or for the supply of any such substance or appliances.'

5 Internal Administration of Hospitals under the NHS

Introduction

Hospitals are interesting organizations to the sociologist, as has been demonstrated by the increasing number of sociologists who have taken to studying them in recent years. Just as physically a hospital is one of the most demanding building types an architect may be called on to design, so as organizations they are most complex. They vary enormously, in size, configuration, the work they do, the technology they employ, the traditions they have inherited. Outsiders sometimes ask the naive question 'Who is in charge of a hospital?' without realizing quite how naive it is, quite how impossible to answer. In most British hospitals the answer is probably 'No one', although a Scot might still be tempted to answer, 'The medical superintendent'; so here we have a phenomenon that many teachers of management assure their students is impossible, an organization that functions reasonably well with no one in charge.

Some see the hospital not as a hierarchy, with management at the top and workers at the bottom, but as an arena, within which different groups and professions compete for influence, power, resources, opportunities. Indeed if we try to impose a hierarchical model on the hospital, we are immediately in difficulties with the medical staff, who in one sense are shop-floor workers, but are also the most prestigious, highly-paid and influential members of the hospital community, often with a seat on the board or committee to which the chief administrative officer is responsible.

Most of the documents cited in this section have been concerned not with finding the appropriate theoretical model for hospital organization, but with smoothing out operational difficulties, and creating a satisfactory career structure for hospital administrators. Once a national service is established, career structures become very important. A national service also brings with it increasing pressures for uniformity and a growing conviction that if two or more ways of doing things are in evidence then one of them must be the right way and the rest of them wrong.

The Bradbeer, Hall, Lycett Green and Farquharson-Lang Reports were all concerned in their different ways with administrative structures and careers—although the Farquharson-Lang Committee showed by far the most lively interest in processes as distinct from structure—while the Platt Report on the Welfare of Children in Hospital (there have been several other Platt Reports) is cited as an examination of an area on the borderline between administration and clinical care, the kind of problem in fact that makes a hospital a hospital.

Report No. 29 of the National Board for Prices and Incomes throws some interesting light on an aspect of hospital management that does not often come into the limelight. That is the necessity to maintain large staffs to clean the buildings, cook the patients' meals, wheel the trolleys down the corridors, and perform the myriad menial tasks that fall outside the scope of the various groups of professional staff but which constitute the essential supporting services for any large residential institution. The fact that there is a good deal of evidence that these supporting services are often badly managed does not mean that the remedies proposed by the NBPI were necessarily the right ones. Attempts to implement them possibly created as many problems as they solved. In 1973 many British hospitals experienced grave difficulties because of a prolonged strike by ancillary staff. It is difficult to know to what extent the increased militancy of ancillary staff unions since 1967 has been fostered by the NBPI Report, but it may well have been a factor.

Finally, the Davies Report looked at what happens when things go wrong in hospitals.

5.1 Report by a Committee of the Central Health Services Council on the Internal Administration of Hospitals (Bradbeer Report)

Published: 1954

Chairman: *Alderman A. F. Bradbeer JP*

Members: *N. A. Ball FHA;* E. C. F. Bird; F. J. Cable FHA; P. H. Constable MA, FHA; A. A. Cunningham MD, MRCP, DPH; Sir Ernest Rock Carling MB, FRCS, FRCP, Hon FFR; H. G. Dain MD, LLD, FRCS; Miss K. G. Douglas SRN, SCM;† Miss L. A. D. Evans SRN, SCM; L. T. Feldon FHA, ACIS; Sir Basil Gibson CBE, JP;‡ J. H. Kitchen; H. Lesser CBE, LLB; Sir Hugh Linstead OBE, FPS, MP;‡ W. G. Masefield CBE, MRCS, LRCP, DPM; J. R. Murray MD, DPM; F. S. Stancliffe; H. Trusson FCIS, FHA; J. Watt MA, MD, DPH; M. Reed and J. P. Cashman (joint secretaries)*

*In place of Sir Owen Morshead, who resigned in March 1952
†In place of Miss C. H. Alexander, who resigned in April 1951
‡Appointed in April, 1951

Terms of Reference (1950): *To consider and report on the existing methods of administration in individual hospitals*, and within Hospital Management Committee groups, *with particular reference to: (i) matters of finance, staff and supplies (ii) the extent to which differences in the work undertaken at different hospitals call for differences in their administrative organization; (iii) the extent to which administrative duties should be undertaken by medical and nursing staff.*

(The words in roman were not in the original terms of reference and were added at the request of the committee.)

The Bradbeer Report dates from the early years of the National Health Service when there was much uncertainty about relationships between hospital management committees and the individual hospitals they controlled; between group officers and administrators of individual hospitals within the group; and between hospital administrators and their medical and nursing counterparts. Some of those called upon to administer the new structure had previously worked for local authorities; others had been brought up in the voluntary system and had been accustomed to entirely different practices and traditions. The former municipal hospitals had often been administered chiefly by a medical superintendent who was responsible directly to the medical officer of health at the town hall. Both the matron and the steward were clearly subordinate to the medical superintendent. In the voluntary hospitals the house governor was responsible for day-to-day administration to the governing body, there was rarely a medical superintendent, and the matron's position was one of prestige and influence. There were many variants to these two basic patterns, and as only the broad outlines of the new administrative structure were laid down in 1948, there were still, by 1950, considerable local differences in practice and interpretation.

The guidance offered by the committee when they reported four years later was based on the concept of 'tripartite administration', a partnership within the individual hospital of medical, nursing and lay elements, but with the lay element supreme at group level in the person of the group secretary, charged with responsibility for implementing the policy of the governing body and for co-ordinating the activities of the group. The committee did not recommend the introduction of group medical superintendents, and set their face firmly against group matrons. Thus the recommendation twelve years later in the Salmon Report, that each group should have a chief nursing officer, was a complete reversal of the view expressed by Bradbeer; just as Salmon's insistence on the clarification of responsibilities through the use of written job descriptions was a rejection of the Bradbeer view that standing orders for individual officers were of little real use.

The Bradbeer Committee emphasized the view that 'to recommend any one rigid pattern of administrative organization would be fatal'. 'We have approached our task', the report stated, 'bearing firmly in mind that throughout the service the administrative pattern must be and remain flexible, so as to fit not only the different circumstances of different groups but also the different circumstances of the same group at different times . . . It is for this reason that many of our recommendations will be found to be expressed tentatively or hedged about with qualifications.'

The Bradbeer Report, 1954

TRIPARTITE ADMINISTRATION

It emerges from this description of the hospital service before 1948 that, at least for the purposes of discussion, hospital administration can be sub-divided into:

(*a*) medical administration;
(*b*) nursing administration; and
(*c*) lay, or business, administration.

Our principal conclusion from our whole study of the subject is that this theoretical sub-division both can and should be translated into practice—in other words, that hospital administration as a whole should be regarded as essentially tripartite. It is amply clear that the borderlines between the three parts cannot be sharply defined, in practice even less than in theory, and that the actual functions to be performed by individual officers or groups of officers must depend on a number of factors—the size of the hospital or group, the state of its development, the nature of the services provided, the hospitals' traditions, even the personal characteristics and capacities of the particular officers available. But we are fully persuaded that the conception of partnership between the three parts of the whole administration should be regarded as fundamental and should determine the lines of all future development, whatever variations of superficial pattern may be necessary to give expression to varied circumstances. . . .

Nevertheless there is one important qualification of the tripartite principle which must be set down at once. We have no doubt whatever—and this view was expressed by several of the bodies who gave evidence before us—that for the efficient administration of the hospitals it controls the governing body must have one officer to whom it can look for securing that its policy is carried out in all hospitals in the group and for co-ordinating and reviewing all group activities. That is to say, at group level—and this includes 'groups' consisting of a single hospital—there must be one chief administrative officer. It is unfortunately true that where this principle is not fully accepted difficulties arise. It must be recognised not only that the governing body has full responsibility for all aspects of the day-to-day administration of its hospitals, but also that the administrative responsibility of its chief administrative officer extends similarly over the whole range of the group's activities. While, therefore, it is in our own view essential to develop a genuinely tripartite administrative organisation at the individual hospital, under whoever is responsible for medical administration, the matron and the unit hospital administrator respectively, it is impossible at group level to visualise any such clear-cut division of function expressed in terms of individual officers. We discuss later on, and recommend against, the appointment of group medical administrators and group matrons. But even if we had found good reasons for these appointments, there would still have had to be one chief administrative officer at group level, not three, with a general co-ordinating function under the governing body.

Except in the 'groups' consisting of a single mental hospital, the chief administrative officer is in practice nearly always a layman. The Ministry of

Health, writing of general and mixed non-teaching hospital groups, has stated that the chief administrative officer 'may be medical or lay, but if medical should not be engaged in clinical work, except in continuance of existing duties.' While agreeing with this view, we regard it as satisfactory that in practice the great majority of chief administrative officers are laymen, since we see little advantage in appointing a medical man without clinical duties to a post of this nature.

We also support the Ministry's view that it is desirable in principle, although not always practicable, that the chief administrative officer should act as secretary of one of the unit hospitals, preferably the largest. If this arrangement is not adopted, there is a very real danger that he will lose the 'feel' of hospital life and get out of touch with the practical problems of its administration.

paras. 20, 22–4

POSITION OF THE HOSPITAL SECRETARY

... We have also considered the relationship between the unit hospital administrator and lay departmental heads in his hospital. The extent to which a departmental organisation—finance, supplies, catering, engineering—is necessary in the unit clearly depends on its size. The King's Fund suggest that 'where departmental heads are appointed, they should be responsible to their unit administrator rather than to their specialist opposite number on the group staff' (which was, we recall, sometimes the arrangement in the local authority service) 'even though in the course of their everyday work they will often be dealing direct with these officers'. The Institute of Hospital Administrators, in their own report on the administration of the hospital service, take the same view— that 'the administrative officer in charge of the individual general hospital must be a qualified hospital administrator of good status, who should have overall charge of his hospital, subject to the higher authority of the group secretary, departmental officers in a hospital being responsible to him for general administrative matters and instructions from various group departmental heads in matters within their technical competence being transmitted through him'. In practice the reverse is sometimes the case: we were told that 'there is sometimes a tendency, particularly where the unit administrator is of junior status, for staff—particularly medical staff—to bypass and hence undermine his authority by making direct approach to the group administrator or specialist officers. It should be established by standing order or otherwise that the normal channel of approach to the group administrator is through the unit administrator'. Some of our witnesses, however, put to us the contrary view. In relation to finance the Institute of Municipal Treasurers and Accountants conceded that individual hospital staff engaged on local financial duties must be under the control and subject to the discipline of the administrative officer but suggested that 'it is equally clear that for the financial part of their duties they should work to the instructions of the chief financial officer and be accountable to him for the financial work, although it is clearly necessary that the administrative officer should be acquainted with the general instructions given to the staff under his control'.

The extent of this particular problem will naturally vary with the extent to which the specialist functions of group administration are centralised at group headquarters. But when these functions are considerably decentralised, as must often be the case for geographical or other reasons, we cannot help feeling that the perhaps gradual establishment of a chain of responsibility from specialist staff at unit level to the corresponding specialist group staff is a natural development. Such a system accords also more closely with the conception of the group as the primary unit of administration and the individual hospital as a sub-unit. And it might reasonably be argued that to make departmental staff at individual hospital level responsible to the local hospital administrator is to encourage the urge for independence of all too many hospitals. On the other hand, we should not like to see the tripartite organisation becoming multipartite and the whole administration at hospital level drifting into fragments. On balance we incline to the view expressed to us by the King's Fund and the Institute of Hospital Administrators and should prefer to see the unit hospital administrator paramount in the lay administration of his own hospital.

paras. 196–7

HOUSE COMMITTEES

One special type of committee to which we have given our attention is the house committee—that is, a committee or sub-committee of the governing body without general functional duties but with duties related to a particular hospital or sub-group of hospitals within the management group. The Ministry's views on the proper functions of these bodies are that in order to avoid fragmentation of the hospital service by breaking down the two-tier system of administration provided for in the Act into a three-tier system, it is undesirable to confer executive functions on house committees—that is, to delegate to them powers of appointing staff, incurring expenditure (other than from non-Exchequer funds) and so on. The Ministry suggests that their value lies rather in the field of overseeing the daily conduct of the hospital and the welfare of patients and staff and of making recommendations to the governing body for them to decide. House committees are valuable also as a link between the local community and the hospital, as an extended opportunity for those interested to take part in hospital work and as a training ground for membership of governing bodies themselves.

We have obtained information from a fairly wide sample of hospital authorities on their practice in the appointment and use of house committees. We are satisfied that house committees perform useful functions, especially in relation to the welfare of patients and staff and in the field of public relations, and that there is a place for them in most groups, particularly to serve the interests of special hospitals where these are grouped with general hospitals. We understand, too, that medical staff, matrons and lay administrators value the existence of house committees to whom they can look for help in their own immediate problems and that where they do not exist a sense of isolation may set in.

We wholly agree with the Ministry's view that it is unsound in principle to give house committees direct power to spend Exchequer money and that it is essential for close control over the estimates to be maintained at group level. We have heard of instances in which house committees have been given unrestricted control of their hospitals' allocation of the group budget but we regard this as objectionable: re-adjustment of the total budget if the committee overspends its share is very difficult to effect. House committees should, however, be kept fully and continuously informed of the finances of their hospital or hospitals. . . .

paras. 233–5

OFFICERS AS MEMBERS

We have given careful thought to a question which has often been raised since the beginning of the health service—the appointment of officers of the hospital service as members of governing bodies and their committees. The Ministry's view is that it is generally undesirable to have officers other than doctors appointed as members of governing bodies and operative committees, even at hospitals other than their own, and with this we agree. Traditionally medical men in the voluntary hospital service served on their own governing bodies and their committees and this fact has been used by various organisations of officers as an argument for similarly appointing not only senior officers like matrons, but representatives even of the humblest grades of hospital staff. It is of unquestioned value to have medical members who can bring their professional knowledge and experience to bear direct on problems that come up for consideration at Board or Management Committee level and many of the staff organisations have argued that the same principle applies to all types of staff. Medical men are, however, in a different position from other officers: they have a statutory right to make recommendations—in the case of Boards of Governors nominations—for membership of their governing body; the senior ones are not, in non-teaching hospitals, directly employed by their governing body; and they not infrequently serve hospitals under more than one governing body. While, therefore, we are in favour of medical staff continuing to serve as members of the governing body, we should deplore any move in the direction of a syndicalist structure which would be the logical and perhaps unavoidable result of extending the principle to other officers. Most objectionable of all would be the appointment to membership of governing bodies of principal officers whose functions are wholly or mainly administrative. It may be argued that such officers have a valuable contribution to make and that they should be allowed to be appointed at least to governing bodies of groups other than their own. But these officers owe undivided loyalty to their own group and should not be put in a position where their loyalty might be in any way divided. While we are prepared to concede that, exceptionally, matrons and other nursing officers might be permitted to serve on the governing body of hospitals other than their own, our conviction is that professional officers other than doctors can best contribute to the work of their own or any other governing body in an advisory capacity. Chief administrative officers, medical superintendents engaged predominantly in administrative work and hospital secretaries should be debarred on principle from membership. . . .

para. 239

5.2 The Welfare of Children in Hospital (Platt Report)

Report of a Committee of the Central Health Services Council

Published: 1959

Chairman: *Sir Harry Platt Bt., MS, MD, FRCS, FACS*

Members: (*Council members*) *P. H. Constable MA, FHA; Miss K. A. Raven SRN, SCM; F. M. Rose MB, ChB; W. P. H. Sheldon CVO, MD, FRCP;* (*non-Council members*) *Professor Norman Capon MD, FRCP, FRCOG; Charles Gledhill MBE, MB, BS, FRCS; Mrs Elizabeth Hollis BSc (Econ.); Miss M. W. Janes SRN, SCM, RSCN; Miss M. E. John AMIA; Miss C. A. McPherson MA; Miss E. Tylden MB, BChir, MRCS, LRCP*

Terms of Reference (1956): *To make a special study of the arrangements made in hospitals for the welfare of ill children—as distinct from their medical and nursing treatment—and to make suggestions which could be passed on to hospital authorities.*

The appointment of a committee on the welfare of children in hospital in 1956 marked a period of growing concern about the possible effects of separating young children from their mothers by admission to hospital and of maintaining this separation by means of restrictive regulations about visiting. The traditional belief of many nurses that children 'settled' better in hospital if frequent visits were not allowed and that in fact visits from parents 'upset' the children had been challenged by research at the Tavistock Institute for Human Relations which appeared to demonstrate that children might suffer permanent psychological harm from this separation. There was also growing concern about the practice of nursing children in adult wards where separate children's accommodation was not available or was not sufficient, and about the effect on young children of the sights and sounds to which they might thus be exposed.

The Platt Report accepted that an unnecessary stay in hospital could be profoundly damaging and recommended that admission should be regarded as a last resort. Even certain simple surgical operations could, it was suggested, be performed at the hospital without the child's being admitted overnight. There were schemes in Rotherham, Birmingham, and Paddington to provide special nursing facilities to care for children in their own homes to avoid admission to hospital, and it was suggested these should be extended. Children should not be nursed in adult wards, but should be nursed in company with other children of the same age group.

Generally, the report urged that greater attention should be paid to the emotional and mental needs of the child in hospital and it came out firmly in favour of unrestricted visiting by parents, in contrast to the visiting at set hours which was still the pattern in most hospitals. For many years after publication of the report, some of the more conservative hospitals ignored this recommendation and had to be repeatedly chivvied by circulars from the Ministry of Health and representations from organizations having the welfare of children at heart.

There were a number of detailed recommendations that made the report almost a minor textbook on the care of children in hospital, and sections were devoted to the needs of such special groups as those in long-stay hospitals; the blind and deaf; those in infectious diseases hospitals; and children in hospital for removal of tonsils and adenoids. The committee were precluded by their terms of reference from looking at matters of medical and nursing treatment or they might have had some comment to make under this last heading. At that time nearly 200,000 operations for removal of tonsils and adenoids were performed each year in England and Wales, and nearly one child in three had his tonsils out before the age of thirteen, yet there were considerable doubts in some medical quarters as to the value of the operation and comparison with other countries, in Scandinavia for instance, where the incidence of such operations was much lower, disclosed no evidence of increased prevalence of the respiratory infections which the removal of tonsils and adenoids were supposed to prevent. Even scientific medicine has its superstitions and perhaps this wholesale removal of tonsils and adenoids was the twentieth century's counterpart to the ritual blood-letting of an earlier era.

5.3 Report of the Committee of Inquiry into the Recruitment, Training and Promotion of the Administrative and Clerical Staff in the Hospital Service (Lycett Green Report)

Published 1963

Chairman: *Sir Stephen Lycett Green Bt, JP*

Members: *A. J. Bennett MA, FHA; Captain H. Brierley CBE, MC; Professor T. E. Chester MA (Econ.), LLD, FCCS; C. R. Jolly Esq., OBE, FHA, ARSH; A. S. Marre CB; R. A. Micklewright OBE, FHA; E. Ag. Norton CBE, MA; Alderman Mrs D. M. Rees JP; M. S. Rigden FCA, FHA; C. C. Stevens LLB; E. D. B. Todd FSAA, FIMTA; Alderman J. Serrell Watts CBE, MA, JP; H. W. Silver (secretary)*

Terms of Reference (1962): *Having regard to the need for maintaining a high standard of efficiency in the administration of National Health Service hospitals, to inquire into the present arrangements for recruitment, training and promotion of administrative and clerical staff in the hospital service, and to make recommendations.*

Hospital adminstrators frequently complained that hospital administration as a career was scarcely recognized by the general public and that the recruitment of able school and university leavers suffered because of this. The complex structure of the National Health Service and wide local variations in practice made it difficult to explain to a member of the general public exactly what a hospital administrator did and exactly what he was responsible for (in one group the group secretary might be virtually general manager, but in some of the more committee-ridden groups he might be little more than committee clerk and office manager). But the Lycett Green Report and the earlier (1957) Report of Sir Noel Hall on the grading Structure of Administrative and Clerical Staff in the Hospital Service made it a little easier to explain what the career structure was. Most of the Lycett

Green recommendations were accepted by the Ministry of Health and subsequently implemented. A National Staff Committee consisting of members and officers of hospital authorities, together with representatives from universities and a representative of the Ministry, was set up to oversee the recruitment, training and management development of hospital administrators and to supervise the arrangements for the making of senior appointments. Regional staff committees were created to exercise similar functions at a lower level and to implement the policies of the National Staff Committee.

A system of planned movement was introduced to enable hospital administrators who had completed their basic training to gain varied experience in different types of work and under different hospital authorities and a system of annual staff reports, based largely on that used in the Civil Service, was brought in for all members and former members of the junior administrative (training) grade and for those officers who had not been through this grade but who wished for advancement in the service and volunteered to be subject to annual reporting with this end in view. The two existing schemes of training in hospital administration—the national and the regional schemes—were merged and shortened from two and a half to two years. This consisted of planned practical experience interspersed with periods—the longest was three months—at a university or at the King's Fund College of Hospital Management. Later changes in the scheme shifted the emphasis still further onto practical experience, and the main theoretical module of thirteen weeks was split into two periods of five and eight weeks. The American example of master's degrees in hospital and health care administration went unheeded in Britain.

Steps were taken towards the standardization of appointments procedures and criteria. The National Staff Committee was made responsible for drawing up short lists of applicants for the most senior posts, although the final choice from the short list was to be made by the individual hospital authority. Regional staff committees similarly drew up short lists for posts of intermediate seniority. National and regional assessors were to take part in the appointment interview for these grades of posts, although they were given no power of veto—this was thought to be unnecessary in view of the role of the staff committees in short-listing candidates in the first place.

The Lycett Green Report disclosed a disquieting situation in the administrative grades of the hospital service. There was a concentration of staff in the age group 40–45 and many of these appeared unlikely to gain promotion beyond the general administrative or senior administrative grades into the designated grades (e.g. hospital secretary in a large hospital—in a small hospital the post would be filled by someone on the S.A. grade; deputy group secretary; supplies officer; etc.). Care had to be taken that these officers were not demoralized by seeing young men jump over their heads into the top jobs, and at the same time provision had to be made for their replacement when they retired in 15–20 years' time. It was against this background, and against the background of problems arising from the fragmentation of the hospital service and the failure of many employing authorities to look beyond their own immediate needs to the needs of a national service, that the committee made their recommendations.

The Lycett Green Report also made recommendations to improve and rationalize the recruitment of clerical staff to the hospital service.

Lycett Green Report, 1963

PROMOTION IN THE HOSPITAL SERVICE
Promotion to administrative posts is normally made after advertisement, short-listing and interviewing by the appointing authority, following the system adopted in local government. The authority usually acts through an appointment or selection committee although some authorities act through the whole board or committee on occasion, particularly when dealing with the most senior appointments. Whichever way the appointing authority acts, the body which makes the effective appointment is expected to include a regional assessor, and for the most senior posts (i.e., posts at or above the level of Group Secretary in a $20\frac{1}{2}/30$ points group, and a Finance or Supplies Officer in a $50\frac{1}{2}/60$ points group), a national assessor.

Persons to serve as national assessors are chosen by the employing authority from a national list of members and officers of hospital authorities selected by the Minister from nominees of hospital authorities, or from Secretaries of Regional Boards, or of Boards of Governors of Undergraduate Teaching Hospitals. Persons to serve as regional assessors are designated by the Regional Staff Advisory Committees. It has been laid down that the national assessor should be from outside the appointing authority to which the appointment in question relates, and that an officer should not be chosen as an assessor from either the national or regional lists unless his own grading is higher than that of the post to be filled.

This system gives, it is claimed, the fairest possible method of selection by open competition, in that under it justice is manifestly seen to be done and that appointments by reason of favouritism or local bias are eliminated. The presence of assessors brings an independent view to bear in the making of appointments, even although it is always open to the employing authority, if it so decides, to disregard the assessors' advice. The system, however, is not without its critics.

It is said, for instance, that the interests of the 'local boy' are invariably favoured, but it is probable that such instances are less frequent than is sometimes believed and, in any event, are, through the influence of assessors, likely to become fewer as time goes on. It must equally be remembered that in some cases the interests of the 'local boy' may be prejudiced where a conscientious committee wishes to show its extreme impartiality. Another criticism is that employing authorities are free to make appointments from outside the Service to the detriment of suitably qualified applicants from within it, and it is again true that there have been occasional well-publicised incidents where this has occurred. We think, however, that attention should be directed to Table 5 of Appendix III which shows that during the $2\frac{1}{2}$ years covered, very few higher posts were filled by entry from outside the hospital service, and that nearly all top posts were filled by promotion. The comparatively large number of appointments from outside the Service to the Assistant Secretary grade in recent years were the result, we think, of appointments made to such positions as Work Study Officers and Training Officers, where persons of the necessary experience were not readily available within the Service.

The chief criticism of the existing method of promotion is, we think, of a different order. We believe that appointing authorities within the hospital service approach their task with a high sense of responsibility which they discharge as conscientiously as possible, and that even in those cases where appointments have been made in disregard of the advice of the assessor or assessors, they have been made in the belief that they are in the best interests of the appointing authority and of the hospitals for which they are responsible. They are not called upon, in their view, to deal with the needs of career planning or the long-term interests of the Service. As a result, there is a widespread tendency for hospital authorities to appoint to positions within their service applicants having the experience of, and coming from, their own type of authority. It is this tendency, this failure to regard the Service as an entity and not just a number of separate units, which, we believe, is at the bottom of the fragmentation of the Service between the various types of authority, to which Sir Noel Hall drew attention in his Report.

We have already mentioned that one of the functions of Regional Staff Advisory Committees is the compiling and maintaining of personnel registers of all officers in the administrative and designated grades, from which factual information can be made available to authorities making appointments. These registers have been set up in most, but not all, regions, but they do not always cover all staff in the general administrative grade and above, and there is little evidence of their being used to provide information to appointing authorities about prospective candidates for their vacancies, as was intended. The general opinion of our witnesses was that the registers, containing as they do only factual information, are of very limited value, and that to be of real use they need to include information about the performance of staff, or to be combined with a system of reports on staff. By no means all of those who gave evidence were in favour of the enlargement of the registers to give the latter information.

paras. 65–70

CAREER PLANNING

We are aware that there are some people in the hospital service, both officers and members of hospital authorities, who ... hold the deep and sincere conviction that any diminution of the present powers of hospital authorities in relation to the control of their staff would destroy their autonomy and that this would be altogether too high a price to pay for any improvement in administrative efficiency which might result. We consider that the threat to the autonomy of hospital authorities is exaggerated. In the first place, it appears to be too easily assumed that the only alternative to their present control of staff is a centralised system of control based upon the Ministry, with hospital authorities compelled to take officers, from chief officers downwards, without being consulted, and with all grades of staff liable to compulsory posting to any part of the country. This system is usually referred to by its critics as 'the Civil Service system', but our own enquiries into the practice of those branches of the Civil Service which maintain large and sometimes numerous offices in different parts of the country, and whose organisation and structure resemble that of the hospital service in certain respects (e.g., the Post Office, the Ministry of Pensions and National Insurance, and the Inland Revenue), have led us to suppose that those who use the term are not particularly clear about the actual practice of such parts of the Civil Service. ... Secondly, the problem of combining central control with local independence is one which is not peculiar to the Health Service, or even to the public service. Enquiries that we have made of banks and large industrial undertakings, many of them with nation-wide or even world-wide ramifications, have revealed that they have been in varying degrees successful in the field of staff selection and training in reconciling the requirements of local independence with central control. It may, of course, be objected that banks and large industrial organisations are not comparable with the hospital service, but in our view there are certain aspects of administration which are common to all large-scale organisations, such as personnel relations and the control of staff, and in these fields there are useful lessons to be learned.

Our proposals respect the close personal relationship which exists between members of hospital authorities and their most senior officers, and we seek to maintain the right of hospital authorities to select these officers for themselves, although we consider that initial reviews at regional or national level are required of the applicants for such appointments. In our view, however, the relationship is much less close in the case of less senior staff, and while we are recommending that hospital authorities should surrender to separate bodies a degree of control over appointments at this level, we do not think that this will involve any real diminution of their autonomy. We hope, indeed, that all hospital authorities will rapidly come to see that this change is but a small price to pay for what we hope will be the higher quality of applicants for appointments to their senior posts by reason of the increased facilities it will give for their proper training in the earlier stages of their careers. We are confident that, after due consideration, those who at the moment fear any further diminution of their authority will realise that such fears are unwarranted and that the measures that we propose are to their ultimate benefit.

Similarly, although we consider wide and varied experience essential for staff, and that suitable staff movement should be encouraged in every way, we are not proposing to go so far as to make liability to move compulsory or a condition of service. We think, however, that it may need to be made clear to staff, especially to new entrants, that their advancement may well depend on their willingness to move to other posts. It is, in fact, an integral part of our proposals that a young administrator should move to a succession of suitable posts, to gain wider experience, during the earlier years following completion of his initial training.

paras. 81–3

We contemplate that the regional staff committee will normally provide planned movement for an officer for up to six years after he completes his junior administrative training and that during this period they will place him in two or three responsible posts of different types. For the selected officers who had not been through the junior administrative grade, the duration and scope of planned movement would be adapted to fit, so far as practicable, their respective ages and needs. We envisage that an officer's movement by the regional staff committee in some instances will be lateral and in other instances will involve his promotion, if the committee is satisfied that his progress justifies a higher grade. An officer undergoing planned movement would not thereby be debarred from applying for a vacant post in a higher grade outside the plan, but would be wise to be guided by the committee's advice.

para. 151

5.4 Report by a Committee of the Scottish Health Services Council on Administrative Practice of Hospital Boards in Scotland (Farquharson-Lang Report)

Published: 1966

Chairman: *W. M. Farquharson-Lang MA*

Members: *Sir Arthur Duncan; T. D. Hunter MA, LLB; R. M. McKenzie MC, MA; J. C. G. Mercer MB, ChB, DCH; A. M. Watson;* J. H. Wright CBE, MD, FRCP; A. A. Hughes (assessor); T. H. McLean (secretary)*

*Mr Watson died in 1965

Terms of Reference (1962): *To study the administrative practice of hospital boards, including the allocation of business to committees and the delegation of responsibilities to officers; and to consider whether, taking account of the practice in other fields, any changes are desirable.*

The Farquharson-Lang Committee were concerned only with the administrative practice of hospital boards in Scotland, and throughout the report it must be borne in mind that Scottish health service legislation and traditions differ in certain respects from those of England and Wales. It must also be remembered that in Scotland the term 'boards' referred to boards of management (i.e. hospital management committees) as well as to regional hospital boards. Nonetheless, the report had an immediate impact in England and Wales, as well as in Scotland, and in a circular to hospital authorities, HM (68) 28, published in 1968, the Minister of Health commended certain of the report's recommendations to authorities in England and Wales; in particular those concerned with the delegation of responsibilities to officers and the streamlining of committee structures. No mention was, however, made in this circular of the recommendation for a 'chief executive'.

The committee summed up their report as follows.

We see as our main conclusion the need for a general reappraisal by all boards of the respective functions of members and officers, to ensure that the best use is made of the particular talents and skills of each category. This will be achieved only if boards concentrate their attention on the wider issues and delegate to officers the maximum degree of responsibility, while retaining their function of overall direction and control. The committee structure, particularly at boards of management, is at present in real danger of becoming so complex that it hinders rather than helps the management function of both boards and officers in carrying out their business efficiently; that is why we are seeking simplification.

At the same time we have concluded that there is a need for a general manager, or 'chief executive' as we have called him. The appointment of such a person with the requisite managerial ability should not only facilitate the practice of boards and committees, but should also lead to more purposeful co-ordination of effort within the organization by providing a clearer channel of management authority. This proposal, coupled with our recommendations for a medical advisory service, should lead to management practice more consistent with that proved to be successful in other spheres, and should, in our view, strengthen rather than weaken the position of the medical experts.

paras. 314–15

The report opened with a critical review of present practice in which hospital authorities were gently chided both for complacency about their existing arrangements, and for occupying the time of boards and committees with trivialities that should have been delegated to officers. Concern was expressed that this not only tended to blur the proper distinction between the work of members and the work of officers, but also to make it difficult to recruit good people, and particularly younger people, to serve on boards and committees. On the one hand, men and women of calibre would quickly lose interest if expected to spend their time discussing trivialities; on the other hand there would be a limit to the time that could be afforded by people still active in business or professional life. It was therefore suggested that voluntary members should not be expected to devote more than twelve hours a month to their duties, although this excluded time for travelling and home reading. The time for chairmen should not greatly exceed this. It was also suggested that members might spend more time visiting hospitals for which they were responsible, and less time at meetings.

Boards of management should not have more than fifteen members (twelve in groups with fewer than 700 beds), the committee thought, and even the largest regional hospital board should not have more than eighteen. The numbers of standing committees should be cut, three should be enough even in large groups, and house committees should be dispensed with altogether.

Much emphasis was laid on the delegation of day-to-day management to officers, both at board of management and regional hospital board level. This should be achieved by defining the functions of boards and committees, and proceeding on the assumption that any aspect of management not reserved to the hospital authority was delegated to officers, rather than by attempting to define the extent of officers' powers. The report was, however, most notable for its firm rejection of the Bradbeer Report's concept of tripartite administration and for its proposal that there should be in each hospital authority a 'chief executive' who would function as a general manager and who might be either a lay or medically qualified person, the determining factor in his selection being his ability and experience as a manager. Scotland, which had retained medical superintendents long after their appointment had been almost entirely discontinued in England and Wales, was thus urged to allow the possibility that a non-medically qualified person might become the 'chief executive' of a hospital authority. In England and Wales, this stress on managerial ability rather than professional qualification was seen as creating an opportunity—at least in theory—for a person qualified in medicine, nursing, or one of the other health professions, to become 'chief executive', rather than a professional hospital administrator.

The report suggested that the possibility of a full-time career in medical administration should be retained by the creation of a medical advisory service. On the nursing side, the Farquharson-Lang Committee suggested to the Salmon Committee (q.v., p. 316), which was then sitting, that it would be preferable to have one source of nursing advice within each hospital group to which the board and its chief officer could turn, rather than a number of matrons of theoretically equal status.

The committee thought—in the face of the opinions of most of the regional hospital boards themselves—that there was scope for more delegation of responsibility from regional boards to boards of management. There also seemed to be room for improvement in communications between the two levels. Relations between regional boards and the Scottish Home and Health Department, however, appeared to be good, and no change was called for. The report also discussed liaison with other parts of the health service and with the universities.

Farquharson-Lang Report, 1966

ATTITUDE OF HOSPITAL AUTHORITIES TO ADMINISTRATIVE
PRACTICE

In terms of experience the service is, relatively, still in its youth, and the scope for development in this field should offer an exciting challenge to authorities and their senior administrators. We were, therefore, somewhat concerned to find, both from written and oral evidence, that so many were content with their existing arrangements, even though they had not modified them since the inception of the service. Nevertheless there were some who had clearly been giving much thought to practice and a number who had been stimulated to critical self-examination as a result of our enquiries.

Again, others, while conscious of the need for improvements in practice, were evidently looking to some external source, such as this Committee, to provide solutions to their more difficult administrative problems. We are sure that, on reflection, they must realise that no external advisory body can do this, having regard to the infinite range and nature of the problems, and that the Committee's recommendations must be confined primarily to matters of principle and of general application. Each authority must ultimately determine its own practice not only on the basis of any general advice available to it but also on its own knowledge of its own special circumstances. . . .

paras. 13–14

DELEGATION OF RESPONSIBILITIES TO OFFICERS

Since the written evidence provided no specific information on the extent of delegation to officers, we decided to examine the minutes, papers etc. of boards and committees. We hoped that the decisions recorded (and discussions leading up to them) would indicate which major matters *members* were reserving for their own discussion in committee. By identifying the general nature of these problems we could then deduce the other—presumably less important—matters which were being left to officers to decide. Unfortunately this examination revealed no distinction. In some instances it seemed entirely fortuitous whether matters were referred to committees or dealt with by officers. Only rarely did minutes indicate any discussion on the more important problems in the running of the service. On the other hand, the records showed mainly discussion on matters of day-to-day management or of minor matters which should, in our view, have been left to officers. (We recognise that some issues which appear trivial on record may have deeper implications, which should be considered by members, but the examples were too numerous for this to be true in every case.) This practice was most prevalent at meetings of house committees, where the great majority of items did not seem to call for decision by members either on grounds of importance or for financial reasons. We cite below one or two examples, which have been drawn from the minutes of boards with differing committee structures and disguised to prevent identification with particular boards:

(a) Various requests from junior staff for leave of absence to sit examinations were granted.

(b) The Committee selected a suitable colour for the cards to be attached to food carriers at..hospital

(c) Following examination of time sheets the Finance Committee agreed that the appropriate extra duty allowances would be paid to four members of staff for two months.

(d) It was resolved that a boiler-house pipe which had burst frequently should be lagged or boxed to prevent a recurrence.

(e) It was resolved that certain glass windows should be replaced and meshed after breakage by truant boys.

(f) The Committee were shown a counterpane which had shrunk to half its proper size. It was resolved to investigate the matter.

(g) The Medical Superintendent suggested that the new staff houses should be called numbers 1 and 2 East Grantlie. The matter was adjourned until the next meeting so that he could consider the Committee's alternative names of Lower and South Grantlie.

Many of the minor decisions would have been covered even by a limited scheme of delegation had this existed. . . .

The reappraisal of the functions of boards and committees calls also for a reappraisal of the delegation of responsibilities to officers. We therefore, recommend that boards should review both aspects of practice concurrently. Notwithstanding the lack of specific evidence, we are of the opinion that far too many matters which could be settled by officers (if need be with subsequent report to committees) are still being referred to board members, thereby diverting their efforts away from what we believe to be their proper functions. This has also the serious disadvantage of delaying action while the matters are processed through the committee machine—a procedure which can take weeks. We think that there is considerable scope for greater delegation and that this applies also to Regional Boards, despite the views expressed to us in evidence that the reasonable limit had already been reached.

We accept the principle that such delegation must be exercised within the general limit of the board's defined policy and its financial responsibilities, but we do not regard these as seriously inhibiting more extensive delegation. Nor do we regard it as necessary or reasonable to restrict it to 'establishment' functions. We should like to see a pattern more on the lines of that within the Civil Service, where administrative officers have a considerable measure of discretion in the interpretation and application of policy, within the general directions laid down by the Cabinet, its Committees and by Ministers in charge of Departments. We should add that, having regard to the general levels of remuneration now obtaining for chief officers, we think that it would be reasonable to expect such delegation at all boards, whether or not it is at present being practised.

One Regional Board pointed out that it would be difficult to extend the present scheme of delegation without bringing into question the relationship between the board and Boards of Management. The board have taken the view that an officer should not have the power at his own hand to reject proposals made by a Board of Management. We think, however, that a rigid adherence to this principle could seriously inhibit a proper exercise of delegation by senior officers and that it is undesirable to establish a distinction between the board and officers acting as agents of the board. In all his activities the officer should be fulfilling the instruction and defined policy of his board, and he should determine in each case whether he should deal with a proposal from a Board of Management in terms of Regional Board policy or refer it to a committee or to the board. If he is confident that his board would support his action, he should take the decision and report later, thus avoiding delay. If, however, the matter is highly controversial, or Regional Board policy is not specific, he should refer the matter to his board. Given such discretion, officers are not, in our view, likely to exercise it capriciously.

We are not disposed to accept the view that the general calibre of existing officers is such that they could not accept their responsibilities even as we now see them, nor do we think that boards should make assumptions about this without putting officers to the test. Experience at management courses for senior administrative officers organised by the Scottish Staff Advisory Committee has shown that many older officers, about whom such assumptions might be made, can show a degree of imagination and initiative when confronted with management problems much greater than their existing limited area of authority allows.

paras. 62, 66–9

'HOUSE' COMMITTEES

We are not in favour of 'house' committees, with or without powers, for the following reasons:

(a) They are wasteful of members' and officers' time and lead to additional delay within the board and committee structure before a decision emerges.

(b) They encourage members to intervene in decisions of *day-to-day* management which we consider should be left to officers. We accept the principle that decisions should be taken as close as possible to the level at which they are implemented but we think that the persons making such decisions should be the officers, unless they are sufficiently important to warrant reference to a group 'functional' committee.

(c) The existence of a system of boards and committees at two levels (region and group), with the functions which we envisage, should enable the voluntary member to make a full contribution. To add a third level (hospital units) is more likely to cause confusion than lead to efficiency, particularly if 'house' committees are given powers. Furthermore, there is the risk that they will cause fragmentation of the group and make the problems of group administration even more difficult.

(d) We doubt whether the existence of a 'house' committee is, of itself, a major contributory factor in morale. But staff must feel confident that they have a channel of approach to the governing body which is accessible and considerate. We suspect that too often the 'house' committee has become a device for covering up defects in internal administration which should be put right at source i.e. by more effective management by officers. We do not think that the extension of activities by members into the internal administration of the hospital will help to resolve these difficulties, since this can lead to confusion of responsibility. We trust that our recommendations in Part V on the allocation of responsibilities among chief officers and on the co-ordination of activities at this level will provide a starting point for reviews of internal administration which are aimed at improving communications and morale.

(e) We, do, however, regard personal contacts between members and officers as of first importance, and in recommending a planned visiting policy (paragraph 75) we have very much in mind the opportunities which this presents for such contacts. We suggest that boards should from time to time review their arrangements, e.g. for consultations through bodies representative of the various staff interests on matters which affect the interests of the staff, or on matters of management to which the staff can make effective contribution. The purpose should be to ensure that the governing body is identifiable, collectively and individually, and that internal management is conveying their policy and decisions effectively to the staff concerned. The morale of smaller units can be helped by such obvious steps as relatively more frequent visiting by members, and the holding of meetings there, at which members can meet staff.

(f) An argument advanced in favour of 'house' committees is that they contribute to a lively local interest in hospitals, and help to encourage voluntary bodies e.g. the League of Friends in their activities and the raising of funds for amenities. Moreover it is pointed out that such bodies can contribute greatly to the welfare and morale of patients and staff alike. We do not agree that 'house' committees are necessary for this. The co-ordination of the efforts of the various voluntary bodies in relation to particular units within the group should be the primary responsibility of officers, although boards may wish to designate individual members or groups of members to act as a liaison between the board and such bodies. Any group activity necessary on the part of members can be achieved through the board and the functional committees.

(g) Lastly, we cannot see how it is possible to establish a compact and efficient committee structure in any group of other than the smallest, if 'house' committees are established.

Accordingly we recommend that boards with 'house' committees should, when reviewing their overall committee structure as recommended in paragraphs 117 to 126, dispense with them but at the same time take steps to ensure that any functions which should be continued are re-allocated between members and officers on the basis of the reappraisal of their respective responsibilities. ....

paras. 115–16

A 'CHIEF EXECUTIVE'

The advantages of a single channel of management and administration seem to us clearly to outweigh the possible disadvantages. We therefore recommend that a chief executive post should be established at each type of board. This post would be filled either by a lay or medically qualified administrator, but the determining factor in his selection should be his ability and experience as a manager, not his professional qualifications. We do not rule out the possibility that administrators with other professional qualifications might be considered for such posts. We recognise that a carefully planned training programme would be necessary, which would ensure that future chief executives not only had had experience at hospital, group and regional level, but also had acquired a broad and thorough understanding of the medical planning and administrative problems by the time that they had reached the deputy or chief executive posts.

para. 212

A MEDICAL ADVISORY SERVICE

The chief executive would not, however, himself have ultimate responsibility for advice to the board and committees on medical matters, even if he had previously been a medical administrator. This would be provided in the various ways to which we refer in paragraphs 233 to 248. The present system of medical administrators should, in our view, be replaced by a medical advisory service on a nation-wide basis, thus retaining the Scottish tradition of full-time medically qualified persons concerning themselves with problems of medical administration, but using them in a different role.

The proposal for a chief executive supported by medical advisers is an important change for the medical staff of boards, and we have therefore considered whether the change presents an opportunity for devising a new career for medical administrators. For lay administrators national recruitment through the junior administrative grade has become firmly established, as have also arrangements for their initial training and planned movement, with the assistance of the Scottish Hospital Administrative Staffs Committee (formerly the Scottish Staff Advisory Committee). Hitherto there have been no co-ordinated arrangements for recruitment to medical administrative posts at group and regional level, but we understand that Regional Boards have such arrangements in view and are invoking the assistance of the Committee, in view of their experience in the field of lay administration. We are not dealing here with training; this is to be examined by a Working Party set up by the Scottish Home and Health Department. But we are concerned to ensure that the effect of our recommendations should be to create an attractive career for the future medical staff of boards. . . .

We suggest, therefore, that the time is now opportune to establish a national service for hospital medical advisers, organised on at least an all-Scottish basis, which would provide the opportunity for young medical men interested in medical administration to enter upon a career in the medical advisory service at about the registrar/senior registrar stage. After initial training, each entrant would then have a series of different assignments throughout the service to give him balanced experience at both groups and regions and also by secondment to the Scottish Home and Health Department. We think that all authorities would benefit by having as their senior advisers persons with this kind of preparation and experience, and that such a service would present a much more attractive prospect to young medical men than the existing arrangements under which there is little room for movement unless an officer is prepared to put himself forward for advertised vacancies.

paras. 213–15

5.5 The Pay and Conditions of Manual Workers in Local Authorities, the National Health Service, Gas and Water Supply

Report no. 29 of the National Board for Prices and Incomes

Published: 1967

Chairman: *The Rt Hon. Aubrey Jones*

Members: *The Rt Hon. H. A. Marquand (deputy chairman); H. A. Clegg; D. A. C. Dewdney; J. F. Knight; R. G. Middleton DSC; Dr Joan Mitchell; Lord Peddie MBE; P. E. Trench CBE; Professor B. R. Williams; R. Willis; A. A. Jarratt (secretary)*

Special members for the purpose of this inquiry: *A. W. H. Allen; J. K. Bottomly*

This inquiry was carried out under the supervision of *Mr R. Willis*

Terms of Reference (as far as the NHS was concerned) (1966): *. . . in pursuance of their powers under section 2(1) of the Prices and Incomes Act, 1966, the First Secretary of State, the Secretary of State for Scotland and the Minister of Health hereby refer to the National Board for Prices and Incomes for examination the question of the pay and conditions of service, and the principles for determining these, of ancillary workers in the National Health Service.*

The National Board for Prices and Incomes was set up by the Wilson Government in 1966 as part of its attempt to control inflation. References to the Board were generally designed to procure an examination of whether particular wage increases, or proposed wage increases, were justified and in accordance with Government economic policy. The reference to the Board of the pay of manual workers in the health service, local government, gas and water supply took place during a period designated by the Government as one of 'severe restraint'. This did not altogether preclude increases in pay, since the Government had set out certain criteria which could be accepted as grounds for an increase, even during this period of severe restraint. Among these were genuine increases in productivity, and the need to improve the lot of the lowest paid workers.

NBPI 29 established that manual workers in the National Health Service were among the lowest paid workers in the country, largely because they did not have the opportunities to earn overtime that existed in industry. It declared, however, that these grades were overmanned and that there were substantial opportunities to increase productivity. In the long term it looked to schemes of measured day work and productivity bargaining, devised on a proper basis of detailed work study, as the solution to the problem. However, as a short-term means of giving some relief to these low-paid workers without imposing an unreasonable burden on the tax and rate payer, the Board suggested what became known as the interim scheme, an admittedly crude agreement to pay a 10 per cent bonus in return for a 10 per cent saving in manpower. The crudity of this device was widely criticized but reading of the report shows that the Board anticipated most of the criticisms. They were, however, unable to see any other way of dealing quickly and simultaneously with the special problem of low pay combined with low productivity which afflicted the health service and local government alike. The emphasis on the introduction of bonus schemes for ancillary staff—laundry workers, porters, domestics etc.—which acceptance of the NPBI recommendations entailed involved the hospital service in the recruitment and training of large numbers of additional work study officers and the diversion of officers already in post from work in other areas to the setting up of bonus schemes. The administration of schemes also involved relatively heavy costs in hospital finance and administrative departments. At the present time it remains to be seen whether all this diversion of effort and resources will pay worthwhile dividends, or whether too much faith has been placed in a rather mechanistic, 'scientific management' type of approach to remedy a deep-seated malaise of management.

Report No. 29 criticized the complexity of the pay structure for the ancillary grades in the health service, and as a result of this a revised structure, based on job evaluation, was negotiated on the Ancillary Staffs Whitley Council and came into effect in November 1969. The new structure provided for wider differentials with only seven grades for ancillary workers and a separate 12-grade scale for supervisors. It was agreed that the structure should be kept under review to ensure that it continued to reflect accurately the levels of responsibility in each grade.

NPBI Report No 29, 1967

LOW PAY AND LOW PRODUCTIVITY

The present pay and conditions of full-time male manual workers in the four industries can be summed up as follows. In local government and the National Health Service average weekly earnings are low, and particularly low in local government in Scotland, compared with those in industry generally. Moreover workers in the National Health Service, unlike those in local government, have been losing ground during the past five years. Secondly, a much higher proportion of the men in these two industries are found at the lowest levels of earnings than is the case in industry generally. There will be a marked improvement in the relative position of manual workers in local government in England and Wales if their current agreement is fully implemented, in which case manual workers in Scottish local authorities and in the National Health Service would clearly be left with the high proportion of lowest paid workers among the industries under reference. One reason for low pay in local government and the Health Service is the relatively low level of skill that is required of most manual workers: another is the small amount of overtime worked. The relative absence of overtime earnings is not materially offset by other elements in pay, such as incentive bonuses and shift allowances. As negotiated rates compare favourably with other industries, the situation may be summarised by saying that it is the earnings opportunities of workers in these industries that are limited.

para. 47

. . . women full-time workers in the National Health Service, who outnumber the full-time men, are better paid in relation to the average for all industries than are their male counterparts. Women full-time workers in local authorities, with fewer opportunities for work at premium rates, are less well placed in relation to the average level of earnings for women generally; their relative position thus corresponds more closely to that of the men in their industry. Comparisons of the hourly earnings of women part-time workers reveal a similar picture to that for full-time workers.

para. 55

There is . . . no immediate answer to the problem of low pay in these services. The root cause of the problem is low productivity and any remedy must be capable of curing the weaknesses of low pay and low productivity at the same time. Its aim should be to raise standards of pay and standards of labour utilisation in step so that the pay of the employees in the two industries can move more closely into line with levels of pay elsewhere because standards of work justify it.

The proper remedy is not in doubt. It is for individual local authorities and employers in the National Health Service to introduce properly worked out and controlled schemes that will directly relate pay to improvements in productivity. . . .

paras. 103-4

MANAGEMENT AND SUPERVISION

There are, in our view, three important prerequisites to securing a closer relationship between pay and more effective labour utilisation. First, we think there is a need for standards of labour management to be raised in both local government and the National Health Service. In local government this will entail much more extensive training in management, which should be embarked upon forthwith. Whilst we cannot make detailed recommendations as these matters are outside our terms of reference, we suggest that one of the main impediments to the efficient running of the present labour force in both services is the present structure of management and perhaps also of the Councils and Committees to which the managers report. We regard this as a matter of the utmost importance and would draw the attention of the Government to our views.

Secondly, there is need for better supervision: it is only through supervisors that higher management can have the effect it desires upon its employees. We have the impression, from our discussions with the industries concerned, that the pay of supervisors may not in general be sufficiently high in relation to the wages of workers to encourage the best men to accept the additional responsibilities of the supervisory grades. . . .

paras. 105–6

Thirdly, in both local government and the National Health Service there is a need for work study in a much wider range of manual tasks. This will mean an increase in the number of work study staff and possibly some increase in the use of outside consultants. In view of the large numbers of workers employed, the extension of work study throughout the two industries will take several years. Thus it is all the more necessary that the appropriate resources should be applied to the task forthwith. As a first step, the facilities for the training of work study staff should be greatly increased.

We turn now to our detailed proposals for raising together standards of pay and of labour utilisation. Most manual workers in local authorities' services and the National Health Service are paid by time. Only 16 per cent of the male manual workers in local authorities' services in England and Wales are paid under incentive schemes and the numbers covered in local authorities' services in Scotland and in the National Health Service are negligible. We believe that most of the work in the two industries lends itself to measurement and therefore to methods of payment which relate the level of earnings to the level of performance. It should perhaps be stressed that incentive bonus schemes in which payment varies directly with some measure of performance are by no means the only method of relating pay to productivity. Another is measured day work whereby a fixed addition to the weekly or hourly rate is paid in return for the achievement of a given performance. Again, in productivity bargaining an increase in pay is normally also of a fixed amount, but here it is usually related to acceptance of a change in methods of work as well as to a fixed standard of performance. In many circumstances, these devices may be more appropriate than a variable bonus, particularly in parts of the National Health Service. However, we emphasise the point not only with the Health Service in mind for it appears to us that local authorities have also so far concentrated their attention too narrowly on the variable bonus type of scheme. All these types of scheme require very careful preparation and should be based on work study. Moreover, if they are not to give rise to undesirable wage drift and cause distortions in the wage structure, they should be kept continuously under surveillance.

We would emphasise that the introduction of such methods of payment in the

National Health Service must not of course be injurious in any way to the well-being of the sick; and need not be so, provided that the scheme selected is appropriate to the work. But where a vital service is overmanned the justification for improving the use of manpower is as cogent as in any other field. Moreover, the tasks of many manual workers in the Service, e.g. in laundries, are some way removed from the direct care of the sick.

paras. 107–9

THE INTERIM SCHEME

Long term developments of this kind, though they provide the most satisfactory answers in the long run both in terms of pay and productivity, do not provide a sufficiently quick answer to the immediate problem. It would be a harsh message for local authority and health service workers to tell them that they are relatively low paid, that the remedy lies in a better use of their labour by their employers, but that many of them will have to wait for several years for the remedy to begin to work. What is needed in addition is a scheme for securing quick increases in pay and productivity even though such increases could not be as large as those to be expected from long term action. We do not want to present such a scheme as an alternative to long term action. It should be seen as a precursor to more thorough developments or as supplementary to such developments.

What more precisely would be the conditions such a scheme would have to meet? It would have to provide a means of relating pay and productivity. It should not require exhaustive expert work study. It should be capable of widespread application. It should not make heavy demands upon standards of management or require widespread re-organisation. It should not make heavy demands for training. It must therefore be a relatively simple device.

We can suggest such a device, namely, a productivity increment which would be paid to the manual workers employed by a local or hospital authority when a predetermined saving in manpower had been achieved. The size of the increment, which might be expressed as a percentage of wage rates—though it would not be added to basic rates for the purpose of calculating overtime and other premia—and the size of the associated saving should be negotiated by the N.J.C. for Local Authorities' Services and, separately, by the Ancillary Staffs Council. To meet the conditions in the previous paragraph, the saving should not be set too high. We consider that a target saving of 10 per cent would be well below the savings possible from properly worked out incentive schemes of payment and should be within the capacity of most authorities. An associated payment to each worker equivalent to 10 per cent of his basic rate of pay would substantially help to close the gap between pay in the two industries and in other industries. It would be advisable to proceed in two stages, each of 5 per cent, in both the saving and the payment.

paras. 113–15

5.6 Report of the Committee on Hospital Complaints Procedure (Davies Report)

Published: 1973

Chairman: *Sir Michael Davies*

Members: *Miss Mary Appleby OBE, JP; Barry Askew; Professor Kathleen Bell; Stanley Berwin LLB, Solicitor; Professor Maurice Kogan; R. M. Mayon-White MD, PhD, FRCP; R. H. Morton, Solicitor; Frank Pethybridge BA (Admin.), FHA, FRSH; Miss Audrey Prime; John Revans CBE, LLD, FRCP; Sir John Richardson Bt., MVO, MD, FRCP; Miss Ann Shearer; Mrs Margaret Stacey; Miss P. A. I. Vick, SRN, SCM, DN; S. M. Wheeler FHA, FCA; Miss Olive Williams MBE; Peter Fletcher (secretary)*

Terms of Reference (1971): *To provide the hospital service with practical guidance in the form of a code of principles and practice for recording and investigating matters affecting patients which go wrong in hospitals; for receiving complaints or suggestions by patients, staff, or others about such matters; and for communicating the results of investigations; and to make recommendations.*

The Davies Committee were appointed at a time when a number of hospital 'scandals', such as those leading to the Ely, Farleigh and Whittingham Inquiries (see pp. 402–9), had suggested that procedures were not always adequate to ensure that when patients were neglected or ill-treated the matter was brought to the notice of the authorities and dealt with in a proper manner, and in addition there was a growing feeling in all walks of life that the interests of the consumer of goods and services, both private and public, required increased protection. Some of the basic points made in the report were that while there was evidence that almost all patients were fully satisfied—and rightly so—with the standard of care and consideration they received from the hospital service, those who had grievances had the right to have them fully and fairly investigated; oral and written complaints should have the same status and receive the same careful handling; and that normally the investigation and satisfaction of complaints is primarily the function of management. It was important to have some external checks, and the existence of such checks would have a healthy effect on the functioning of the basic procedures, but normally an external agency would only come into the picture when the basic procedures operated by management had failed to give satisfaction or had broken down. The chief of the external checks discussed in the report, apart from the courts, were the Health Service Commissioner (see p. 177), the Community Health Councils to be set up under the reorganized health service (see p. 174), the Hospital Advisory Service and the possibility of special inquiries such as those that investigated Ely, Farleigh and Whittingham Hospitals. The Davies Committee did not let their terms of reference preclude them from suggesting how these various institutions might function most effectively.

The most difficult category of complaints to deal with in the hospital service had always been those involving medical treatment and care. If a patient believed a doctor had been negligent, then he could pursue the matter in the courts, but for many this was a remedy that existed only in theory. In fact the Davies Committee believed that few patients with a grievance of this kind were motivated by a desire for revenge or punitive damages; more often they merely wished to ensure that other patients did not have similar experiences in the future. The committee suggested that a system of investigating panels should be set up by regional health authorities. Each would have an independent lawyer as chairman, and independent members, and would have among its functions the investigation of complaints regarding medical treatment and care, in cases where the complainant did not intend to go to law, but had not been fully satisfied by the health authority concerned.

The report was accompanied by a code of practice which it was suggested should be adopted by all health authorities and which set out in detail the steps to be taken in dealing with various types of complaint, suggestion, or comment on the service. In supplying this code the committee were complying with their terms of reference, but flying in the face of the view expressed to them by the legal advisers of regional hospital boards. In their evidence, the legal advisers argued that it would be inappropriate to lay down one mode of procedure to be followed by all authorities in dealing with all types of complaint. The committee should lay down principles, leaving procedures to be developed according to local circumstances. The committee, however, commented:

> At some point 'principles' have to be translated into actual procedures and evidence of current practice from hospital authorities and other organizations ... shows clearly that 'principles' are not generally translated

into 'procedures' by the hospital authorities themselves. What tends to happen is that staff at all levels are left with only 'principles' of a most general kind to guide them, and complaints are dealt with *ad hoc*.

The Davies Report represented a bold attempt to be detailed and specific in the field in which it would have been easy to take refuge in generalities. With so many conflicting interests to be resolved, it would have been impossible to escape criticism. The committee members themselves were aware that they would have failed if their report were regarded either as an anti-staff 'patients' charter', or as an anti-patient code for the protection of staff. On the other hand, whilst trying to close loopholes that had in the past made it all too easy for administrators and authorities to evade the proper investigation of complaints, they had to guard against setting up procedures so formal that patients and their relatives would be deterred from using them. The committee were probably helped in these respects by an unusual diversity of membership. Apart from the lawyers, doctors and other health service professionals, Mr Askew and Miss Shearer were journalists who in their time had been vigorously critical of health service authorities, Miss Appleby was director of Mind (National Association for Mental Health), Professors Bell and Kogan and Mrs Stacey were academics in the field of sociology and social administration, and Miss Prime a trade union official.

Davies Report, 1973

LETTERS FROM MEMBERS OF THE PUBLIC
When we were first appointed our Chairman wrote to the national and provincial press, and to many periodicals, and spoke on the radio, appealing to the public to write to the Committee if they had information or suggestions about the procedure for dealing with suggestions and complaints in hospital, which they thought would help us in our work. The Committee received 859 letters in response to this appeal. Some were about health services or other matters outside our terms of reference; some asked for information or an interview; some praised the services which our correspondents or their relatives had received in hospital; and some came from people who were mentally disturbed. Most of the letters however contained specific complaints about hospital services, sometimes from people who thought, mistakenly, that we would investigate them. Only a minority actually made suggestions about the hospital complaints procedure.

We did not invite members of the public to write to us about individual complaints, although we were glad to receive these letters which have increased our understanding of some of the matters that trouble patients and cause them distress. It was clear from most of them that these former patients (or, in a few cases, their relatives or friends) were dissatisfied complainants; they had raised their complaints with somebody in authority but were not satisfied with the outcome. We believe that the large number of unresolved complaints we received,

Subject of letter	Number of letters
Suggestions about the hospital complaints procedure	132
Letters containing individual complaints about hospital services ..	512
Letters of praise of hospital services	30
Letters from mentally disturbed people	39
Requests for information or interview, etc.	66
Outside terms of reference	80
TOTAL LETTERS RECEIVED	859

either because of misunderstanding about the information we were seeking or simply because of a strong sense of grievance, is a measure of the need for improved internal procedures and for a system of external review of complaints.

para. 5.11

COMPLAINTS ABOUT MEDICAL TREATMENT

Most of the 500 or so letters that made individual complaints mentioned more than one subject; altogether 512 letters raised 836 subjects of complaint. The subjects most frequently mentioned were:

Subject	Number of letters	Percentage of all (512) letters in category
Medical treatment	160	31%
Waiting time	93	18%
Staff attitudes	89	17%
Lack of information about treatment ..	80	16%
Food	67	13%
Accommodation	64	12%

Complaints about medical treatment head the list by a clear margin. This is not surprising; according to reports by hospital Boards to the Department of Health and Social Security 'clinical' complaints (which may include some listed under the second, third and fourth headings above) account for nearly half of all written complaints. Complaints about medical treatment figure even more prominently in the (46) letters from former patients who both made individual complaints and sent suggestions for improving the complaints procedure. In four-fifths of these letters, a suggestion for improving the procedure was linked to the writer's experience of the way in which a complaint about medical treatment had been handled. Here are two examples, the first representative of a number of letters we have received, and the second from a Chairman of a Hospital Management Committee in a personal capacity.

'I nearly lost my son due to a young houseman's incompetence. It was very near indeed (he was saved by another hospital). I did not wish to take it to

Court—much too dramatic, and I know doctors have a code of defending their colleagues. But, on the other hand, I did not wish other children to die as mine so nearly did. What can one do in these circumstances? In my experience there is very little—what we need is a private committee to whom I could have written. They would listen, or read letters stating the position and mistakes made. Then the doctor could be politely corrected—the press need not hear of it, but just as important, the doctor could learn from his mistakes. In my case I wrote to the hospital but had no reply. Did the doctor learn his lesson, or have other children died because my letter had no effect? This hospital is famous and rich, so it isn't just the small or inadequately staffed ones who make mistakes. In other walks of life—the Civil Service, Army, etc— senior staff are corrected. Why should doctors be regarded as infallible?'

'Obviously, written complaints are received by the Hospital Management Committees from time to time about the conduct of medical treatment. Normally, in my experience, the consultants concerned are very co-operative in the investigation of written complaints, assisting the administration in the framing of an appropriate reply. However, there are some consultants who absolutely refuse to co-operate, insisting on handling the complaints, usually by way of interview, themselves, dealing direct with the patient. In such cases, I am afraid that in practice the powers of a Hospital Management Committee and of a Regional Board, who are the employing authority and are really responsible, can prove inadequate to alter the situation, which has to be accepted as the best procedure available in difficult circumstances. This is clearly unsatisfactory to the public, since the doctor is seen to be the judge in his own court. In my view, any new code should lay down an enforceable requirement that the Hospital Management Committee (or the Area Health Board) should handle the complaint, dealing direct with the public and being seen to do so.'

Many of the letters giving details of complaints about medical treatment show how the fear of litigation can inhibit investigation. In some of these cases, the complainants had no wish to take civil legal proceedings, and claimed to have said so when making the complaint. What they were seeking was full and fair investigation and a way of avoiding possible repetition of the failures they alleged in the interest of others. The first extract in the previous paragraph is an example of this. The evidence we have makes it abundantly clear that many complainants feel the fear of possible litigation means their complaints are not satisfactorily dealt with. We do not under-rate the real difficulties of handling complaints of this kind, but we are not in any doubt that there is considerable scope for improvements. We return to the subject in Chapter 8, and make recommendations.

Another conclusion we have drawn from these letters about medical treatment is that many of these complaints might have been settled satisfactorily, and some of them might not have arisen, if there had been better communication between the patient and his doctor. This is one of the themes of a recent Rock Carling lecture in which Dr C. M. Fletcher, a consultant physician at a large teaching hospital, said: 'In giving information the first requirement is that doctors should overcome any unwillingness to tell patients what they want to know and recognise that failure to do so is the commonest reason for their patients being dissatisfied with the care they have received.' Failure of communication is not, of course, at the root of all complaints about medical treatment, but we have formed the impression that even some of the most serious complaints drawn to our attention could have been settled if more information or better explanations had been provided. The survey of hospital patients we commissioned included questions on information about illness and treatment and about one-fifth of them felt they were not given enough information. One-seventh did not feel they could ask the doctor to tell them what they wanted to know, either because doctors were too busy (27%), not readily available (15%), 'aloof' or 'unapproachable' (14%), or because they may give 'reassurance' but not a straight answer (8%). Other replies could not be readily classified but indicated that the patient simply found it difficult to communicate with doctors. These findings show that a sizable minority of patients want more information about illness and treatment and that many of them do not feel able, or lack the opportunity, to ask for it. We believe that many of the misunderstandings which lead to hospital complaints would not arise if patients and their relatives felt more free to ask hospital doctors about diagnosis, prognosis and treatment and that better communication would result in more satisfied complaints. If patients do not recognise and exercise their right to question the doctor, doctors themselves should take the first step in the dialogue, to avoid unnecessary complaints and bring greater satisfaction to all concerned.

paras. 5.14–16

6 The Medical and Dental Professions

Introduction

This section concentrates heavily on the period from 1946 onwards, and but for the scene-setting opening section on the 1858 Medical Act might well have been entitled 'Doctors and the National Health Service'. Some reference to the part played by the medical profession in the debates leading up to the National Insurance Act, 1911, and the National Health Service Act, 1946, can be found on pages 76–7 and 135–40 respectively.

Topics for discussion which arise out of this section include the position of the doctor in society; the nature of a profession and the extent to which this is affected by a situation in which the State is almost the only significant employer of members of the profession; the part the medical profession can and should play in the management of the health service; the impact of technology and changing disease patterns on medical training and organization; how many doctors does Britain need?

A recurring theme over the last 140 years has been the struggle of the general practitioner for status and recognition. The BMA was founded to give him a voice, and has fulfilled that function very adequately. The first suggestion for a Royal College of General Practitioners came about 1840, although the College was not founded until 1952 (it became Royal in 1967). In spite of their experience of working within a legislative framework since the 1911 National Insurance Act, it was general practitioners who were most reluctant to co-operate with the Government in the setting up of the National Health Service, and who for many years after 1948 were in a state of simmering discontent over their pay and conditions of service.

Several documents not cited here, including the 1954 Cohen Report on General Practice Within the National Health Service and the 1963 Annis Gillie Report on the Field of Work of the Family Doctor, tried to grapple with their problems. However, if in 1963 general practitioners still saw themselves as the Cinderellas of the medical profession, by the early 1970s their position was clearly a much more comfortable one, both in financial terms and in terms of professional standing and self-esteem. The new deal agreed between the Government and the BMA in 1965 gave them the opportunity to earn as much as all but the most successful members of the consultant branch of the profession, and the Todd Report recognized general practice as a specialty in its own right, even if it had to stand logic on its head to do so.

A still unsolved problem which does not receive the prominence it deserves in this section is that of hospital junior medical staffing. Britain is now heavily dependent on overseas medical graduates to staff the junior hospital grades, although this varies regionally. Increased militancy on the part of junior doctors has brought some improvement in their lot, but in the early 1960s they could argue that they were the most exploited group in the NHS, nurses not excepted. The long-term solution to this problem may come not only from improvements in pay and conditions, but as the numbers of medical graduates being produced by the medical schools increase, and as the number of consultant posts grows in accordance with official policy, much of the pressure on these grades may be relieved.

The 1969 Working Party Report on the Responsibilities of the Consultant Grade made it clear that if consultant numbers were to increase, this would mean that consultants would have to meet personally more of the service needs of their patients, and delegate less to junior staff. This has some interesting implications for the position and status of the consultant. For an early discussion of consultant status the reader should turn to the 1937 BMA Report on a General Medical Service for the Nation, of which some account is given on pp. 121–6.

The relationship of doctors to the health service is a peculiar one. The service cannot function without them, and they are about the only group of which this is absolutely true. This fact is well known to the Government, to the public, and to the doctors themselves. They thus have enormous power and influence, but they have carefully avoided too intimate an involvement with the administration of the service. The 1967 Cogwheel Report was an attempt to get some harmonization between doctors' clinical decisions and activities and their administrative implications. Such an attempt flew in the face of a tradition in which the doctor saw the hospital as his workshop, and the business of the administration as providing him with the tools to do his job in whatever way he saw fit. Further assaults on this individualistic approach to the practice of medicine were made in the 1972 Hunter Report, and in the various proposals for the future organization of the National Health Service discussed in Part 4.

It is unfortunate that the number of documents competing for inclusion in this part has not allowed me to do justice to the dentists as a separate group sharing many of the problems of the medical profession, but having nonetheless characteristics, a history, and problems of their own. As it is, those passages of the Pilkington Report which apply to them have had to suffice.

6.1 Medical Act, 1858

The 1858 Medical Act established the pattern of state regulation of medicine which still obtains at the present time. It set up a General Council for Medical Education—which later became known simply as the General Medical Council—with powers to supervise the training of doctors, to maintain a medical register and an official pharmacopoeia and to administer a disciplinary code which enabled them to strike off the register any doctor convicted of a criminal offence or proved guilty of infamous conduct in a professional respect. The Act was, however, as remarkable for what it did not do as for what it did. It did not prohibit the unqualified practice of medicine. Even today it is still possible for a person to practise medicine without any qualifications as long as he does not represent himself to be a registered medical practitioner. Many appointments, including all medical appointments in the public service, are open only to registered medical practitioners, and only a registered medical practitioner may prescribe dangerous drugs or sign death and certain other statutory certificates, but many osteopaths, for example, are not medically qualified (although some are) and are perfectly entitled to treat members of the public who entrust themselves to their care.

Secondly, the Act did not establish a uniform medical qualification, a single portal of entry to the profession. Unlike the later General Nursing Council, the General Medical Council was not set up as an examining body, and never became one. Its task was to maintain a list of qualifications considered to reach the standard required for registration and to admit to the register those who held such qualifications. Thirdly, although the General Council was constituted in such a way as to leave the government of the profession in medical hands, there was no provision to ensure that the membership of the Council would be representative of the profession as a whole. Members were to be appointed by the Crown, by the universities and by the medical corporations, and the average doctor had very little chance to influence these nominations. Only after the amending Act of 1886 was an elected element introduced on the Council and then it was provided that five members should be elected by a ballot of registered medical practitioners.

The 1858 Act was preceded by no fewer than fifteen unsuccessful medical reform Bills and two select committees on medical education, which reported in 1834 and 1847. Most of the unsuccessful Bills failed either because they attempted to suppress unqualified practice, which in the current state of the medical profession would have left a large proportion of the population without a doctor at all, or because they were opposed by the Royal Colleges of Physicians and Surgeons. In the 1840s only about one-third of those who were practising medicine were qualified by examination. This did not mean that the rest were quacks. Many of them had served a sound apprenticeship or had walked the wards of a hospital under a well-known physician or surgeon. Such men were at least as skilled and competent as some of the graduates in medicine of the older universities, and parliament was not prepared to see them put out of business. On the other hand, the Royal Colleges had vested interests to protect and were well placed to protect them, since it was their members who looked after the health of the well-to-do and influential

One of the most vocal groups in favour of reform was the Provincial Medical and Surgical Association, founded at Worcester in 1832 and later to become, in 1856, the British Medical Association. The PMSA had been founded to counterbalance the influence of the London-based Colleges and to give the provincial doctor, and particularly the provincial general practitioner, a voice in the affairs of his profession. There was plenty to reform. In the early nineteenth century there were three recognized classes of medical practitioner, the physicians, the surgeons and the apothecaries. The physicians, the licentiates of the Royal College of Physicians, were graduates and regarded themselves as gentlemen. Their College had been founded in the sixteenth century and given a monopoly of medical practice in London. Fellowship of the College was achieved by election, not examination, and the government of the College was exclusively in the hands of the Fellows.

The Royal College of Surgeons was slightly less exclusive. It had been founded in 1800 (this is the London College, the Edinburgh and Irish Colleges were founded earlier), an event which reflected the rise of the surgeon to social significance in the eighteenth century. By the mid-nineteenth century consulting surgeons were generally drawn from the same social class as the physicians. The largest group numerically were the apothecaries. The Apothecaries Act 1815 gave to the Society of Apothecaries the right to examine and license apothecaries throughout England and Wales, and the licentiateship of the Society of Apothecaries became the most common qualification among general practitioners. Those who wanted a surgical as well as a medical qualification usually took the Membership of the Royal College of Surgeons.

Nothing has yet been said of university degrees in medicine. Before 1858, and for some time afterwards, the universities were much less important as qualifying bodies than the professional corporations. The hospital-based London medical schools generally encouraged their students to take the professional rather than the university examinations, and when in 1836 the new University of London was given the right to grant medical degrees, the degree in surgery did not confer the right to practise. Once again the medical corporations had moved to protect their interests, and they consistently opposed the development of medical schools in provincial cities. A medical school was founded at Manchester in 1814, quickly followed by others at Liverpool, Leeds and Birmingham, but the Royal College of Surgeons did not recognize the right of the provincial schools to prepare students for its membership examination until 1839.

The Bill which became the Act of 1858 was drafted by John Simon, at that time medical officer to the Board of Health. The President of the Board was W. F. Cowper, but by the time the Bill was ready there had been a change of government, and Cowper had to introduce the Bill in the Commons as a private member. Simon would have preferred a more radical measure, and indeed as originally drafted the Bill would have given the General Council on Medical Education large powers to regulate the standard of the qualifications which would carry the right of admission to the medical register. However, in order to gain the support of the new Conservative Government for his Bill, Cowper had to compromise. The controversial clause 4 was dropped. Under the Act as passed, if the General Council was dissatisfied with the standard of the qualification awarded by any of the licensing bodies, all it could do was request the Privy Council to suspend the right of that body to have its qualifications registered.

Even as drafted, the Bill was a compromise measure. Simon had shown a certain ingenuity in his settlement of the controversies surrounding the composition of the General Council, but the result was a Council on which the medical corporations were strongly represented and one which was therefore unlikely to press home reforms affecting those bodies. Simon quickly became disillusioned and exasperated. The General Council operated under the supervision of the Privy Council and in 1858 Simon had become medical officer to the Privy Council. By some fairly bare-faced manipulation he got the General Council to propose that the 1858 Act required some amendment. Once again Simon drafted the Bill, making it a considerably tougher measure than the General Council had in mind. The General Council was, however, persuaded or browbeaten into accepting it, and into accepting the principle which it embodied of one portal of entry to the medical register. That portal would be a single examination in medicine and surgery conducted by a conjoint board under regulations laid down by the General Council.

There was widespread support for the Bill in medical circles, but in spite of this the British Medical Association opposed it because it made no provision for direct representation of the body of the profession on the General Council. The BMA's opposition ensured the defeat of the Bill. Thus perished one of the twenty-three amending Bills which were introduced between 1858 and 1882. Eventually, after a select committee and a Royal Commission had reported on the affairs of the medical profession, the amending Act of 1886 was passed. It introduced the principle of direct representation, it provided that medical students must qualify in medicine, surgery and midwifery before admission to the medical register, and it strengthened the powers of the General Council to ensure that registrable qualifications were of a proper standard.

In spite of the slender powers entrusted to the General Council in the early years, the medical corporations had been slowly putting their houses in order. In 1861 the Royal College of Physicians reorganized the Licentiateship examinations so that the LRCP became a basic qualification which could be combined with Membership of the Royal College of Surgeons to meet the requirements for registration. In 1884 the two Colleges formed a Conjoint Board to grant the LRCP MRCS qualifications jointly. The qualification awarded by the Society of Apothecaries also became a dual diploma, the Licentiateship in Medicine and Surgery of the Society of Apothecaries (LMSSA).

The basic requirements for registration established in 1886 remained the same until 1950, when a further Medical Act laid down the requirement that after passing his qualifying examinations a doctor must spend a year working under supervision in hospital before being granted full registration and becoming entitled to practice independently. The Acts of 1858 and 1886 provided a framework that allowed medical education to develop freely, whilst enabling the public to distinguish between qualified and unqualified practitioners. The more rigid system favoured by Simon might not have served the profession and the public as well.

Medical Act, 1858

ADMISSION TO THE MEDICAL REGISTER
Every person now possessed, and (subject to the provisions herein-after contained) every person hereafter becoming possessed, of any one or more of the qualifications described in the schedule (A.) to this Act, shall, on payment of a fee not exceeding two pounds in respect of qualifications obtained before the first day of January one thousand eight hundred and fifty-nine, and not exceeding five pounds in respect of qualifications obtained on or after that day, be entitled to be registered on producing to the registrar of the branch council for England, Scotland, or Ireland, the document conferring or evidencing the

qualification or each of the qualifications in respect whereof he seeks to be so registered, or upon transmitting by post to such registrar information of his name and address, and evidence of the qualification or qualifications in respect whereof he seeks to be registered, and of the time or times at which the same was or were respectively obtained: Provided always, that it shall be lawful for the several colleges and other bodies mentioned in the said schedule (A.) to transmit from time to time to the said registrar lists certified under their respective seals of the several persons who, in respect of qualifications granted by such colleges and bodies respectively, are for the time being entitled to be registered under this Act, stating the respective qualifications and places of residence of such persons; and it shall be lawful for the registrar thereupon, and upon payment of such fee as aforesaid in respect of each person to be registered, to enter in the register the persons mentioned in such lists, with their qualifications and places of residence as therein dated, without other application in relation thereto.

S. 15

The several colleges and bodies in the United Kingdom mentioned in schedule (A.) to this Act shall from time to time, when required by the general council, furnish such council with such information as they may require as to the courses of study and examinations to be gone through in order to obtain the respective qualifications mentioned in schedule (A.) to this Act, and the ages at which such courses of study and examination are required to be gone through, and such qualifications are conferred, and generally as to the requisites for obtaining such qualifications; and any member or members of the general council, or any person or persons deputed for this purpose by such council, or by any branch council, may attend and be present at any such examinations.

Any two or more of the colleges and bodies in the United Kingdom mentioned in schedule (A.) to this Act may, with the sanction and under the direction of the general council, unite or co-operate in conducting the examinations required for qualifications to be registered under this Act.

In case it appear to the general council that the course of study and examinations to be gone through in order to obtain any such qualification from any such college or body are not such as to secure the possession by persons obtaining such qualification of the requisite knowledge and skill for the efficient practice of their profession, it shall be lawful for such general council to represent the same to Her Majesty's Most Honourable Privy Council.

It shall be lawful for the Privy Council, upon any such representation as aforesaid, if it see fit, to order that any qualification granted by such college or body, after such time as may be mentioned in the order, shall not confer any right to be registered under this Act: Provided always, that it shall be lawful for Her Majesty, with the advice of her Privy Council, when it is made to appear to her, upon further representation from the general council or otherwise, that such college or body has made effectual provision, to the satisfaction of such general council, for the improvement of such course of study or examinations, or the mode of conducting such examinations, to revoke any such order.

After the time mentioned in this behalf in any such Order in Council no person shall be entitled to be registered under this Act in respect of any such qualification as in such Order mentioned, granted by the college or body to which such order relates, after the time therein mentioned; and the revocation of any such Order shall not entitle any person to be registered in respect of any qualification granted before such revocation.

In case it shall appear to the general council that an attempt has been made by any body, entitled under this Act to grant qualifications, to impose upon any candidate offering himself for examination an obligation to adopt or refrain from adopting the practice of any particular theory of medicine or surgery, as a test or condition of admitting him to examination or of granting a certificate, it shall be lawful for the said council to represent the same to Her Majesty's Most Honourable Privy Council; and the said Privy Council may thereupon issue an injunction to such body so acting, directing them to desist from such practice, and, in the event of their complying therewith, then to order that such body shall cease to have the power of conferring any right to be registered under this Act so long as they shall continue such practice.

Where any person entitled to be registered under this Act applies to the registrar of any of the said branch councils for that purpose, such registrar shall forthwith enter in a local register in the form set forth in schedule (D.) to this Act, or to the like effect, to be kept by him for that purpose, the name and place of residence, and the qualification or several qualifications in respect of which the person is so entitled, and the date of the registration, and shall, in the case of the registrar of the branch council for Scotland or Ireland, with all convenient speed send to the registrar of the general council a copy, certified under the hand of the registrar, of the entry so made; and the registrar of the general council shall forthwith cause the same to be entered in the general register; and such registrar shall also forthwith cause all entries made in the local register for England to be entered in the general register; and the entry on the general register shall bear date from the local register.

No qualification shall be entered on the register, either on the first registration or by way of addition to a registered name, unless the registrar be satisfied by the proper evidence that the person claiming is entitled to it; and any appeal from the decision of the registrar may be decided by the general council, or by the council for England, Scotland, or Ireland (as the case may be); and any entry which shall be proved to the satisfaction of such general council or branch council to have been fraudulently or incorrectly made may be erased from the register by order in writing of such general council or branch council.

The registrar of the general council shall in every year cause to be printed, published, and sold, under the direction of such council, a correct register of the names in alphabetical order according to the surnames with the respective residences, in the form set forth in schedule (D.) to this Act, or to the like effect, and medical titles, diplomas, and qualifications conferred by any corporation or University, or by doctorate of the Archbishop of Canterbury, with the dates thereof, of all persons appearing on the general register as existing on the first day of January in every year; and such register shall be called 'The Medical Register'; and a copy of the medical register for the time being, purporting to be so printed and published as aforesaid, shall be evidence in all courts and before all justices of the peace and others that the persons therein specified are registered according to the provisions of this Act; and the absence of the name of any person from such copy shall be evidence, until the contrary be made to appear, that such person is not registered according to the provisions of this

Act: Provided always, that in the case of any person whose name does not appear in such copy, a certified copy, under the hand of the registrar of the general council or of any branch council, of the entry of the name of such person on the general or local register shall be evidence that such person is registered under the provisions of this Act.

If any of the said colleges or the said bodies at any time exercise any power they possess by law of striking off from the list of such college or body the name of any one of their members, such college or body shall signify to the general council the name of the member so struck off; and the general council may, if they see fit, direct the registrar to erase forthwith from the register the qualification derived from such college or body in respect of which such member was registered, and the registrar shall note the same therein: Provided always, that the name of no person shall be erased from the register on the ground of his having adopted any theory of medicine or surgery.

If any registered medical practitioner shall be convicted in England or Ireland of any felony or misdemeanor, or in Scotland of any crime or offence, or shall after due inquiry be judged by the general council to have been guilty of infamous conduct in any professional respect, the general council may, if they see fit, direct the registrar to erase the name of such medical practitioner from the register.

S. 18–29

6.2 Report of the Committee to Consider the Future Numbers of Medical Practitioners and the Appropriate Intake of Medical Students (Willink Report)

Published: 1957

Chairman: *Rt Hon. Sir Henry Willink Bt., MC, QC*

Members: *J. T. Baldwin MB, ChB; Sir Harold Boldero DM, FRCP; Sir John Charles KCB, MD, FRCP, DPH; The Lord Cohen of Birkenhead MD, FRCP, JP; Sir Andrew Davidson MD, FRCP (Ed.), DPH, FRS (Ed.); A. B. Davies MB, ChB; J. P. Dodds CB; Professor Sir Geoffrey Jefferson CBE, MS, FRCP, FRCS, FRS; L. G. K. Starke CBE, FIA; A. B. Taylor DLitt; Philip Muston (secretary)*

Terms of Reference (1955): *To estimate, on a long term basis and with due regard to all relevant considerations, the number of medical practitioners likely to be engaged in all branches of the profession in the future, and the consequential intake of medical students required.*

The Willink Report has gone down in history as a classic miscalculation. In the early 1950s it became clear that the medical staffing structure in the hospital service was out of balance. The grades of registrar and senior registrar were supposed to be training grades for potential consultants. A doctor was expected to hold a post as registrar for two years, and as a senior registrar for three. By that time he should have his appropriate higher qualification and be eligible for appointment as a consultant, at the age of perhaps thirty-five, although the Spens Committee had envisaged appointment to a consultant post at the age of thirty-two. What was happening by 1950, however, was that time-expired senior registrars were unable to get consultant jobs. There were 2,800 doctors in the registrar and senior registrar grades, which were supposed to turn over completely every five years, and only twice that number of consultant posts in the entire health service. There were also another 2,000 doctors in the grade of senior hospital medical officer, a sub-consultant staffing grade, and some of these would from time to time compete for the limited number of consultant vacancies.

The Ministry of Health tried to deal with what was fast becoming a crisis by requiring hospital authorities to discontinue the employment of time-expired registrars and senior registrars who had failed to secure higher posts, but an angry reaction from the medical profession forced them to redesignate the registrar grade as a staffing rather than a training grade, to increase the tenure of senior registrars from three years to four, and to allow time-expired senior registrars to be retained on a year-to-year basis while they looked for jobs. One remedy that was not adopted was to increase radically the number of consultants posts. The Ministry's measures eased, but did not resolve, the situation. No long-term planning was taking place, and in the prevailing climate of concern at the unexpectedly high costs of running a National Health Service, remedies that might prove expensive were unlikely to be welcomed.

The Willink Committee were faced with two opposing views: (1) that if the medical services were to be adequately manned and to be as comprehensive and rapidly expanding as they should be, then too few doctors were being trained; and (2) that too many doctors were being trained and that in future the number of doctors was likely to exceed the number of available posts. Their terms of reference were not restricted to the National Health Service, but extended to all branches of medical practice, taking account of doctors who trained in Britain but subsequently worked overseas as well as those who settled and took up practice in Britain having trained elsewhere.

The first task was to determine the existing number of doctors and estimate how many would be required to offset future losses by death and retirement. Then followed the assessment of the expansion likely to occur in various fields of medical practice and the number of additional doctors required to meet this expansion. Finally it was necessary to assess how many students needed to enter the medical schools in order that the number of qualified doctors might meet the requirements arrived at under the first two parts of the exercise. The committee decided to take their calculations up to 1971 but no further. This would be ten years beyond the date up to which the output of graduates from the medical schools had already been determined by the numbers of students who had already commenced the six-year course.

There were from the start difficulties in getting sufficient information from official statistics. No official body had details of the total numbers of doctors in practice in Britain and the BMA had to come to the rescue with its register of doctors who would be available in an emergency. Eventually the committee arrived at an estimate of the numbers of doctors required annually to offset deaths and retirements and maintain the number of active doctors at the 1955 level. The figures were: 1955–60, 1,150 annually; 1960–5, 1,180 annually; 1965–70, 1,230 annually; 1970–5, 1,260 annually. It was then estimated that compared with the 1955 figure of 18,817, an extra 625 principals would be required in general practice to bring the average list size down to an acceptable level, and that in addition an annual increase of seventy-five would be necessary to make reasonable provision for the effect of population changes. In the hospital service the number of specialists would need to increase at the rate of 160 a year until June 1965 and about eighty a year thereafter, and there would need to be similar increases in junior staff. No significant expansion was required in the number of doctors engaged in the public health service, but about twelve extra doctors a year should be allowed for expansion of university medical teaching and research. After considering also the requirements of industrial medical services, the pharmaceutical industry and central government departments, the committee decided that 780 extra doctors were needed to meet deficiencies existing in 1955 and that the annual numbers of additional doctors needed to meet further likely expansion in civilian practice were: 1955–60, 465; 1960–5, 440; 1965–70, 280; 1970–1, 280. Consideration of the requirements of the armed forces did not modify these figures, since the armed forces were at that time contracting rather than expanding.

The next section of the report considered medical migration and arrived at the conclusion that the net 'export' of doctors was at that time in the region of 200 annually and that it was likely to decrease steadily over the next sixteen years. The main factors which appear to have impressed themselves on the committee were the diminishing opportunities for British doctors to be employed in the self-governing Commonwealth countries and in the colonies, and the limited requirements of the medical missionary societies. Migration to North America was not mentioned. Summing up, the committee declared that British medical schools had not been producing too many doctors in the past, but they soon would be, and the annual intake of medical students should therefore be reduced by 10 per cent. This recommendation was accepted in principle but in fact the numbers of medical students had already started to decline. By 1961 it was sufficiently clear that the Willink Committee had made a monumental miscalculation for the Minister of Health to announce that the number of places should be increased by 10 per cent. However, as it took six years to train a doctor the effects of the Willink Report were felt throughout the 1960s in a severe shortage of junior medical staff.

The main factors of which the Willink Committee had not taken sufficient account were the deficiencies of official statistics, emigration of doctors dissatisfied with conditions in the NHS to North America and other developed countries, population trends, and developments in medical practice and technology which called for more junior staff. The question of medical emigration became highly controversial in the early 1960s, when Dr John Seale published a paper in the *British Medical Journal* suggesting that about one third of British medical graduates went overseas. The Minister of Health, Enoch Powell, attacked Dr Seale's figures in a public speech—and as Dr Seale was at that time only a senior registrar he must have been honoured to be taken so seriously. However, it became clear that both the Ministry of Health and the medical establishment took his statistics as a criticism of the NHS and of the existing structure of the profession. Dr Seale was only vindicated when an independent study directed by Brian Abel-Smith confirmed that the rate of medical emigration was much more substantial than had hitherto been realized, although Abel-Smith and his colleagues put it at nearer one-quarter of the annual output of doctors rather than one-third. There was evidence to suggest that many of the migrating doctors were disgruntled senior registrars who had failed to get consultant posts and did not view general practice as an attractive alternative or one that would put to use their lengthy specialist training.

6.3 Report of the Royal Commission on Doctors' and Dentists' Remuneration (Pilkington Report)

Published: 1960

Chairman: *Sir Harry Pilkington*

Members: *Sir David Hughes Parry, QC; Sir Hugh Watson; Professor John Jewkes; Samuel Watson CBE; John Henry Gunlake CBE, FIA, FRSS; Kathleen Mary Carver Baxter; Arthur Desmond Bonham-Carter TD; Ian Donald McIntosh MA; W. A. Fuller and J. B. Hulme (joint secretaries)*

Terms of Reference (1957): *To consider (a) How the levels of professional remuneration from all sources now received by doctors and dentists taking any part in the National Health Service compare with the remuneration received by members of other professions, by other members of the medical and dental professions, and by people engaged in connected occupations; (b) What, in the light of the foregoing, should be the proper current levels of remuneration of such doctors and dentists by the National Health Service; (c) Whether, and if so what, arrangements should be made to keep that remuneration under review: And to make recommendations.*

Two years before the 1946 National Health Service Act came into effect the Government set up three committees under the chairmanship in each case of Sir Will Spens to report on what ought to be the range of incomes of general medical practitioners, general dental practitioners, consultants and specialists in the new service. The three committees worked independently, but all expressed their recommendations in terms of the 1939 value of money, leaving 'to others the problem of the necessary adjustments to present-day values of money'. This clear indication that doctors should be protected against the effects of inflation was to cause problems later.

The Committee on General Practitioners, after taking into account the estimated level of general practitioner incomes before the war, and the need to prevent a drain from general practice at a time when entry into specialist practice was to be made rather easier than it had been in the past, recommended a scheme which would have ensured that the average general practitioner's income was £1,111 a year in 1939 values. The British Medical Association estimated that the translation of this figure into post-war money values would mean that the average general practitioner should be paid £2,222, a betterment factor of 100 per cent. The Ministry of Health, suddenly awakened to the full implications of their acceptance in principle of the Spens formula, offered an average income 60 per cent above the £1,111 recommended by Spens. After prolonged argument the dispute was, in 1951, referred to a High Court judge for arbitration, and Mr Justice Danckwerts found in favour of the doctors. The Danckwerts award was accepted by the Conservative Government in the following year.

The Danckwerts award also had implications for the system by which general practitioners' pay was calculated. General practitioners had rejected any form of salary, and held out for a system of payment based on capitation fees for patients on their lists, a system familiar to them from experience of the 1911 National Health Insurance scheme. However, apart from capitation fees, general practitioners could earn additional fees for maternity work, and for part-time work for the local health authority or in hospital, as well as from private practice, and the average earnings of the Danckwerts award were intended to take account of all these sources of income.

The system therefore became very complicated. An agreed average net income was multiplied by the number of doctors and an agreed amount for practice expenses was added to this total pool. Deductions were then made for general practitioners' estimated earnings from other sources, and the money that was left was distributed in the form of capitation fees and supplementary allowances of various kinds. The complexities of this system were to lead to a great deal of trouble later on.

As the three committees worked independently, it is difficult to know what significance to attach to the fact that the income figures suggested by the Spens Committee on Consultants and Specialists were considerably higher than those envisaged by the Committee on General Practitioners. There had traditionally been an income gap between the two branches of the profession, although it had been narrowing between the two world wars. However, the Committee on Consultants and Specialists had to face rather more squarely the problem of the spread of earnings among consultants themselves. It was obviously impossible to assure to the whole consultant body incomes equivalent to those that had been earned before the war by the most successful consultants, largely in private practice: equally it would have been impossible to secure the co-operation of the profession if a ruthless levelling down had been proposed.

The solution arrived at was the ingenious, and in a public service unique, device of distinction awards. All consultants were to be paid according to the same basic scale, or a proportion of that scale if they worked part-time. A national committee would, however, be set up with the task of selecting individual specialists whose outstanding distinction merited a higher reward. There would be three grades of award and the top award would have the effect of doubling the basic salary. The Spens committee proposed that the national committee to be set up should be 'predominantly professional'; in fact it was set up with a membership consisting entirely of leading members of the medical profession. The value of the awards was adjusted from time to time to take account of changes in the value of money and in consultant remuneration generally.

The Committee on Consultants and Specialists also made recommendations for the pay of specialists in training. The recommendations for these grades (those which eventually became known as senior house officer, registrar and senior registrar) were based on the belief that they had been substantially underpaid in the past.

The Committee on General Dental Practitioners, like the Committee on General Medical Practitioners, expressed their recommendations in terms of average incomes, but in this case they had to be translated into fees for items of service, as that was how it had been decided dentists should be paid. The dentists' committee envisaged an average income for a general dental practitioner slightly below that envisaged for general practitioners.

Now the Danckwerts award had slightly reduced the gap between the incomes of consultants and general practitioners that had been envisaged by Spens and thus somewhat soothed the ruffled feelings of the general practitioners. So in 1956 the general practitioners and the consultants set up a joint negotiating committee and submitted directly to the Minister of Health a claim for a 24 per cent increase all round, the claim being based, for the most part, on rises in the cost of living. The Government rejected the claim but set up a Royal Commission on Doctors' and Dentists' Remuneration. The British Medical Association saw this as a delaying tactic and made militant noises, but while the BMA were threatening to call on doctors to resign from the National Health Service, the Royal College of Physicians threw a spanner in the works. The president of the College, Sir Russell Brain, later Lord Brain, was chairman of the profession's joint negotiating committee, and after receiving certain reassurances from the Government he disowned the BMA's policy of non-co-operation.

When the Royal Commission reported in 1960 they recommended a general increase of about 21 per cent, together with certain changes in the method of calculation of the general practitioners' 'pool'. They also suggested the setting up of a small Standing Review Body, outside the National Health Service, to keep doctors' and dentists' pay under review and to make recommendations from time to time. The Royal Commission recommended that the existing relationship between consultants' incomes and general practitioners' incomes should remain unchanged—the ratio was about 3 : 2. This, not surprisingly, precipitated more trouble with the general practitioners.

In the first decade or so of the health service, the general practitioners had been very conscious of the need to improve their status, and one expression of this concern was the founding in 1952 of the College (later Royal College) of General Practitioners. In this they were declaring themselves the equals of the consultants. Incidentally, they outnumbered the consultants by about three to one. They were also declaring that in a world where medicine was becoming increasingly specialized, general practice was itself a specialty, and not simply what was left when the specialists had taken their pickings, or, worse, simply a sorting office for the specialists.

The original award of the Royal Commission was supposed to last for three years, until 1963, but early in 1962 the Review Body which the Royal Commission had recommended was set up to prepare for its future role. The chairman was Lord Kindersley, a banker, and the Review Body was to report, not to the Minister of Health, but to the Prime Minister. The members included an eminent lawyer, an actuary, two university professors and two financiers, but, since the Review Body was to be entirely independent, no doctors.

The Review Body asked the doctors to prepare a document setting out their claims. Significantly, it asked for one document for the whole profession, not separate documents for consultants and general practitioners. The BMA agreed to this and announced that they considered it vitally important that the profession should speak with one voice. A committee was set up to prepare the profession's case, consisting of two general practitioners and three consultants.

Up to a point all went well. The Review Body's first report, in 1963, recommended a general increase for all doctors of 14 per cent. Both the BMA and the Government accepted the recommendation in principle. However, the complexity of the 'pool' system meant that while consultants got a straight 14 per cent increase in pay, the result of a 14 per cent increase in the figure used as a basis for the calculation of the pool (net income of the average general practitioner) was that individual doctors would only receive increases amounting to 7 or 8 per cent. The wrath of the doctors broke not so much over the Government and the Review Body as over the BMA. There were stormy meetings in various parts of the country; the Medical Practitioners' Union was active in organizing protest, and a new organization, the General Practitioners' Association, came into being and quickly recruited 6,000 of the 22,000 general practitioners.

As a result of futher pressure from the BMA, making desperate efforts to preserve the unity of the profession, the Ministry set up a working party on the problems of general practice, under the chairmanship of Sir Bruce Fraser, then permanent secretary. The Review Body deliberated on a memorandum submitted by the BMA demanding, with consultant support, a further increase for general practitioners. The doctors were asking for an extra £18 million a year, but when the Review Body reported it offered them £5½ million. The BMA's reaction was to draw up a Charter for the Family Doctor which, if implemented, would cost the Government £40 million. When the Minister agreed to consider the Charter, the doctors postponed their threatened resignations from the NHS. Negotiations went on throughout the summer of 1965. Eventually agreement was reached, not on the terms of the Charter as originally set out, but on a new system that met the demands of the doctors virtually in full and which was referred to the Review Body for pricing. At the same time proposals were agreed for increasing the pay of junior hospital doctors. The total cost was estimated at £39 million p.a.

The new system of payment for general practitioners was based on a capitation fee for treatment of patients during working hours (8 am to 7 pm with a half day on Saturday and a day off on Sunday), a basic practice allowance, and supplementary payments for out-of-hours work, for patients over 65, seniority, group practice, and service in areas designated as under-doctored. At the same time, progress was reported on the question of full direct payment of reasonable practice expenses. For the time being at least, this agreement brought peace to general practice.

As far as dentists were concerned, the Royal Commission's report offered cold comfort. The dentists had been the victims of the kind of manoeuvre that is known in industry as 'rate-cutting'. They were paid by item of service, and the payments had been fixed with the intention that they should result in the average dentist earning rather less than the average family doctor. There was, however, a shortage of dentists, and the dentists worked longer hours than the Government had expected them to, and got through rather more work during these hours than it had been thought they could do. The result was that they achieved very high earnings, enough to upset the intended differential between dentists and family doctors. This kind of behaviour is known in trade union circles as 'rate-busting' and it had the usual result: the Government cut rates to a level where dentists were more likely to earn what they had been intended to earn. Against this background the Pilkington Report recommended that for the time being there should be no change in the rates of payment for dental services.

Although the setting up of the Review Body was the major long-term achievement of the Pilkington Commission, they deserved credit for the painstaking examination to which they subjected the question of doctors' and dentists' earnings in relation to other professions and occupational groups. The report included not only this comparative information, carefully analysed, but full discussion of the methodology. Surprisingly, very little of the information already available from published or central government sources was of use for the purposes of the Royal Commission. For example, published rates and scales of pay for doctors and dentists gave a fairly good picture of the earnings of full-time salaried doctors, but little idea of the total earnings of the large and important group of part-time consultants. The information available from central sources on general practitioners' pay gave no indication of the variation of earnings between one doctor and another, or their relationship to different types of practice or stages in a doctor's career. Similar problems were encountered with regard to the other professions with which it was wished to draw comparisons. Much of the information could of course have been obtained from the Inland Revenue, but the Board of Inland Revenue were prevented by their rules of confidentiality from imparting it.

The Royal Commission therefore had to undertake extensive investigations, which included sample surveys of members of the medical and dental professions, and of accountants, actuaries, barristers and advocates, solicitors, architects, surveyors, engineers and in university teachers. In addition to these questionnaire surveys, the Royal Commission approached a selected sample of large firms for information on the earnings of graduates in industry. Evidence was also obtained from various sources on the earnings of a number of other groups, including salaried professions within the National Health Service, veterinary surgeons, ministers of religion, the civil service, clerks of local authorities, and officers of the armed forces.

There was little wonder that the Royal Commission commented: 'We were appointed nearly three years ago to carry out a task that was then expected to be simple, and short. It has turned out to be neither.' The wealth of information derived from the various inquiries was set out either in the body of the report or in a number of valuable appendices. Bound with the report was a Memorandum of Dissent by Professor John Jewkes, who did not sign the main report. Professor Jewkes wanted general practitioners to be given rather more than his colleagues had recommended, together with a 30 per cent increase in the value of consultants' distinction awards and in fees for their domiciliary visits. He also preferred the term 'Advisory Council' to 'Review Body' and wanted that body to have rather wider powers than his colleagues suggested, and to include one or more eminent members of the medical profession.

Pilkington Report, 1960

THE POOL SYSTEM

The pool system, though unusual, has a number of practical advantages. The main element of a general practitioner's earnings is capitation, and this requires him to have a list of patients in respect of whom he is paid. When, however, the numbers of patients on the lists of all general practitioners are added together they amount to a total which exceeds the whole population. The explanation is that the lists have been inflated in various ways, for example, by a number of people having been placed on one list without being removed from another. If there were a system of capitation without a pool the consequence would be that the Exchequer would have to pay for medical attention to more people than exist in the country. Under the present pool system, however, the profession as a whole is paid a certain sum without reference to the total number of patients and it is only in the division of this sum among practitioners that the size of each doctor's list becomes a factor; inflation may thus work some small injustice as between one doctor and another but imposes no burden on the Exchequer. A further advantage of the pool system is that it facilitates negotiation on adjustments of remuneration. The pool is budgeted for as a lump sum, and changes which involve only a redistribution of the same total can be negotiated between the profession and the Health Departments in an easier and less formal manner than would be necessary if, as in a salaried service, each item were separately budgeted and required Treasury consent for any alteration. Finally the pool system makes it possible to ensure that, although payment is not by way of salary, the intended level of average earnings will be exactly realised, neither more nor less. Experience gained in the payment of dentists, whose intended level of average remuneration has seldom been realised . . . emphasizes the value of this feature.

Because of the practical advantages described in the preceding paragraph and because the profession is accustomed to it and on the whole likes it, we recommend a continuance of the pool system, but not in precisely its present form.

paras. 327–8

RECOMMENDED LEVELS

In Chapter V we explained the considerations which we think should govern the earnings of doctors in general, and indicated the extent to which total career earnings between the ages of 30 and 65 should, in our view, be increased above the 1955/56 level. We have now to recommend precise figures for the realisation of those aims so far as general medical practitioners are concerned. We have recommended two major changes in the calculation of the pool, namely, that the deductions hitherto made in respect of private earnings (£93 per doctor in 1955/56) and of the Exchequer contribution for superannuation (£165 per doctor in 1955/56) should not be made in future. We have also recommended three minor adjustments, namely, that in future inducement payments should be, and group practice loans should cease to be, provided from the pool, whilst practitioners over 70 years of age should be removed from the calculation.

Taking all these matters into account we recommend that as from 1st January 1960 there should be paid into the pool the sum of £2,425 per annum in respect of every practitioner below the age of 70 providing unrestricted General Medical Services.

para. 338

DISTINCTION AWARDS

The origin of the awards system is to be found in the Spens Committee's report. It stated that, 'if the best possible recruits are to be attracted to specialist practice, there must remain for a significant minority the opportunity to earn incomes comparable with the highest which can be earned in other professions'. The Spens Committee also considered that 'there is a far greater diversity of ability and effort among specialists than admits of remuneration by some simple scale applicable to all. If the recruitment and status of specialist practice are to be maintained, specialists must be able to feel that more than ordinary ability and effort receive an adequate reward'. While they did not discuss the question whether there should be only one specialist grade, they clearly assumed that it was not possible to take account of the diversity of ability and effort by having some kind of hierarchy among specialists, or at least some grading of posts within the specialist group. It followed from this assumption that differentiation of pay could not be secured by promotion to posts with higher salary scales. The Committee, therefore, suggested that a predominantly professional Committee should select 'individual specialists whose outstanding distinction merits additional reward', that 4 per cent of all 'consultants' eligible should be selected for conferment of the first distinction (£2,500 a year), 10 per cent for the second (£1,500) and 20 per cent for the third (£500). (The Spens Committee used the words 'consultant' and 'specialist' interchangeably.) They also emphasised strongly that 'whilst it would in our view be impracticable to distribute these distinctions on the basis of a specified quota for each hospital region, they should not be allowed to gravitate towards a few large teaching hospital centres; and we wish to stress that, in making awards as between those who on other grounds appear to have equal claims, regard should be had to the desirability of spreading such awards over the country, as well as over different branches of specialist practice'. The awards system introduced when the National Health Service was brought into being followed exactly the lines recommended by the Spens Committee.

para. 213

Awards are paid by Boards of Governors and Regional Hospital Boards after receiving instructions from the Health Ministers. The Health Ministers in turn act on the advice of an Advisory Committee under the Chairmanship of Lord Moran with the following terms of reference:

> To advise the Minister of Health and the Secretary of State for Scotland which specialists engaged in the National Health Service should receive awards for professional distinction, having regard to the desirability that 4 per cent of the number eligible should receive the highest award (at the rate of £2,500 a year) 10 per cent the second award (£1,500 a year) and 20 per cent the third award (£500 a year).

We understand that soon after they were established the Committee decided that 34 per cent of consultants in England and Wales should receive awards, and similarly 34 per cent in Scotland. It was further decided that a Scottish Sub-Committee, consisting of the Scottish members of the main Committee with the addition of a number of other consultants co-opted for the purpose, should consider the position in Scotland and make recommendations to the whole Committee. Since the procedure adopted for deciding which consultants should be recommended for awards is different in the two countries we now describe the arrangement in each country separately.

ENGLAND AND WALES

We understand that in the first instance the Ministry of Health calculate the total number of vacancies to be filled annually arising from deaths, retirements and the steady increase of the total consultant establishment. This number is then divided approximately equally between the ten provincial regions on the one hand and the four metropolitan regions on the other, and the provincial share is then subdivided between the regions in proportion to the number of consultants in each region. This subdivision is given to the Committee and used by them as a starting point. The number of new awards finally given in any region may vary slightly from the purely arithmetical allocation of vacancies.

Lord Moran described to us in some detail the way in which the Committee obtain names for consideration. He and the one lay member of the Committee visit all hospital regions in England and Wales and consult selected advisers about the quality of the consultants in the region. The exact nature of these local informal consultations varies as between one region and another according to the availability of suitable local advisers, the number of large hospital centres in the region, and other local factors, but Lord Moran always seeks a number of independent opinions on each recommendation. Lord Moran consults, as he considers necessary, leading members of the Colleges and specialty associations in London. Having as a result of these intensive enquiries drawn up a list of possible candidates he lays this before the Committee for consideration, and the Committee decide on the names to be recommended to the Minister.

He also described his practice of holding open meetings in the regions, at which he explains to all consultants who care to attend the whole process involved in the selection of consultants to receive awards.

Since the origin of the system is the need for a differentiation of income in a professional group in which there is no hierarchy of appointments, we first considered whether it was inherent in the nature of consultant practice in hospitals in the National Health Service that such a hierarchy was impossible or at least undesirable. There have been suggestions from various quarters that instead of linking awards to individuals, differentiation of income could be obtained by giving higher remuneration to the holders of posts of special responsibility. We asked the Health Departments whether, in their view, the organisation of hospital work in England and Wales on the one hand and Scotland on the other (we understood that there were certain long-standing differences in staffing arrangements between England and Scotland) made it possible to identify such posts. The Ministry of Health told us that 'they found it impossible to obtain any worthwhile lists of posts with special responsibility, and generally our enquiries of Boards have merely confirmed the statement in the Government's evidence that in England and Wales there is no easily discernible hierarchy of responsibility among consultants.' . . .

paras. 215–22

For our part, we agree that some considerable differentiation of income among consultants is necessary in order that good work may be encouraged and rewarded and that there may be a spread of income among consultants comparable to that in other professions. Two common methods of securing differentiation in other fields are not open to the consultant so far as his Health Service work is concerned. Unlike some professional men in private practice he cannot vary his fees in accordance with his professional standing; and unlike the salaried employee in most fields he cannot look forward to promotion. In these circumstances we consider the awards system is a practical and imaginative way of securing a reasonable differentiation of income and providing relatively high earnings for the 'significant minority' to which the Spens Committee referred. We therefore unreservedly support the continuation of the system. . . .

para. 224

REVIEW MACHINERY

We have considered the following five possible ways in which medical and dental remuneration could in future be kept under review:

(*a*) Direct negotiation between the Health Departments and the medical and dental organisations.

(*b*) Negotiation through Whitley Councils.

(*c*) Arbitration in cases of unresolved dispute.

(*d*) The use of a formula of some kind by reference to which remuneration could be more or less automatically adjusted in changing circumstances.

(*e*) The establishment of an advisory body composed of persons of standing to make recommendations to the Government about doctors' and dentists' pay.

The first three are methods used at present. The third is not an alternative to the others, but an arrangement used along with (*a*) or (*b*).

para. 411

Having considered the various arrangements set out above, we have reached two conclusions.

The first is that the existing arrangements for negotiation in respect of the doctors and dentists with whom we are concerned are generally adequate for the consideration and settlement of minor matters, and we recommend that they continue to be used for this purpose. There is some evidence, however, that the Whitley Committee for the hospital service does not work as quickly and efficiently as it might, and we recommend that the two sides jointly consider what action might be taken to improve its procedures.

The second conclusion is that none of the four methods considered above is adequate for dealing with major matters. We have decided that the most appropriate form of machinery would be the appointment of a Standing Review Body of eminent persons of experience in various fields of national life to keep medical and dental remuneration under review and to make recommendations about that remuneration to the Prime Minister.

An arrangement of this kind was suggested for the consideration of salaries in the higher Civil Service by the last Royal Commission on the Civil Service, and a Committee under the Chairmanship of Lord Coleraine was appointed to carry out this task. There are, of course, a number of important differences between the settlement of remuneration for civil servants on the one hand, and doctors and dentists on the other. But we are satisfied that the appointment of such a body is the only means of achieving the three aims to which we referred at the beginning of this chapter—the settlement of remuneration without public dispute, the provision of some assurance for the professions that their remuneration is not determined by considerations of political convenience and the provision of some safeguard for the community as a whole against medical or dental earnings rising higher than they should.

The members of the Review Body should be appointed by the Government after consultation with representatives of the medical and dental professions. It should consist of a Chairman and six other members, all of whom should be persons of eminence and authority. They should be selected as individuals able to bring a wide variety of experience and wisdom to bear on the problems involved and should not be regarded as the representatives of any interest. No members of the medical or dental professions should be included. The Chairman should be able to devote a substantial part of his time to the work of the Review Body, and in order to secure a man of the right calibre the Government might have to pay him a substantial sum.

We recommend that the terms of reference should be:

> To advise the Prime Minister on the remuneration of doctors and dentists taking any part in the National Health Service.

We do not think it desirable to define exactly the factors of which the Review Body should take account in making its recommendations. It would be presumptuous on our part, after recommending the appointment of persons of eminence and authority, to seek to tie their hands for years ahead in circumstances of which we are not at present aware. While it should be left to them to decide which factors might be relevant at any particular time and the weight to be attached to them, we expect that three factors which would always be relevant would be changes in the cost of living, the movement of earnings in other professions, and the quality and quantity of recruitment in all professions.

We consider that the deliberations of the Review Body should be conducted in private in order to avoid the appearance of arbitration between two opposing points of view. We would expect that normally the Review Body itself would initiate consideration of possible changes in remuneration and then make its recommendations to the Government. The Government may, however, on occasion wish to take the initiative, and in these circumstances would ask the Body for its advice. While its function will be to advise the Government, and therefore only the Government ought to have the right formally to approach it, the Government ought to give the professions a firm undertaking that they would always pass to the Body any views or representations which either of the professions might make.

In order to be able to make its judgments the Body must have information, as up-to-date as possible, about general economic circumstances, recruitment to the professions and particular sections of them, and the earnings of members of the medical, dental and other professions. It should have little difficulty in obtaining sufficient information under the first head from all the material which is regularly published. Information on the second can be obtained from time to time from employers (including the Health Departments) and professional associations. There are, however, very considerable difficulties involved in obtaining comprehensive factual information under the third head, and we deal with this problem in a special section at the end of this chapter.

Although its proposed terms of reference are wide we would expect that the Body would concern itself only with major matters. For example, it might consider the desirable levels of remuneration of general medical and dental practitioners and the spread of incomes within these groups. It might also think it necessary to relate its recommendations about general dental practitioners to the hours worked. So far as the hospital service is concerned 'major matters' might well include the scales to be paid to members of the various grades and the number and value of awards to be paid to consultants. It might also be necessary to consider from time to time the relative advantages and disadvantages of whole-time and part-time service so that the numbers of doctors and dentists employed on these two bases are reasonably related to the needs of the service.

There may in practice be doubt whether a particular question is of 'major' or 'minor' importance. The decision should be left to the Review Body itself. In order to adhere to the principle that it should concern itself only with major matters, there should be no appeal or recourse to it in cases where minor matters cannot be resolved elsewhere.

paras. 426–35

6.4 First Report of the Joint Working Party on the Organisation of Medical Work in Hospitals (Godber or 'Cogwheel' Report)

Published 1967

Chairman: *Sir George Godber KCB, DM, FRCP, DPH*

Members: *J. O. F. Davies CBE, MD, MRCP, MRCS, DPH, QHP; H. G. Hanley MD, MB, ChB, FRCS, LRCP; Mrs J. A. Hauff (succeeded T. B. Williamson in February 1967); T. Rowland Hill MD, MB, BS, FRCP, MRCS;* H. H. Langston MB, BS, FRCS, LRCP; T. L. T. Lewis M.B, BChir, FRCS, FRCOG, (designated successor to Sir Arthur Porritt in May, 1967); R. M. Mayon-White MD, FRCP, MB, BS, PhD, DCH (succeeded Dr T. Rowland Hill in April 1967); G. McLachlan CBE, BCom, FCA; G. A. Phalp TD, BCom, FHA; Sir Arthur Porritt Bt, GCMG, KCVO, CBE, MA, BM, MCh, FRCS;† Sir John Richardson Bt, MVO, MA, MD, BChir, FRCP; K. Robson CBE, MD, FRCP; T. B. Williamson;‡ H. Yellowlees MA, BM, BCh, MRCP; I. T. Field MB, BS, and Gillian R. Ford MA, BM, BCh (joint secretaries)*

*Died in April 1967
†Appointed Governor General of New Zealand in January 1967
‡Retired from the Joint Working Party because of illness in February 1967

Terms of Reference (1966): *To consider what developments in the hospital service are desirable in order to promote improved efficiency in the organization of medical work.*

The Godber Report—more familiarly known as the 'Cogwheel Report', from the device on the cover—is here considered together with the Brotherston Report, which represented the deliberations of a Scottish working party on identical terms of reference. The two reports were published, by the Ministry of Health and the Scottish Home and Health Department respectively, on the same day, the English report running to twenty-four pages and costing 2s. 9d. (14p) the Scottish report to seventy-nine pages and costing 6s. 3d. (31p). Admittedly the Scottish report examined in fair depth some aspects of the brief that the English report only touched upon, but a comparison of the two reports would dispel any lingering notions about Scottish economy, at any rate where words were concerned.

The English working party was 'joint' in the sense that it was appointed jointly by the Minister of Health and the Joint Consultants Committee, each nominating six members. (The JCC was a BMA-dominated committee representing consultant medical staff in the hospital service.) Presumably the use of the word 'joint' in the title of the Scottish working party indicated that it was set up on a similar basis, although this was not made clear. An interesting difference, however, was that the Godber working party included two members who were neither doctors nor civil servants: Gordon McLachlan, secretary of the Nuffield Provincial Hospitals Trust, and Geoffrey Phalp, then secretary to the board of the United Birmingham Hospitals. There was no such element on the Scottish working party.

The main recommendations of both reports were on similar lines. Specialties falling into the same broad medical or surgical categories within a hospital or hospital group should be grouped together to form divisions. Each division should carry out constant appraisals of the services it provided, deploy clinical resources as effectively as possible, and cope with problems of management arising within its clinical field. Each division should have a chairman, elected in the Scottish report, appointed by the regional hospital board or board of governors in Cogwheel. (In the event this was not a very significant distinction, since many English hospital authorities let it be known that they would appoint whoever the medical staff elected.) Cogwheel proposed a medical executive committee composed of representatives (not necessarily the chairman) from each division; in Brotherston a committee consisting of the chairmen of divisions was recommended. Cogwheel envisaged the chairman of the medical executive committee as a clinician with time in his contract for administrative duties and for serving both as a part-time medical administrator and as chief medical spokesman for the hospital or group of hospitals. The continuing position of the medical superintendent in Scottish hospitals prevented the Scottish working party from recommending that the chairman of the committee of chairmen should take a substantial administrative role, although the slightly bewildering prospect was held out that doctors elected to this position might from time to time be summoned by regional hospital boards to attend meetings of chairmen of committees of chairmen.

Both reports accepted that the continued division of the health service into three parts was a hindrance to effective working and looked forward to eventual legislation to overcome this. Meanwhile, the Cogwheel Report suggested that the medical executive committee should number among its duties that to 'provide effective liaison with the community services outside the hospital'.

Both reports were careful not to suggest anything that might seem to undermine the individual doctor's freedom to treat his patients as he thought best, but the Brotherston Report set its foot firmly in clinical places with a recommendation that American medical audit procedures should be examined and introduced in Scottish hospitals, with any necessary modifications, as 'patient care evaluation'. 'Audit', the working party felt, suggested supervision by an outside authority, which was not the principle they wished to see introduced. The role of the outside authority should be simply to process the information provided by the hospital and to present it to the medical staff in a meaningful form for their evaluation.

Again, there was the suggestion in the Scottish report that work study and operational research techniques should be extended, on an experimental basis, into the clinical field, and that junior medical staff should be encouraged to undertake operational research in the same way as they were already encouraged to undertake clinical research. Equal weight, it was urged, should be given to either field when considering suitability for promotion. Consultants, too, should be encouraged to carry out operational research studies and should be granted relief from routine duties for short periods to enable them to do so.

While these suggestions were undoubtedly useful steps towards solving what Professor R. W. Revans has described as 'one of the most obstinate of all hospital problems—the cult of individualism among the medical staff', no direct attack was made, in either report, on one of the principal buttresses of the castle of anarchy, the system of bed allocation to individual consultants. The Cogwheel Report made some tart remarks about worshippers at the false shrine of 100 per cent bed occupancy who kept their patients in hospital 'regardless of the adverse effect on turnover and actual bed use, and with no consideration for the desire of the patient to return home as quickly as possible'. It also criticized consultants who kept 'acute' patients in so as to avoid the bed becoming available for a 'chronic' patient who might block it for a long period. But the report's recommendations went no further than the pooling of emergency beds, although a further paper on effective bed use was promised at a later date.

The Brotherston Report discussed at length a number of 'alternatives to traditional systems of hospital care'. It, too, recommended the pooling of emergency beds, and argued that this should enable routine admissions to hospital to be planned in advance. In this case patients who were admitted to hospital on an elective basis should reach hospital only after all the investigations and treatments which could reasonably be done on an out-patient basis had been completed, and the hospital organization should be designed to ensure that any additional investigations and treatment were started as soon after admission as practicable.

Pursuing the theme of 'alternatives to traditional systems of hospital care', the Brotherston Report declared that intensive nursing care areas (concentrating expensive equipment and skilled staff in one place) were desirable in all general hospitals; short-stay beds, including overnight and observation beds, should be part of all new acute hospital developments. An experiment on five-day wards (avoiding the need to provide staff at weekends) should be carried out in an existing large hospital. Experiments should be carried out with pre-discharge wards, and to determine the need for hostel beds associated with a large hospital. Day hospitals, planned early discharge in close collaboration with community health facilities, and the extension of community screening, were also mentioned.

Both reports discussed the need for management training for clinical staff and the English report in addition discussed the need for organized training for professional medical administrators. Both reports spoke of the value of bringing clinicians together with non-medical administrators and nurses in multi-disciplinary management courses. However, while the English report did not discuss the length of such courses, the longest course envisaged in the Scottish document was 'of perhaps two weeks' duration'. It is possible to wonder how much even doctors could be taught of management in two weeks.

In a circular to hospital authorities, HM (68) 67, which accompanied the publication of the Cogwheel Report, the Ministry of Health asked hospital authorities to encourage their medical staffs to organize themselves along the lines of the report. Subsequent progress was uneven, with marked regional variations, as was noted in the Second Report of the Joint Working Party (1972). A Third Report, which discussed the future of the Cogwheel system in the reorganized health service, was published early in 1974. This report was marked by particular emphasis on collective review by consultants of the quality of care provided to patients. It came at a time when the medical journals were showing growing interest in the technique of medical audit as practised in the United States and elsewhere.

Godber Report, 1967

THE ROLE OF THE CLINICIAN IN MANAGEMENT
For very many years the question of hospital administration has produced over generalized and emotional debate often clouded by the question of whether or

not the chief administrators should be medically qualified. A number of questions need reconsideration. What is meant by medical administration? How important should be the clinician's contribution to management? How can the clinician's participation in management be made more effective?

para. 28

Again, there is a range of problems which need corporate medical consideration and for which a strengthening of medical administration is necessary. It is simple to lay down standing orders or rules governing admission to a hospital bed. But is the whole medical process as it is deployed for the benefit of each individual patient effective? Is it achieving the best possible results? How efficient is the co-ordination of general, specialist and after-care services as it relates to an episode of illness? The answers to these questions are sought all too infrequently, and too often an individual consultant engages in his own immediate and highly responsible tasks without seeking or even having a ready opportunity, to discover how they fit into the general pattern of the hospital.

para. 38

Although the hospital has the central and most dramatic part in medical care arrangements, it is only a part of the broad based social welfare service each part of which must co-ordinate its functions with the others if anything like integrated action is to be achieved. Some areas have active, functioning, maternity and psychiatric liaison committees with representatives from each of the different sectors providing care. However, co-operation between the local authority and hospital services is uneven and both services suffer in consequence. Still less is there sufficient opportunity for general practitioners to express their views on the best deployment of specialist services for the population as a whole. Nothing exists at the hospital or group level for examining the waiting lists for particular diagnoses (for example tonsils and adenoids, hernias, cataract, certain of the paediatric conditions) with the practitioners who are the source of referral. Equally, there is often no machinery for the consultants and general practitioners to consider jointly how to make use of hospital facilities for postgraduate education.

para. 40

A REVIEW OF NEEDS IN CERTAIN SPHERES

Hospital beds.—There is inefficiency in the use of beds in hospitals. Without reasonable flexibility some wards become chronically over-crowded, while others are permanently underfilled. The development of specialisation and the tradition that consultants have a fixed number of beds completely and permanently at their disposal, have tended in many hospitals to make for inflexibility in the deployment of beds. With the increase in number of consultants and the present lack of a system for continuous review it is difficult to achieve a satisfactory policy for the admission and movement of patients to make the best use of all beds, unless there is exceptional goodwill between all members of the staff. A number of investigations undertaken in recent years have suggested that at any one time a substantial number of hospital beds are occupied by people who could have been discharged at an earlier date, who would be more appropriately cared for in a long stay ward or in welfare type accommodation as provided by local authorities, or need never have been admitted at all. A recent Ministry survey of 6,000 self-care patients who were ambulant and able to wash, dress and feed themselves indicated that 1,321 were being retained in hospital for other than medical reasons.

A number of factors may lead to a patient being retained in hospital for longer than necessary and the pursuit of high bed occupancy as an end in itself is certainly one of these. The bed occupancy figure alone cannot be used as a measure of efficient bed use, but in spite of much public comment in recent years, this fact is still insufficiently appreciated. Administrators, and members of Hospital Management Committees and of Boards, often tend to give undue weight to occupancy figures. As a result, patients may occasionally be kept in hospital for longer than necessary out of a misplaced desire to improve occupancy figures regardless of the adverse effect on turnover and actual bed use, and with no consideration for the desire of the patient to return home as quickly as possible.

Some consultants, in order to prevent allocation of a bed to a patient with a chronic illness who might 'block' it for a long period, have adopted the practice of retaining a patient who could have been discharged, until the bed can be filled by a patient with an 'acute' illness. This misuse could be prevented by improved arrangements for transfer of patients with chronic illness not requiring the same facilities to other accommodation. While it is appreciated that the necessary alternative accommodation is not available in all areas, improved bed management on a group basis and better liaison between hospitals and local authorities such as could be achieved through an effective executive committee of the medical staff, could do much to improve the position.

Arrangements for emergency admission can be a major cause of inefficient use of beds, particularly in hospitals where these are made on a rigid 'firm' and specialty basis and each unit keeps some of its beds empty to take possible emergencies. Such arrangements result in far more beds being kept empty than would occur if a system of beds for common use or a special admission ward were available. Another instance is the way in which obstetric beds are kept empty for patients who may be admitted in labour. A certain amount of bed wastage here is inevitable, but it can be reduced by different hospital staffs coordinating their admissions so that one hospital when full, may have assistance from another hospital nearby where there are empty beds. The most important requirement is an agreed area plan for maternity work with a recognised booking policy, well understood by hospital and home care services.

It will be necessary to prepare a separate paper to deal comprehensively with the problems of effective bed use and the contribution which could be made by efficient medical management in this field, but some indication of this has been given above. The use of 5-day wards, overnight hostel facilities and out-patient treatment units are among the many other measures which could lead to improved bed use, and which could be investigated and exploited by an active executive committee of medical staff.

Organisation of out-patient and in-patient services—There is good reason to believe that patients spend longer in hospital than is necessary because planning of their requirements is not carried out in advance. For example, they may have to lie in bed awaiting X-ray examination because at short notice the X-ray department cannot provide an appointment. Many forms of X-ray examination are nowadays elaborate and preliminary preparations have to be made. While individual administrators may tackle this problem with zeal there is a tendency to leave this too much to chance; a better medical organisation would keep the issue fresh and make timely adjustments. The practical problems might be eased further by employing an efficient and possibly expanded secretariat who could co-ordinate new and previous examinations and procedures before the actual date of admission, in co-operation with the general practitioner. Such a secretariat would need adequate permanent accommodation within the hospital,

paras. 43–8

Review of clinical practice.—The normal therapeutic regime for quite common conditions will vary considerably between one hospital and another, or between one consultant and another in the same hospital. The treatment of hernia well demonstrates the wide differences in the length of stay of the patients in different hospitals, or under different consultants in the same hospital. This is a material point, for over one million patient days are used a year for patients with hernia, and these patients also suffer a mean waiting time of 15·6 weeks. Moreover, absence from work may precede admission, with consequent loss of earnings to the patient and in manpower to the nation.

Further examples where, at the present time, clinical practice and opinion differ in a variety of situations are the treatment of varicose veins and after-care in meniscectomy; tonsillectomy; and fenestration. A specific instance concerns the after-care of meniscectomy patients at a certain hospital where the average length of stay was 13 days. Because of the length of the waiting list some patients were referred to another hospital with more available operating theatre time, where the operation was carried out by the members of the medical staff from the general hospital. Five years later it was realised that the average stay at the second hospital was 18 days, while the length of stay at the general hospital remained the same. This chance finding in the preparation of a paper then led to the appropriate action. No-one at present has the specific duty to suggest what may be done in such circumstances or even to institute appraisal of current practice.

paras. 50–1

THE DIVISIONAL SYSTEM

It seems to the Working Party that no matter how the hospital sector of the health service is organised, the medical efficiency and the organisation of clinical functions of each individual hospital, large or small, is a problem unique to that hospital. In order to find the structure in which such appraisal of the hospital's function would be feasible, the Working Party found it necessary to look closely at the basic medical organisation of the hospital service. The 'firm' system as it operates at the moment has something to be said for it within a limited field, but members of the 'firm' do not necessarily have the opportunity—nor always the will—to communicate with colleagues within the same broad sector of activity and having similar or related organisational problems. For example all the surgical specialties tend to have lengthy waiting lists and make demands on anaesthetic services and theatre time. *Taking the district general hospital complex as the basic unit it is suggested that the grouping together of specialties would allow an organised approach to many of the problems which medical staff should be facing and so establish effective medical administration in hospitals.* Some of the specialties fall naturally into single or composite groups within either broad medical or surgical categories. Others—such as neurosurgery—represent both medical and surgical interest. The number and size of specialty groups or 'Divisions' would be influenced to a great extent by the size and pattern of the existing group hospital services. Divisions might be formed from the medical specialties, the surgical specialties, the laboratory services, radiology and radiotherapy, psychiatry, obstetrics and gynaecology or some combination of specialties deriving from a specific development at a particular hospital. The division would include all the consultants and their junior staff and would meet regularly to review its work. Suitable information could be placed before the meeting covering work done, results, facilities required and any question of mutual assistance. In such a system the substantial contribution of junior staff—especially registrars—to the organisation of the work could be more fully recognised. One of the present frustrating factors for many capable young doctors is undoubtedly their lack of opportunity to influence the management of their own work in order to improve efficiency.

The Working Party examined the theoretical application of the divisional system to two areas. In one the natural grouping of specialties gave rise to six divisions and in the other to nine. One of these exercises was applied in a region which already had a system whereby clinicians are grouped together. There is no written constitution for these groupings but they represent the working arrangements for clinicians in an area to come together for discussion. This region was therefore conditioned to grouping by specialties and accepting one member as spokesman for the rest of the group. This small number of *services* or *divisions* would result in a small number of representatives and it is suggested that these should form an *executive committee* which would be less cumbersome than the present medical advisory committee.

The functions of a 'division' have been indicated in a general way in paragraphs 42 to 53; namely the review of hospital bed usage against the background of community needs, the organisation of out-patient and in-patient services, the review of clinical practice, vocational training and postgraduate medical education. Under these broad main headings will be included the study of data on waiting lists, out-patient waiting times, time spent in hospital by patients awaiting operation or investigation and supervision of medical records. The use of resources, manpower, both medical and ancillary, and equipment will need to be considered by divisions and the optimum use of these worked out. This will involve liaison with other divisions and with non-medical groups. Liaison activities with other divisions and with other departments and committees within the hospital group, with general practitioners and with medical officers of health, to name only a few, will form an important part of the division's duties. Postgraduate activity should cover both informal inservice training schemes for junior staff with more formal clinico-pathological conferences and programmes for all the doctors practising in the area (including those in general practice and local authority service). Association with the other community services, particularly home nursing, should make possible the integration of care for groups such as the very old and the very young and should also lead to the development of policy on subjects such as out-patient surgery, early discharge after delivery, and rehabilitation.

paras. 56–8

6.5 Report of the Royal Commission on Medical Education (Todd Report)

Published: 1968

Chairman: *The Rt Hon. the Lord Todd DSc, FRS*

Members: *The Rt Hon. the Lord Platt MD, FRCP; Sir Edward Colling-wood CBE, ScD, FRS; Sir Brian Windeyer FRCP, FRCS, FFR; Sir Peter Medawar CBE, DSc, FRS; Professor A. G. R. Lowdon OBE, FRSE;* J. R. Ellis MBE, MD, FRCP; Miss Josephine Barnes DM, FRCP, FRCS, FRCOG; Professor G. M. Carstairs MD, FRCP (Ed.); G. F. Dixon MA; Professor Andrew W. Kay MD, ChM, FRCS; J. N. M. Parry FRCS, FRCGP; Professor J. R. Squire MD, FRCP;† Professor R. M. Titmuss CBE; E. M. Wright DPhil;‡ Professor F. G. Young DSc, FRS; J. N. R. Barber; Mrs E. M. Chilver MA; Professor C. M. Fleming CBE, MD, FRCP (Ed.); Professor G. M. Wilson MD, FRCP; M. W. Hodges (secretary); W. G. Hammerton (assistant secretary)*

*Died September 1965
†Died January 1966
‡Resigned because of ill-health, August 1967

Terms of Reference (1965): *To review medical education, undergraduate and post-graduate, in Great Britain, and in the light of national needs and resources, including technical assistance overseas, to advise Her Majesty's Government on what principles future development (including its planning and co-ordination) should be based; in particular, in the light of those principles and having regard to the statutory functions of the General Medical Council and the current review by that Council of recent changes in the undergraduate curriculum, to consider what changes may be needed in the pattern, number, nature or location of the institutions providing medical education or in its general content; and to report.*

The Todd Report was the first comprehensive review of medical education since the Goodenough Committee nearly twenty-five years before.

It concerned itself with both undergraduate and post-graduate education; with the number of medical school places required; and with the provision and organization of medical schools. Recommendations were based on a study of existing trends and the likely future pattern of health services in Great Britain, and it was felt that these indicated a need to more than double the annual intake to the medical schools (from 2,430 to 5,000) by 1990. This massive expansion was to be achieved by the planned growth of existing schools and the creation of new ones at such places as Southampton, Leicester, Nottingham, Swansea, and possibly later at Stoke-on-Trent, Hull, Norwich and Coventry. In addition it was proposed that the Universities of Aston, Salford and Strathclyde should provide pre-clinical teaching leading to the clinical courses offered by the Universities of Birmingham, Manchester and Glasgow respectively.

A separate chapter was devoted to the problems of the London medical schools and probably more heat and controversy was generated by this section of the report than by any other. It was recommended that the twelve London undergraduate medical schools should be merged in pairs to form six medical schools each functioning as the medical faculty of a multi-faculty university institution. Thus the hitherto independent medical schools of the London Hospital and St Bartholomew's Hospital would merge to become the medical faculty of Queen Mary College. The various post-graduate medical institutes of London should, it was suggested, become linked with and ultimately become parts of the six combined medical schools.

The basis of the Royal Commission's proposals for undergraduate and post-graduate medical education was the conviction that the aim of the undergraduate course should be to produce not a finished doctor but a broadly educated man who could become a doctor by further training. Every doctor who wished to exercise a substantial measure of independent clinical judgment should be required to follow a substantial course of post-graduate training planned in relation to the field of medicine in which he wished to work. This would apply as much to general practice as to the hospital specialties and indeed the report recognized general practice as a specialty in its own right, including in its use of the term 'specialist' a doctor who had completed a course of post-graduate vocational training for general practice.

The suggestion that there should be two grades of fully responsible doctor, the specialist and the consultant, was another of the more controversial recommendations. The existing system was one in which a doctor who aspired to consultant status might have completed the required time in the registrar and senior registrar grades and have achieved his Fellowship or Membership but yet have to wait a number of years before appointment to a consultant post. Todd envisaged that a doctor who completed his vocational training and passed the necessary examinations and assessments would at once be graded as a specialist, entitled to treat patients on his own responsibility. His name would be entered in a vocational register as entitled to practise independently in the specialty in which he had trained. The grade of specialist would be a career grade although the more able specialists would later achieve promotion to the consultant grade. In addition there would be provision for accelerated promotion to the consultant grade for doctors who showed exceptional promise during the early years of their post-graduate training.

Post graduate training would be divided into two phases: three years of general professional training, much of which would be common to all or a number of specialties, followed by a further period, normally of two years, of supervised practice as a junior specialist. The three years' general professional training would be preceded by an intern year in which the young doctor would not so much undergo formal training as gain his first taste of clinical responsibility. The five-year undergraduate programme would also be divided into two parts: three years of pre-clinical studies leading preferably to a bachelor's degree in medical science followed by two years of clinical training (in place of the two pre-clinical and three clinical years which were then usual). The aim in the pre-clinical period would be to train the student in scientific method and to give him a grounding in the appropriate disciplines. Particular attention was paid in the report to the need for teaching in the behavioural sciences, sociology and psychology, and in such areas as genetics, statistics and epidemiology. It was suggested that the course be designed on a modular basis, with a wide range of options from which the student could choose those most relevant to his future career intentions.

In order to broaden the field from which medical students were selected the Todd Report proposed that the requirements for entrance to a medical school of three A level science subjects should be relaxed and the 1st MB examination should be abandoned.

The published report included a number of useful appendices; some were excerpts from evidence submitted to the Royal Commission; others recorded the results of surveys specially carried out for the Royal Commission; and Appendices 8, 10 and 11 set out specimen curricula to illustrate the Royal Commission's thinking.

Todd Report, 1968

POSTGRADUATE TRAINING

In our view the years immediately following the intern year present the most urgent problems, both because of the number of trainees involved and because of the present disorganised state of training during those years. The present provision of separate and unrelated courses for specialist qualifications takes up a great deal of teachers' time and although important differences of interest, knowledge and skill will no doubt remain between specialties, at least for a long time to come, we think that if adequate training is to be made available for all doctors every effort must be made to find and emphasise the common features, which are often substantial, rather than the differences. The training of the future general practitioner, the Consultant physician and the paediatric specialist, for example, need not differ greatly, particularly in the early stages. Courses common to a number of specialties could be arranged in clinical science, e.g., biochemistry and pulmonary physiology, and some further knowledge of clinical pharmacology is essential for all who prescribe drugs. Pathology plays an important part in postgraduate training in many branches of medicine; the facilities and staffing of many pathology laboratories must be improved if they are to make their proper contribution to professional training. There are many branches of clinical medicine in which a greater than average knowledge of community medicine is desirable . . . ; opportunities should be created for interested young clinicians in all specialties to get experience in epidemiological research methods, training in the epidemiological and statistical aspects of their own specialties, and a simple introduction, in courses provided by universities, to the principles of management and operational research. Consideration should be given to providing, in all large hospitals, formal instruction in this subject and in psychiatry, to be open to all first-year trainees irrespective of the field in which their current appointment is held. Most doctors will at some time be expected to undertake some form of teaching; accordingly, in addition to the valuable part already played by scientific societies in providing young doctors with experience of public speaking and constructive criticism of their performance, the availability of short simple courses of basic teaching techniques would be useful to all doctors.

Common elements such as those mentioned in the preceding paragraph should, together with the elements specifically appropriate to each specialty, be incorporated into systematic three-year schemes of general professional training available to all doctors in Britain, including graduates from overseas. An essential feature of the new training scheme would be the trainee's progress through a planned series of six-month or twelve-month appointments. For each specialty training appointments of certain kinds would be essential and others optional. In Appendix 5 examples are given of the appointments which might be regarded as compulsory and optional in certain specialties. Many kinds of appointment would, we think, be recognised as equally appropriate for a number of specialties; thus, if the career plans of a young doctor were to change, much of the training he had already undertaken could be credited towards what was required for his new choice. All the appointments would usually be held within one geographical area, to avoid the annual job-hunting and concomitant upheaval which at present beset the trainee. He should not be forced to move unless the training he needs cannot otherwise be provided. On the other hand, he should not be prevented from moving to another centre during the general professional training period if he so wishes.

During these three years young doctors should be allowed, if they show the aptitude, to undertake worth-while research without being penalised financially;

if a trainee spent part of his general professional training period in approved full-time research, he should be allowed to pursue his research interest thereafter on a part-time basis. Any research done should be taken fully into account in the assessment at the end of the period (*see* para. 93). We hope very much that any who show enthusiasm and ability for research will be encouraged to begin some original work at this stage: new ideas and quests for fresh horizons are essentially qualities of youth. The three-year series of appointments would also allow a trainee to be seconded overseas during the period with the knowledge that he had a position in this country to which he could return.

paras. 74–6

The general professional training scheme would be vocational rather than academic in nature and would be based on a series of appointments in which the young doctor would render professional service simultaneously with his training. Nevertheless, emphasis should be placed throughout on applied scientific methodology. With the help of universities, the practical training should be accompanied by systematic education and training, with lectures, seminars and demonstrations based as far as possible on features common to different specialties or fields of practice (*see* para. 74). The trainees should have sufficient time for these educational activities and to assimilate their experience and knowledge. . . .

Training appointments should not be limited to hospitals. Many doctors will benefit from short appointments during this period as trainees in general practice, in research or in administrative posts. Prospective medical teachers and others whose interests and capacities make academic appointments or long university courses a desirable part of their training should be allowed to count these, to the extent that they are relevant, towards general professional training requirements. Flexibility should be possible without losing the administrative convenience of the trainee's being regarded as an employee of the hospital authority through the general professional training period. . . .

paras. 78–9

One of the principles which we firmly hold is that in the assessment of general professional training there is no place for a single major 'pass or fail' examination. Trainees should be assessed on a progressive basis throughout the three-year period, so as to relate the assessment closely to the trainee's particular experiences, to avoid some of the unreliability inherent in a once-for-all review covering the whole of the training, and to provide a basis for a reappraisal of progress and plans at intervals during the training period. Some form of general check should therefore, we think, take place at intervals—perhaps at the end of each year. As we have said in paragraph 86, some form of selection may in any case be needed in the first year in order to decide which trainees may be allowed to continue training in the more popular specialties. The final assessment should include a review of the interim assessments. Provision should also be made for full account to be taken of any special experience the trainee may have had, e.g. in overseas service or in research. The trainee might himself offer this for consideration. If, as we hope, the early postgraduate phase ceases to be dominated by preparation for formal examinations, many more trainees than at present should be able to take part in research.

para. 93

Professional training for the hospital specialties is inevitably bound up with the hospital staffing structure. We have therefore given very careful consideration to the latter, and particularly to the opportunities it offers for a doctor to make a career in his chosen specialty. Until recently only the Consultant grade was acknowledged as a proper aiming-point for the young doctor training for a hospital career. The Medical Assistant grade was introduced some years ago in recognition that the hospital service needed in permanent responsible positions, and could offer adequate careers to, many more doctors than could expect to become Consultants; and also in recognition that hospital posts which did not offer satisfactory training should not be filled on a temporary basis by doctors nominally in training. For reasons we discussed briefly in Chapter 2 the Medical Assistant grade has not become popular; we think it will be superseded with advantage by a new grade . . . which for convenience we shall call the 'Hospital Specialist' grade. We envisage that the doctor who has successfully completed his professional training in a hospital specialty will make his career as a Hospital Specialist or, if he shows high ability, as a Consultant.

We recommend, therefore, that on completion of general professional training all doctors seeking a career in the hospital service should enter a single career grade of Junior Specialist. When they had had the prescribed experience as a Junior Specialist they would be eligible for vocational registration . . . and could expect promotion to Specialist, in which capacity they would exercise a substantial degree of independent clinical judgment. The registered Specialist in the hospital service would, like all other hospital doctors, be a member of a team, holding a gradually increasing personal responsibility but looking to a Consultant for guidance and help in unusually difficult cases. Promotion to the Consultant grade would be based on demonstrated ability.

We expect that a good proportion of Junior Specialists and Specialists will be part-time; the grade should attract many women who, because of family commitments, are not able to give full-time service to medicine but have been able to complete their general professional training, perhaps over an extended period. . . . The Specialist grade should also offer a means of providing part-time hospital appointments for suitably trained doctors whose main interests lie in other branches of medicine, and especially for general practitioners.

paras. 102–4

TRAINING FOR GENERAL PRACTICE

As we have explained in Chapter 2, we think that primary medical services in this country will, for the foreseeable future, continue to be based on general practice but in a form very different from that of the traditional single-handed practice or small partnership. We believe that general practice will be a satisfying and challenging specialty. We see in the future a general practitioner providing care for the families and individuals in the local community, working with a group of colleagues (each, probably, with a personal interest in a particular specialty) aided by proper diagnostic services, ancillary staff and efficient practice organisation; and cooperating closely with other agencies. We see him, moreover, playing a responsible part in the hospital and other health services, and recognised as a specialist in his own right by virtue of his unique and essential contribution to medical care. This vision will become a reality only if general practice, like

hospital practice, is based on organized professional training of the kind we
have proposed. . . .

para. 114

Professional training in general practice should, we think, aim at producing
a first-rate clinician in the field of internal medicine, with a good knowledge of
preventive medicine and with special knowledge of the problems—both clinical
and organisational—associated with family doctoring and with the role of
general practitioner as 'doctor of first contact' in the community. We should like
to see, in accordance with our recommendations for other specialties . . . all
would-be general practitioners undertaking a three-year period of general professional training, comprising a series of six-month, or perhaps twelve-month,
rotating appointments. One of the compulsory appointments, early in the period,
would be spent in general practice, somewhat on the lines of an appointment in
the present Trainee General Practitioner Scheme, but would if possible include
some time with the local authority and perhaps also some study of occupational
health. A six-month appointment in obstetrics and gynaecology would be highly
desirable. The next most important subjects to be included are general medicine,
paediatrics and psychiatry. Other subjects for which training appointments
should be arranged where possible are anaesthetics (including general dental
anaesthesia), dermatology, geriatrics, ophthalmology, otorhinolaryngology and
physical medicine; concurrent experience of two or three of these subjects
could often be provided in a single training period. A sound and up-to-date
knowledge of therapeutics is essential for all general practitioners; great emphasis
should be placed on training in therapeutics during general professional training
and opportunities should be provided for attendance at lectures and courses in
clinical pharmacology. . . . On satisfactory completion of this general professional training, signified by the award of a certificate based on progressive
assessment of the trainee's performance . . ., trainees would, we hope, be considered eligible for membership of the Royal College of General Practitioners.

para. 119

After the period of general professional training the young doctor should have
two years' further professional training as an Assistant Principal in general
practice; during this time he would be responsible for the treatment of patients
to a Principal in the practice. We do not think that the posts or supervisors
required in this period of further professional training could be or need be as
highly selected as those appropriate for the trainee during his general professional training. The young doctor would still need guidance and advice, but
would now have sufficient experience to carry a considerable amount of clinical
responsibility. During this period there should be ample opportunities for
further education outside the practice, including attendance at courses offered
by university departments and professional organisations, and for suitable
attachments to hospitals, local authorities and other general practices where
possible. We should particularly like to mention the importance for the young
general practitioner of instruction in the good administration of general practice;
introductory courses on this subject, or extended courses on the lines of those
which have been held in Canterbury and in Wessex, would be very useful. We
recommend that the second year of further professional training be spent in a
practice in a different environment from that of the first. After satisfactory

completion of his professional training the doctor should be competent to exercise independent clinical judgment as, in effect, a 'Specialist' in general practice. He should therefore be eligible for inclusion in the vocational register for general practitioners ... and for appointment as a Principal in general practice in the National Health Service.

para. 121

VOCATIONAL REGISTRATION

Possession of a certificate and evidence of appropriate subsequent experience will not in themselves, however, be a sufficient guarantee to the public, or to others concerned, of the competence of the doctor. Present registration arrangements are a necessary complement to a sound system of undergraduate education and initial experience: they provide an authoritative endorsement of a doctor's primary qualification, and an easily accessible means of identifying those who have acquired it. The time has now come, in our view, for the establishment, on similar lines, of a system of vocational registration as the necessary complement to a proper system of professional training; we recommend that the General Medical Council should be the vocational registration authority. Vocational registration need not introduce undue rigidity into training or into appointment procedures. Unusual experience, or overseas professional training, should be eligible on its merits for consideration by the Council, after consultation with the appropriate college or other professional body. As with the registration of primary qualifications, vocational registration would be informative: it would signify that in the opinion of the profession the trainee had had the training and experience that would normally be expected to make a doctor sufficiently competent to exercise a substantial measure of independent clinical judgment in his chosen field.

Vocational registration should cover general practice and community medicine as well as the hospital specialties. Such registration could help to ensure that no doctor became a Principal in general practice in the National Health Service who had not received adequate training, and would achieve this object without either introducing a rigid requirement for one particular form of training or, on the other hand, leaving standards to be decided by individual executive councils. Vocational registration would also inform the public which doctors, whether or not they were in the National Health Service, had been recognised as suitable for the full responsibilities of general practice.

Vocational registration should therefore cover every doctor with a substantial measure of independent clinical or administrative responsibility, including general practitioners, hospital specialists and doctors engaged in community medicine. Vocational registration would signify a reasonable minimum of informed competence in a specified field, and should therefore be granted on the basis of general professional training and a specified period of further training and experience. The length of the latter period would be prescribed separately for each specialty, in consultation with the college or other professional body concerned, and would no doubt depend on the complexity of the particular specialty, on the type of training and whether it had been undertaken full-time; as a general rule the period ought not to be less than two years. . . .

paras. 158–60

6.6 The Responsibilities of the Consultant Grade (Godber Report)

Report of a Working Party appointed by the Minister of Health and the Secretary of State for Scotland

Published: 1969

Chairman: *Sir George Godber KCB, DM, FRCP, FRCOG, DPH*

Members: *J. R. Bennett MD, ChB, MRCP; Dr Katherine Bradley MB, ChB; J. H. F. Brotherston MA, MD, DPH, Dr Ph, FRCP (Ed.), FRCP (Glas.), FRSE; A. A. Driver MD, ChB, DPH; M. A. R. Freeman BA, MD, BCh, FRCS; J. H. Friend MD, BS, MRCP; N. G. C. Hendry MB, ChB, FRCS; W. P. U. Kennedy MB, ChB, MRCP; W. Lewin MS, MB, FRCS; Sir John Richardson Bt, MVO, MA, MD, BChir, FRCP; H. Yellowlees MA, BM, BCh, MRCP; I. Field MB, BS, and M. R. P. Gregson (joint secretaries)*

Terms of Reference: *No formal terms of reference were published but the foreword by the chairman stated: 'The Working Party was appointed in 1968. . . . The object of the Working Party was to consider the problems of the consultant grade, and our report is presented to Ministers in the hope that it may be used as a working document for discussion.'*

In spite of the various changes in the hospital medical staffing structure that followed the recommendations of the Spens and Platt Reports the problem of an imbalance between the number of doctors in the training grades of registrar and senior registrar and the number of consultant appointments falling vacant had persisted. The Todd Report's solution to this and other problems was to propose two grades of fully responsible doctor, the specialist and the consultant, appointment as a specialist to follow automatically on completion of the required post-graduate training. The Working Party, whilst accepting the Todd concept of vocational or specialist registration, rejected the arguments for two fully responsible grades and suggested instead an increase in the numbers of the existing consultant grade, and steps to bring the number of training posts more definitely into line with the number of expected vacancies in the consultant grade.

These measures would, of course, have the effect of obliging consultants to undertake more of the care of their patients themselves, with less opportunity to delegate routine service work to junior but nonetheless relatively experienced doctors stuck in a promotion bottleneck. The work of junior doctors would be more closely related to their training needs.

After prolonged discussions with the medical profession the Department of Health announced in the summer of 1971 that the numbers of consultants would be increased by 4 per cent a year and the number of junior staff by only 2·5 per cent a year, with the aim of bringing training posts and consultant vacancies roughly into balance at the end of ten years.

6.7 The Organisation of Group Practice (Harvard Davis Report)

Report of a Sub-Committee of the Standing Medical Advisory Committee of the Central Health Services Council

Published: 1971

Chairman: *R. Harvard Davis MA, DM, MRCGP*

Members: *K. F. G. Day OBE, MRSH; R. W. Elliott MD, MSc, DPH; J. A. S. Forman OBE, MB, BChir, FRCGP; R. G. Gibson CBE, LLD, FRCS, FRCGP; W. G. Harding MRCP, FRCS, DPH; Miss J. I. Jones SRN, SCM, HG Tutor Cert, QN; D. H. Kay BA, MB, BChir, DObst RCOG; Professor J. Knowelden JP, MD, MRCP, MRCS, DPH; H. L. Matthews MD, MRCP; R. M. Mayon-White MD, PhD, FRCP, DCH; J. S. Norell MB, BS, MRCS, LRCP, LMSSA; G. W. Page MB, BChir, MRCGP; Professor G. A. Smart MSc, MD, FRCP; H. Steinman OBE, FPS, FBOA; Mrs A. M. Carpenter, E. W. Craddock, and Miss C. M. Douthwaite (secretariat)*

Terms of Reference (1968): *To review the working and organization of group practice, with particular reference to health centres, and to make recommendations.*

The traditional pattern of general practice in the UK was that of the doctor who worked on his own, from his own premises, with the minimum of secretarial or nursing help—often his wife kept the practice records and accounts. The limitations of this form of practice were recognized by the Dawson Report (*see* pp. 111–20) of 1920, which recommended that general practitioners should work in groups based at health centres; by the National Health Service Act of 1948, which required local authorities to provide health centres (*see* p. 139); and by the Gillie Report of 1963, which set out the advantages to both doctors and patients of practising in groups.

Until the late 1960s the reluctance of doctors to work in health centres was matched only by the reluctance of local authorities to build them, but group practices based on doctors' own premises steadily increased in number. The number of fully-fledged general practitioners practising in partnerships of three or more increased from 23·4 per cent in 1952 to 52·7 per cent in 1969, although at the latter date only 257 GPs (1·3 per cent of the total) were practising from health centres. The 1966 agreement between the Government and the medical profession on a 'Charter for the Family Doctor Service' (see p. 233) resulted in the offer of special payments to doctors who combined into groups using common premises and employing ancillary staff, and at the same time it was becoming common for local authorities to attach home nurses, health visitors and midwives to general practitioners to care for the patients of the practice rather than, as hitherto, for patients who happened to live in a defined geographical area.

The 1960s therefore saw the emergence of the concept of a group practice team composed of doctors, nurses and in some cases social workers, supported by secretarial staff, working from common premises. Towards the end of the decade the increasing cost of land and building persuaded many doctors, particularly younger doctors, to revise their attitude towards health centres provided by the local authority and by the end of 1969 there were more health centres under construction than had been built in the whole of the previous twenty-one years.

By the time the Harvard Davis Committee were appointed it was also clear that unification of the health service under one administrative organization would take place within the next few years, and many hoped that this reorganization would make possible a shift of emphasis, in the provision of care and in financing, from the hospital to the community health services. Some ambitious schemes had been advanced to make this possible, including the concept of a 'community care unit', a group practice centre large enough to serve a population of at least 50,000—this would mean that at least twenty doctors would work there—and having its own pathological and radiological services. Consultants would come and conduct weekly or fortnightly outpatient clinics at the centre instead of in the outpatient department of the district hospital, thus promoting closer contact between consultants and GPs and saving patients' travelling time.

The Harvard Davis Committee rejected the suggestion that laboratory and x-ray services should be decentralized in this way, and felt that rather than duplicate expensive equipment GPs should be given full access to these facilities at the district hospital. The report was also doubtful whether the time was yet ripe to recommend the establishment of such very large centres, in which the number of people working—doctors, nurses, secretaries etc.—might be as many as 100. The problems of administering such a centre were no doubt not insuperable, but they required careful examination and research. However, the Harvard Davis Committee set out a number of advantages which they saw in what they termed 'multiple group practice centres' (to distinguish them from the more ambitious 'community care units'), in which more than one group of doctors would work and from which a population upwards of 30,000 might be served.

Such centres would make the use of more sophisticated equipment economically justifiable; serve as a focus for vocational and continuing education; make it possible for a specialist in community medicine to work from the centre and supervise such activities as immunization schemes, health education and the monitoring of morbidity; provide a base for rehabilitation services and for some of the professional workers, such as dentists and pharmacists, allied to medicine; justify the holding of consultant outpatient clinics in the major specialties; and make it feasible for the GPs to undertake much of the minor work currently undertaken in hospital casualty departments, as well as to admit their own patients requiring only very simple nursing care to beds provided at or near the centre.

The potential disadvantages of scale were that patients would have to travel further to see a doctor and that larger premises might lead to an impersonal atmosphere. These, it was felt, could be avoided by careful siting and design, and by ensuring that all staff were aware of the importance of the personal doctor/patient or nurse/patient relationship.

The Harvard Davis Report fell into two sections: Chapters I and II, and Chapters III–XIII. Chapter I considered briefly the background to the report, arguing the need for a general practitioner providing primary and continuing care in the community, and the need for him to be supported by nurses and other colleagues in order to work efficiently. The aim, it was said, should be the provision of a high-quality service based upon the general practitioner so that as far as possible people could be cared for out of hospital, and when admitted to hospital returned to their homes at the earliest possible moment. A health service based upon the general practitioner was likely to be less costly than a hospital-based service, and would free hospital beds and highly specialized staff for work which demanded their facilities and skills. It was recognized that in the absence of positive medical indications for admission to hospital, patients might have to be given institutional care simply because changing employment patterns meant there would be no one to care for them at home.

In Chapter II it was argued that there were overriding advantages in doctors and nurses working together in groups from the same premises, and in subsequent chapters the committee discussed the requirements of group practice in terms of the nurses, social workers and secretarial staff who would be needed and how they might work as a team. Chapter VI was concerned with premises, Chapter VII with equipment, services and organization, Chapter VIII with record systems, and Chapter IX with

'Group Practice and the Community Physician'. The 'community physician' was a concept described in the first Green Paper (1968) (*see* p. 166) on health service reorganization, and in Chapter IX the Harvard Davis Committee considered his role in relation to general practice. In Chapter X the implications of group practice for other disciplines and professions were considered, and Chapter XI was devoted to consideration of the relationship between the hospital and group practice. This chapter included discussion of the vexed question of whether GPs should have hospital beds, and introduced the concept of the 'nursing unit' to which could be admitted patients who did not require the facilities of the district hospital but who could not be nursed satisfactorily in their own homes. The Bonham-Carter Committee (1969) had spoken in similar terms of their 'peripheral hospital units', but saw these as outposts of the district hospital. The Harvard Davis Committee questioned the validity of this concept and argued that the nursing units should be closely linked with local group practices or health centres.

Finally Chapters XII and XIII dealt with education and research in group practice.

Like most committees on which the medical profession were heavily represented at this time, the Harvard Davis Committee were critical of the setting up of local authority social service departments, as recommended by the Seebohm Committee (*see* pp. 448–56) and of the government's decision that these should not be integrated in the reorganized health service. They doubted whether the administrative separation of health and social services would be satisfactory, and held that the social and clinical aspects of medical care could not be divorced. However, accepting that they were for the time being faced with a *fait accompli*, they suggested that the community physician would be the appropriate person to co-ordinate the activities of the two services. Both social workers and home helps, they thought, should be attached to and operate as part of the group practice team. It was recognized that at present the training of social workers did not equip them for work in general practice, and that doctors were inadequately trained in the social aspects of care, but the recommendations of the report were based on the assumption that improvements in the training of both professions could be looked for in the future.

The profession doctors are most accustomed to working with is of course the nursing profession, and the Harvard Davis Report had a good deal to say about the role of the nurse in general practice. A great deal of work undertaken by GPs could be delegated to suitably trained nurses, and it was argued that suitably trained nurses might be used to screen patients before they were seen by the GP (as distinct from carrying out procedures delegated by him after he had seen the patient). Experiences in the use of nurses in this way, and in undertaking primary home visits for the GP to see if it was necessary for the doctor himself to call, had been reported in the medical press, and some doctors claimed that such a system enabled them to make better use of their time and give better service to the patients they did see, but the issue was still a contentious one when the Harvard Davis Committee reported.

Harvard Davis Report, 1971

THE CONCEPT OF THE NURSING UNIT

From a consideration of the evidence we conclude that, whilst we agree with the recommendations of the Bonham-Carter Committee that as many as possible of the hospital services should be concentrated at one point, there is also a need for more continuous nursing care in the community than exists at present. The patients for whom this is required are those who, for domestic reasons, cannot be treated at home but who do not need consultant management. They could be cared for in nursing units. These, though similar to the present cottage hospital, would not contain the sophisticated resources appropriate to a district general hospital. Such evidence as we possess suggests that they would be economically justifiable and indeed would represent a considerable asset because they would avoid unnecessary admissions to district general hospitals. They would provide medical and nursing care in quieter and more intimate surroundings and would maintain the link between the patient and the group practice team whom he knows. In this way we believe these units would provide an effective and acceptable service more related to the specific needs of the patient. They would realise the nursing potential in the community without prejudicing recruitment to the hospital and would enlist local goodwill. They would increase the range and quality of work of general practitioners. These factors almost certainly explain some of the public concern that is being expressed at the closure of smaller hospitals.

Without doubt, one of the major reasons in favour of the closure of these small hospitals is that they are said to be extravagant to maintain. This may be because there has been a tendency for some of them to produce a service to satisfy general practitioners and patients in a manner unrelated to the requirements of modern medicine in the community concerned. Examples of this are the provision of diagnostic radiology and surgical facilities which are not economically used. We were unable to obtain accurate national figures for direct comparison of the cost of hospital beds with only nursing care, with that of beds where the full range of sophisticated hospital treatment would be available, but we believe that units providing simple nursing care only, must, a priori, be less expensive than beds in a large hospital. Figures we have seen for the Ipswich area demonstrate that the cost of providing a bed with full diagnostic and surgical facilities is nearly double that of one providing only nursing care. A study of the New Zealand hospital statistics would seem to confirm this. There is an imperative need to produce figures for this country.

The term cottage hospital has a connotation of simplicity and economy and conveys a feeling of warmth and homeliness. Moreover the cottage hospitals of this country have established an honourable tradition of care and service that should not lightly be discarded. Consequently we were tempted to advocate the retention of the term 'cottage hospital', but we think that the term Community Nursing Unit more adequately describes the function of the sort of place that we have in mind.

Although some cottage hospitals might provide the base for nursing units and headquarters for the group practice team, we can also see the need for experiments in the provision of similar beds in purpose-built premises in close proximity to group practice centres. The establishment of nursing units in close proximity to group practice centres, as at Hythe (Hants) and Witney, might become the pattern of the future, with the advantage that the nurses of a group practice, supplemented by some others, could undertake the care of patients there.

paras. 192–5

DISTRICT HOSPITAL BEDS

Some general practitioners have expressed the desire to undertake the entire clinical control of their patients in the district general hospital. Even if this expressed need could be fulfilled by the hospital services it seems unlikely for various reasons that many general practitioners could undertake this responsibility adequately. Ready availability and provision of adequate deputies are implicit in providing such care. It would be unusual for many general practitioners to be so fortunately placed and, even if they were, it is unlikely that they could give adequate total patient care without a large measure of involvement of the full-time junior hospital medical staff.

There is quite a different contribution which general practitioners can now, and will probably increasingly wish to make to the hospital service: participation in hospital work as a member of the hospital team. Here the final responsibility lies with the consultant while the continuity of care is provided by the team. General practitioners living many miles from a hospital undertake work of this kind on a sessional basis. The mutual benefit to all concerned of this kind of arrangement is already so well established that it is clear that progress along this line must continue.

The need of general practitioners for direct access to obstetric beds has been increasing over the years and has, to a varying extent, been met by the provision of general practitioner obstetric units. The Peel report, on the future of domiciliary midwifery, has recommended that 100 per cent hospital delivery should be aimed for, although recognising that this cannot be wholly achieved. It also stated that, in the future, only those general practitioners specially trained in midwifery should take part in the domiciliary midwifery service and should use beds in general practitioner/consultant obstetrics units. If these proposals are adopted it would mean the eventual closure of those general practitioner obstetric units not conjoined with consultant obstetric services. The arguments for and against such proposals are outside the context of these paragraphs, but it is relevant to emphasise that, should the recommendations of the Peel report be adopted, then more general practitioner obstetric beds will have to be provided in the joint general practitioner/consultant units which are envisaged to be sited in the district general hospitals of the future.

There is little information regarding the need for general practitioners to have direct access to beds for the long stay chronic sick. Where he does have such access, the beds are usually associated with cottage hospitals where the whole of the medical staff is drawn from the local general practitioners. It seems unlikely that well-organised in-patient geriatric services provided in large conurbations would benefit by having some of their patients admitted directly, and cared for by the patient's own general practitioner, and we received little evidence that general practitioners as a whole feel a great need for this facility. As with beds for obstetrics and acute medical care, general practitioners who undertake this work, should do so as clinical assistants and as an integral part of the geriatric team. Ideally, as in obstetrics, each group practice will have a doctor whose special interest lies in the field of geriatric medicine and rehabilitation. In this way continuity of care by group practice can be maintained.

For obvious reasons the precise need and location of the beds referred to in the preceding paragraphs will vary from area to area. There is also a need to experiment with different methods of providing the nursing care in the community that will avoid the admission to the District General Hospital of some patients.

paras. 196–200

CONSULTATIVE OUTPATIENT CLINICS

The holding of consultative clinics in group practice centres has been enthusiastically advocated by Draper. The Bonham-Carter report, although more guarded, did agree that this possibility should be considered. The need for peripheral clinics or diagnostic centres, where consultations can be undertaken locally, was expressed in the Hospital Plan of 1962, but the implication was that such centres should be an extension of the hospital rather than being within premises which are primarily community orientated. The advantages of holding consultative sessions in group practice centres are numerous:

(i) Patients would be able to receive specialist advice in the same place at which were concentrated the other community medical services. This would be not only convenient for the patients but also reassuring, since the consultation would occur in a setting already familiar to them.

(ii) The necessary personal contact would be promoted between hospital and community personnel at the most logical time, that is at the time of referral.

(iii) By such contact the two groups of people would have a greater understanding of each other's problems with opportunities for mutual education and professional improvement.

(iv) The theme of continuity and interdependence within the health service would be fostered.

(v) The close collaboration between the consultant and the general practitioner, which has been shown to be so necessary if schemes for day surgery or short stay medical treatment are to be successful, would be ensured.

The disadvantages would include:

(i) The need, initially at least, to persuade hospital personnel of the advantages of such schemes that go against accepted hospital out-patient tradition.

(ii) The possible charge that it would lead to dispersal of consultants' time and effort.

(iii) The fact that many consultants consider that out-patient consultative clinics involve not only the consultant but other members of the medical or surgical team. In these circumstances it would be impractical for the team as a whole to be outside the hospital, since it is desirable especially for middle and junior grades of hospital medical staff to be available within the hospital to meet the contingencies of everyday hospital work. The increasing complexity and intensification of hospital work is likely to increase the need for those possessing high skills to be available at short notice.

(iv) The argument that the introduction of community-based consultative services would necessitate an increase in hospital medical staff of all grades, especially of consultant grade.

(v) The widely held view, supported by the Bonham-Carter report, that consultants' time is better used when concentrated in one locus of activity.

In considering these advantages and disadvantages, we have had little help from those with practical experience of such types of consultation because so few schemes are in operation. Those who have described their experiences have been enthusiastic. In particular, Wade and Elmes (1969) have demonstrated that out-patients sessions conducted in a health centre save the patient as much as two visits to the hospital; that the time taken over a consultation is significantly reduced; and that most of the investigations which were necessary could be arranged by the general practitioner before the consultation took place, provided he had access to these facilities. On balance, we feel that the advantages outweigh the disadvantages and recommend that, initially at least, pilot schemes of community-based consultative clinics should be established. The experience gained from these should lead to a better appraisal of their worth and give a lead to future policy. The most suitable specialties would be general medicine, dermatology, psychiatry, paediatrics, obstetrics and some aspects of geriatrics.

paras. 202–3

6.8 Report of the Working Party on Medical Administrators (Hunter Report)

Published: 1972

Chairman: *R. B. Hunter MBE, MB, ChB, LLD, FRCP (Ed.), FRCP (Lond.), FACP, FInst Biol, FRS (Ed.)*

Members: *Professor B. Abel-Smith MA, PhD, R. T. Bevan MD, BCh, MRCS, LRCP, DPH; J. P. Cashman; W. Edgar MB, ChB, DPH, DCH; H. W. S. Francis MA, MB, BChir, DPH; F. Hampson MA, DM, BCh, FRC Path; Professor E. G. Knox MD, BS, MRCP; W. J. E. McKee MA, MD, BChir, MRCS, LRCP;* Professor I. H. Mills MA, MD, PhD, BSc, BChir, FRCP; Professor J. N. Morris MA, DSc, FRCP, DPH; J. A. Oddie DSC, MD, BS, MRCS, LRCP;† G. A. Phalp CBE, TD, BCom, FHA; K. R. D. Porter MBE, MRCS, MRCP, LDSRCS (Eng.), DPH; J. J. A. Reid TD, MD, BSc, FRCP (Lond.), FRCP (Ed.), DPH; K. A. Wood MB, BS, DObstRCOG, MRCGP; H. Yellowlees CB, MA, BM, BCh, MRCS, FRCP; Dr Elizabeth Shore, C. H. Wilson and J. H. Lutterloch (secretaries)*

*Appointed January 1971
†Resigned August 1970

Terms of Reference (March 1970): *To define the scope of the work of medical administrators at regional, area and district levels in a reorganized health service, and to indicate how training and retraining for such doctors could be provided. Revised Terms of Reference (July 1970): To review the functions of medical administrators in the health services and to make recommendations regarding the provision required for their training.*

In the early years of the NHS the post of medical superintendent virtually disappeared as far as general hospitals in England and Wales were concerned (it persisted, however, in Scotland); during the 1960s it became uncommon even in psychiatric hospitals. This left three groups of doctors practising medical administration, viz. local authority medical officers of health and their subordinates; senior administrative medical officers of regional hospital boards and their subordinates; and just over 120 doctors working in the Department of Health and Social Security and the Welsh Office.

The largest group were the local authority doctors; a BMA survey in 1971 showed that there were nearly 1,200 doctors holding administrative posts with local authorities. They were the heirs to the great tradition of nineteenth-century medical officers of health, from Duncan and Simon onwards, who had made such an enormous contribution to creating a healthier environment, but the nature of the work had changed. Much of the day-to-day responsibility for the control of environmental hazards to health had passed into other hands, infectious diseases were no longer the menace of earlier days, and successive waves of legislation had created a number of services which it had fallen to the lot of medical officers of health to administer. It was therefore the case that while the training of public health doctors (for the Diploma in Public Health, the statutory qualification) was often based on the assumption that epidemiology, or the monitoring of community health needs and problems, was their primary concern, most of their time was in practice taken up with the routine administration of services, including at times nursing services.

A number of the regional hospital board and Department of Health doctors were former local authority doctors, or had at least taken the DPH, but again day-to-day administration took up much of their time, although the involvement of RHB doctors in the planning of clinical services (e.g. the siting of regional specialist units, the approval of additional consultant appointments in particular specialties) and in the hospital building programme gave them the opportunity to try to relate future developments to apparent community needs.

The proposed reorganization of the health service, however, not only meant that the traditional role of the medical officer of health would disappear, it also brought with it the suggestion that the proper role of the medical administrator was not the routine administration of services but the continuous monitoring of the need for and the outcome of clinical and preventive services. This was touched on in the first Green Paper and expanded in the second and in the Consultative Document, and the term 'community physician' came into use to describe this role. The Todd Report had already referred to both epidemiologists and medical administrators as specialists in 'community medicine' and had recommended a common post-graduate training on a level with that proposed for other specialties.

The Hunter Committee were set up by Richard Crossman as Secretary of State for Social Services and the widening of their terms of reference followed the change of government in 1970 and his being succeeded by Sir Keith Joseph. The committee quickly decided that they preferred the term 'specialist in community medicine' to 'medical administrator' and used it throughout the report, making it clear nonetheless that they did not see the community physician merely as an adviser to the health service administration, but as part of the administration, with a recognized role and a position of some authority. At that time the future management structure of the new health authorities was still an open question, but the Hunter Committee assumed that each regional and area authority would have a chief administrative medical officer, and that there would also be community physicians working at district level. 'We do not think it essential for the proper discharge of his duties,' they wrote, referring to the area chief administrative medical officer, 'that he should be appointed as the chief executive officer to the authority, though should such posts be created, we think he would be a strong contender for them.' This was talk to send shivers down the spines of the non-medical administrators in the health service, but it was by no means extravagant talk bearing in mind that the role of the community physician was seen in the first place as identifying needs, and thus powerfully influencing the deployment of resources, and in the second as monitoring performance, and thus indicating where corrective action was required. The report also laid emphasis on the need for medical men to have a more than advisory function in administration in order that the administration should command the confidence of the medical profession generally.

The membership of the Hunter Committee was naturally well packed with medical administrators and it may be that they were taking a slightly optimistic view of the attitude of their clinical colleagues towards their specialty. Not only had the work of the medical administrator changed since the days of John Simon, but his standing within the medical profession had declined. The jibe of 'failed clinician' was frequently heard and so it was not surprising that the Hunter Report should devote some attention to ensuring that career prospects in community medicine should equal those in the clinical specialties. The career grade should, it was suggested, be comparable in status to the clinical grade of consultant. Community physicians should also be eligible for the distinction awards which offered clinical consultants the opportunity, in some cases, of doubling their basic rate of pay. The report was silent on the effect this would have on the traditional relationship between the pay of medical and non-medical administrators in the health service.

The main Hunter Report was preceded in October 1970 by an interim report on 'the urgent need for the short term introduction of training courses in medical administration'. The argument of the interim report was that in a reorganized health service there would be medical administrators whose previous experience had been entirely in a regional hospital board, local authority, university or in central government, and that in addition many of the necessary 'analytic and investigative skills' that

would be required by the community physician of the future had developed
in recent years, since many of these doctors had completed their formal
training. There was therefore an urgent need for a retraining programme,
and an early decision to set up such a programme would incidentally
provide much-needed reassurance for those medical administrators whose
morale had been affected by uncertainty about their future role and by the
loss of certain functions to the new local authority social service departments, following the implementation of the Seebohm recommendations.

The immediate proposal was for six to eight weeks' training provided
in the form of two separate courses at a limited number of centres. In the
main report the discussion on training was expanded to incorporate
proposals for basic training in community medicine, further specialized
training in such fields as medical information science for those who wished
to specialize, and the opportunity after basic training for doctors to attend
courses in health services management which were also open to other
health service professions.

The Hunter Report opened with two short chapters, an introduction
and a discussion of community medicine in a unified service; Chapter III
discussed the community medicine specialist at a regional level, Chapter
IV at area level, and Chapter V at district; Chapter VI dealt with training
and career structure; and Chapter VII presented broad conclusions. The
appendices included statistical information on medical staff in administrative posts in the health service, and a brief account of the work of
medical administrators in the existing health service and in the central
government departments. The interim report was also reprinted as an
appendix.

Hunter Report, 1972

MANAGEMENT ROLE OF THE COMMUNITY PHYSICIAN

It is often suggested that there must be conflict between the administration and
the medical profession on the management of resources. This is based on a
misunderstanding, as the aim of both is better patient care. Those who stand to
gain most from the better management of resources are patients, whose doctors
need, for example, new equipment or more staff to do a better job by the most
up-to-date methods. We see no conflict between management and the profession
collectively, although there may be difficulties to be resolved for particular
specialties which no longer need the same facilities—beds, equipment and staff—
which were allocated to them in the past. For example, with the changing
pattern of medicine there has been a sharp reduction over the past two decades
in the need for certain categories of beds, such as those for infectious diseases.
A considerable redeployment of resources has taken place, but it has not pro-
ceeded as far or as fast as we consider would have been desirable. One reason is

because there is at present no doctor at what will be area or district level with a clear responsibility to ascertain where medical resources could be saved and better deployed. We see this as an important responsibility of specialists in community medicine, though it will not rest with them alone to decide how resources should be deployed; this will be a matter for area or district management, and clinicians will continue to carry responsibility collectively and individually for resources allocated to them.

The community medicine specialist's two main tasks in relation to management will be:

i to monitor and evaluate the operation of all health services, including their working relationships with related services provided by central and local government and by voluntary bodies; and

ii to promote improvements in the organisation and delivery of health services within available resources.

These functions will be carried out in relation to all services within the area, for example, in promoting the adoption by the authority of new area policies in particular sectors in the development of better primary care services. The community medicine specialist will not, of course, have sole responsibility for these matters. The deployment and responsibilities of community medicine specialists will depend to some extent on the nature of the management structure at area and district levels and the place of the professional advisory machinery in management. However, it seems to us that in areas containing more than one district, there will need to be a broad division of general management functions between area and district; we assume that a district management team will be responsible for the day-to-day operation of most services, and that the job of the area chief officers will in the main be to recommend policies for adoption by the authority, to allocate resources, and to monitor the effectiveness of district management in carrying out agreed area and district policies. There may be some services which are organised and provided on an area basis, but most services concerned directly with people will be carried out in operational units, which we assume will fall under the supervision of district management. Much of the work we describe below would therefore fall to the community medicine specialist working within the district—the district community physician.

In the district, as at the area, the health information system will be used to monitor services. Because of his training and skills, the community medicine specialist must take a lead in building this up, and in the systematic development of indices to measure the performance of health services. This will require community medicine specialists to work closely with the clinicians concerned in the collection and interpretation of data, and reinforces the need we see for a community medicine specialist at district level who can establish a good understanding with clinicians both inside and outside the hospital. A complementary role will be the promotion of improvements in the delivery of health services, which again will involve close working relationships with clinicians.

In the early years of the re-organised service, community medicine specialists will be looking particularly for ways of improving services through integration. The key sector in this process of integration will be general practice, which, possibly, has suffered most from the divided structure of the health service.

Over the past decade, more and more general practitioners have been pressing their demands for the supporting facilities needed to do their job really well. Despite the progress made in recent years, probably only about one in four of general practitioners work in purpose-built or specially adapted premises; in 1970 only about a half had home nurses working with them in attachment or liaison schemes and less than half were teamed up with health visitors. It is still very rare for consultants to hold sessions with general practitioners in the latter's premises. Though there has been a trend for general practitioners to work together in large groups, in 1970 almost a fifth of general practitioners were still working single-handed, and nearly a half in groups of two or three. The Royal Commission on Medical Education favoured groups of 12 in urban areas and the recent report by a sub-committee of the SMAC favoured groups of five or six.

General practitioners are independent contractors, and thus have the right to fulfil their contracts in single-handed practice and to work in isolation from health visitors and nursing staff if they wish to do so. In remote rural areas, single-handed practice may be imposed by the facts of geography. But what is wrong is that the organisation of the health service should make it difficult for general practitioners who wish to do so to develop domiciliary teams or work together in larger groups in purpose-built premises. The establishment of an integrated health service will reduce the administrative barriers in the way of such developments. It will be necessary for the community medicine specialist to ascertain the wishes of local general practitioners and to work out plans with others concerned, for example, the chief nursing officer, by which they can be met as far as possible, within the limits of the manpower and financial budgets of the area authorities. He will liaise with appropriate local organisations to provide where necessary the medical assessments required to establish priorities in cases where requests cannot be met in full. Some general practitioners may wish to conduct their own negotiations with other practitioners and to acquire their own premises. Even here the knowledge and experience of the community medicine specialist can be of value, through his knowledge of wider developments being planned for the area, including the deployment of the personal social services. Other general practitioners may be glad to have the community medicine specialist explore the various alternatives on their behalf and provide a plan which they, as independent contractors, are free to accept, amend or reject.

Contact between general practitioners and community medicine specialists will extend far beyond help with obtaining suitable premises and the attachment of staff. The community medicine specialist will come to know the special interests and skills of particular practitioners so that they can be fully used in the work of the area authority. He will know those who have interests in research, and will be in a position to assist with access to relevant research and computer facilities, and to offer help and advice; or to put the practitioner in touch with those better equipped to advise or act as collaborator. An important aspect of his work will be to provide, or help general practitioners provide, on an adequate basis of mutual confidentiality, the epidemiological and other statistical data they will need.

General practitioners will need the support not only of the local health services but also of the personal social services. They will also need to work closely with local social workers who are also advising the same families. While general practitioners will channel their own requests to social services departments, there will be occasions when services which appear to be essential for their patients are not provided, and where co-operation appears to be breaking down. In such circumstances, the general practitioner will be able to pass on those difficulties which he is unable to resolve himself to the community medicine specialist, who will be able to make direct representations to social services departments.

The establishment at district level of a medical committee on which all doctors are represented will be an important step in establishing closer contact between consultants and general practitioners. The further development of continuing education by the area and the region, in association with the university, will also help to bring together doctors practising primary care and those in the hospital. It will be the task of the community medicine specialist to advise on what further links can be forged by appointment of general practitioners in hospital and by sessions held by consultants in health centres and group practice premises. Under a unified service there should be more opportunities for the general practitioner and consultant to work together, particularly by pooling their skills and knowledge and by devising together treatment plans for individual patients.

So far as general practice is concerned, the community medicine specialist will in many areas have to start virtually from scratch in building up the health information which area and district management will need. Within the hospital, on the other hand, a considerable amount of information is already collected on a routine basis and is expanding rapidly through, for example, the introduction of hospital activity analysis. There is also a lot of statistical material available in local authority health departments. It will be the task of the community medicine specialist to marshall this information in a form suitable for decision making. He will have a special responsibility for assessing the outcome of medical care services generally and for initiating local studies to throw more light on critical areas.

Consultants frequently complain that their beds are blocked by patients no longer needing the services of a particular unit or of a hospital. At present, consultants are often expected to resolve these problems unaided while continuing with their heavy responsibility for providing a clinical service. In the future, the community medicine specialist will learn of the problems encountered by particular consultants and attempt to find solutions. Similarly, he will be able to work out with consultants what would be required to extend the scope of out-patient surgery, to develop a day hospital, or to try out an early discharge policy and monitor the medical, social, psychological and economic effects of that policy as compared with existing methods.

Redeployment of resources may be needed to improve quality of care. It will be many years before each district has rationalised the grouping of its hospital resources. Many authorities will have to continue to manage their district services in a number of different hospital units of varying size. Medical work of a particular kind may need to be channelled to only one of the district's hospitals, and this may involve the redeployment of medical manpower within the district.

It will be the task of the community medicine specialist to ascertain where greater concentration of patients and the resources needed to treat them is required to secure an even quality of care at as high a standard as possible within the resources allocated to the area.

In addition to their main responsibilities in monitoring and promoting improvements in health care generally, we think that, at least in the evolutionary early years of the re-organised service, community medicine specialists should be responsible for the organisation of those personal health services (excluding the nursing services) which are at present the responsibility of local health authorities but which will be transferred to the new area health authorities, and also for the medical services provided at present as a part of the school health service. . . . We also think that community medicine specialists should see that the necessary measures are taken to discharge the area health authority's responsibility for the prevention of communicable diseases through specific prophylaxis and treatment (control of communicable disease generally will be the responsibility of the new local government district authorities). . . .

Community medicine specialists will not be personally concerned in the clinical work involved in these services; for example, at child health clinics or in school health inspections. The pattern of organisation and delivery of these services varies considerably; a significant part of the clinical work will no doubt continue to be performed for some time to come by the doctors currently employed on clinical work by local authorities, often on a part-time basis. Such doctors will doubtless transfer to the new health authorities. There is a trend towards greater participation by general practitioners in these services which we welcome and hope will continue. In recent years too there has been a growing interest amongst hospital paediatricians in the wider aspects of child health care. We do not know how in the long term these services will evolve, but for the foreseeable future it will be a part of the community medicine specialist's remit to promote the development of an integrated child health service, including the school health service.

Similarly, specialists in community medicine should carry a prime responsibility within the unified service for the planning and organisation of programmes for the promotion of health and the early detection of disease, including medical advice on health education (which will be a responsibility of both the area health authorities and the new county and district authorities). In this work he will need to work closely with clinicians, including those in general practice, and with colleagues in other health and social service professions, nurses, midwives, health visitors, social workers and teachers.

paras. 62–76

7 The Nursing and Midwifery Professions

Introduction

Nursing is a much reported profession and only a few selected documents have been included in this section. Nursing and midwifery are usually bracketed together and there has only been space here for one document relating specifically to midwifery, but it is worth bearing in mind that midwifery has certain professional characteristics which set it apart from nursing in a category of its own. Midwives have an independent clinical responsibility, in practice and at law, that nurses have yet to achieve.

Florence Nightingale brought nursing up in the world, and it has been climbing steadily ever since. University degrees in nursing, chairs of nursing at the Universities of Edinburgh and Manchester, an increasing emphasis on research, and a place in the sun for the nursing administrators following the implementation of the Salmon Report, are the latest manifestations of nursing's onward and upward progress. Currently the nursing organizations are fighting for parity with their colleagues for the nurse members of the district and area management teams in the post-1974 reorganized health service. It is a curious development that since the implementation of the Salmon Report, a high proportion of the top administrative jobs in nursing have gone to men—in a profession that was once virtually a wing of the women's rights movement. There are far more male nurses at the top of the profession than the number of men in the profession as a whole would justify on a proportionate basis, even taking into account the high proportion of men in psychiatric nursing.

The practice of nursing, too, has developed apace since Florence Nightingale. Nursing was relatively homogeneous in her day. Now it is immensely varied. In the last three decades the two most significant developments have been the impact of technology, so that some nurses now spend their time working alongside doctors at the frontiers of medical science, and the changing age structure of the population, so that large numbers of nurses are required to provide care of a very basic kind to patients with degenerative and chronic diseases. Belated official recognition of the fact that nursing could make use of the full range of abilities found in the population at large came with the Briggs Report.

Documents for which there was not room in the section included the Midwives Act, 1936, which placed on county and county borough councils the duty of ensuring that an adequate domiciliary midwifery service was available in their areas; the Royal College of Nursing's Wartime Nursing Reconstruction Reports (Horder Reports); the Nurses Act, 1943, which implemented the Athlone recommendation for the recognition of a second grade of nurse; the Nurses Act, 1949, which implemented some of the less controversial recommendations of the Wood Report by setting up area nurse-training committees and empowering the GNC to approve experimental schemes of nurse training; the 1949 Stocks Report, which considered the implications of the Wood Report for midwifery; the Platt Report on Nursing Education, which in 1964 voiced the professional aspirations of nurses for full student status and the establishment of independent schools for nursing; and Report No. 60 of the National Board for Prices and Incomes which dealt in the Board's usual sweeping fashion with pay, conditions of service, and various matters of organization and management. For perhaps somewhat arbitrary reasons the Jameson Report on Health Visiting—and in spite of certain tensions and leanings in the direction of social work, health visitors are still regarded as part of the nursing profession—has been included in Part 2 (p. 53).

7.1 Midwives Act, 1902

The Midwives Act of 1902 created the modern profession of midwifery —interestingly enough some seventeen years before nurses achieved state registration. The Act followed the setting up in 1881 of a Midwives Institute (later the Royal College of Midwives) with the object of raising the general standard of midwifery and the status of midwives, and reports by two select committees, in 1892 and 1893, which had recommended state regulation of the profession and practice of midwifery. The select committees had taken evidence on the abuses practised by unqualified midwives—including the time-honoured practice of sedating the labouring mother with gin—and on their reluctance to call a doctor when complications occurred. It was argued that many maternal and infant deaths and much unnecessary suffering resulted from lack of skill and failure to observe elementary precautions against infection.

In 1869 the Obstetrical Society of London undertook an inquiry which showed that the majority of working-class confinements were attended by midwives but that generally these were untrained and displayed 'not merely a want of any special education, but gross ignorance and incompetence, and a complete inability to contend with any difficulty that may occur'. On the other hand, Forence Nightingale had seen the need to provide training for midwives as well as nurses, and in 1861, a year after the establishment of the Nightingale School of Nursing at St Thomas's Hospital, she launched a training for midwives at King's College Hospital London. This scheme worked successfully for six years, but was abandoned in 1868, following an epidemic of puerperal sepsis. One of Miss Nightingale's blind spots was her failure to accept the germ theory of disease. However, she went on in 1871 to compile her *Introductory Notes on Lying-in Hospitals* and to put forward proposals for an institution to train midwives and maternity nurses. As a result of the 1869 inquiry the London Obstetrical Society decided to conduct examinations and to award a diploma to midwives who could demonstrate a minimum standard of efficiency. The society did not itself provide training, nor did it have any powers to limit the activities of those midwives who did not hold its diploma.

In 1879, and again in 1884, Bills were drafted on the subject, but not introduced. The first Bill to be introduced was in 1890, and further Bills were introduced in 1891, and then annually from 1895 to 1900, but, partly through opposition from the medical profession, who saw in state registration for midwives a threat to their own position, none of these succeeded in getting on the statute book. This was what the Stocks Working Party in 1949 referred to as the 'era of legislative miscarriages'. In 1902 a Midwives Act at last received the Royal Assent. It protected the title 'midwife', reserving it for those certified under the Act, and set up a Central Midwives Board consisting of four doctors and five other persons, one of whom was to be appointed by the Royal British Nurses' Association, the body which was most active in the campaign for the registration of nurses. The Act laid down that when it came fully into operation no women should, habitually and for gain, attend women in childbirth otherwise than under the direction of a qualified medical practitioner, unless she be certified under the Act. The Act eventually came into full operation, and unqualified practice for gain was thus prohibited, in 1910. Penalties were laid down for breach of this provision.

The Act required the Central Midwives Board to maintain a Roll of Midwives, and to prescribe conditions of training. At local level supervision of the practice of midwifery was entrusted to county and county borough councils, who became known as the Local Supervising Authorities. Every certified midwife beginning to practice had to notify the Local Supervising Authority for her area. At this time midwives worked either as private practitioners, collecting fees from their patients, or for voluntary associations set up to provide nursing and midwifery services for the poor. The position of existing midwives was protected under the Act by providing that the Board should grant a certificate to any woman who could produce satisfactory evidence that she had been in *bona fide* practice as a midwife for at least one year when the Act was passed, and that she was of good character.

The Midwives Act was of importance beyond its immediate purpose of raising the standard of midwifery and protecting the health and lives of mothers and babies. It provided significant encouragement and a precedent for the nurses in their struggle for state registration. It created a separate profession of midwifery which although closely related to nursing was not subordinated to it as a mere specialty within a wider field. It established the midwife as the colleague of the doctor, with certain important responsibilities of her own. Unlike the nurse, who technically always works under the direction of a doctor, the British midwife is a practitioner of normal midwifery in her own right. The doctor only takes over as of right when complications occur. The midwife thus occupies a level of clinical responsibility intermediate between that of the state registered nurse and the registered medical practitioner, a position which at present has no parallel in this country, although it might well form a useful precedent to meet certain emerging needs in medical practice which in the USA are being partly met by the creation of a grade of 'physician's assistant'.

Midwives Act, 1902

THE TITLE OF MIDWIFE

1.—(1) From and after the first day of April one thousand nine hundred and five, any woman who, not being certified under this Act, shall take or use the name or title of midwife (either alone or in combination with any other word or words), or any name, title, addition or description implying that she is certified under this Act or is a person specially qualified to practice midwifery or is recognised by law as a midwife, shall be liable on summary conviction to a fine not exceeding five pounds.

(2) From and after the first day of April one thousand nine hundred and ten, no woman shall, habitually and for gain, attend women in childbirth otherwise than under the direction of a qualified medical practitioner, unless she be certified under this Act; any woman so acting without being certified under this Act shall be liable, on summary conviction, to a fine not exceeding ten pounds; provided this section shall not apply to legally qualified medical practitioners, or to any one rendering assistance in a case of emergency.

(3) No woman shall be certified under this Act until she has complied with the rules and regulations to be laid down in pursuance of this Act.

(4) No woman certified under this Act shall employ an uncertified person as her substitute.

(5) The certificate under this Act shall not confer upon any woman any right or title to be registered under the Medical Acts or to assume any name, title or designation implying that she is by law recognised as a medical practitioner, or that she is authorised to grant any medical certificate, or any certificate of death or of still-birth, or to undertake the charge of cases of abnormality or disease in connection with parturition.

S. 1

LOCAL SUPERVISING AUTHORITIES

8. Every council of a county or county borough throughout England and Wales shall, on the commencement of this Act, be the local supervising authority over midwives within the area of the said county or county borough. It shall be the duty of the local supervising authority—

(1) To exercise general supervision over all midwives practising within their area in accordance with the rules to be laid down under this Act;
(2) To investigate charges of malpractice, negligence or misconduct on the part of any midwife practising within their area, and, should a prima facie case be established, to report the same to the Central Midwives Board;
(3) To suspend any midwife from practice, in accordance with the rules under

this Act, if such suspension appears necessary in order to prevent the spread of infection;

(4) To report at once to the said Board the name of any midwife practising in their area convicted of an offence;

(5) During the month of January of each year, to supply the secretary of the Central Midwives Board with the names and addresses of all midwives who, during the preceding year, have notified their intention to practise within their area, and to keep a current copy of the roll of midwives, accessible at all reasonable times for public inspection;

(6) To report at once to the Central Midwives Board the death of any midwife or any change in the name or address of any midwife in their area, so that the necessary alteration may be made in the roll;

(7) To give due notice of the effect of the Act, so far as practicable, to persons at present using the title of midwife.

The local supervising authority may delegate, with or without any restrictions or conditions, as they may think fit, any powers or duties conferred or imposed upon them by or in pursuance of this Act to a committee appointed by them and consisting either wholly or partly of members of the council; and the provisions of subsections one and two of section eighty-two of the Local Government Act, 1888, shall apply to every committee appointed under this section and to every council appointing the same; and women shall be eligible to serve on any such committees.

S. 8

7.2 Nurses Registration Act, 1919

'I dare say it may be justified, but for myself I always dislike to see any legislation passed into law which closes a profession or narrows down the avenue through which people can approach that profession.' That was the comment of one MP, Col Wedgwood, on the Nurses Registration Bill. But Col Wedgwood was in the minority. Most MPs were in favour of the principle of registration, even if they had reservations about some features of the Bill. Some of them may have thought of Shaw's words 'All professions are conspiracies against the laity', as they listened to the Minister whose Bill it was explain why it had been necessary to introduce a government Bill, but they were all aware that the measure was the outcome of close on forty years' campaigning by prominent nurses, and that then, as now, the nurses had the sympathetic support of the public. Ever since Florence Nightingale and her small band had brought some kind of order and humanity into the chaos of British army administration in the Crimea, the man in the street had had a soft spot for nurses. If a group of them turned out in uniform to support a candidate at election time, it was worth a good many votes.

The Minister responsible was Dr Christopher Addison (later Lord Addison), a former professor of anatomy who that same year had become Britain's first Minister of Health. The new Ministry had been created following the Haldane Report on the Machinery of Government, and replaced both the National Health Insurance Commission (*see* p. 77) and the Local Government Board (*see* p. 50), of which Dr Addison had been president. One of the first problems with which Dr Addison had to deal was the fact that the nursing profession was split firmly down the middle on the mechanics of registration and professional government, and each faction had found a sponsor for their own Bill. The Bill drafted by the College (later Royal College) of Nursing was introduced in the House of Lords early in 1919, and the Bill drafted by the Royal British Nurses' Association in the House of Commons. Dr Addison tried to bring the two organizations together, but neither would give way to the other, and eventually both withdrew their Bills when the Minister promised to introduce one of his own.

At this time Florence Nightingale had been dead for nine years. She had never been in favour of registration, but even her immense prestige had been unable to counter the influence of the 'lady nurses' who felt that without registration to indicate to the public that they were fully trained professional women they might be confused with the relatively untrained practical nurses who still gave the bulk of the care in workhouse infirmaries. The cause of nurses' registration was also caught up in the movement for women's rights, and Mrs Bedford Fenwick, leader of the Royal British Nurses' Association, was an admirer of Mrs Pankhurst. The conflict between The RBNA and the College of Nursing came about partly because the RBNA were unwilling to compromise on standards in order to ensure that the hospitals had enough nurses to care for their patients, while the College were prepared to be more realistic, but also because the two organizations were engaged in a contest for supremacy and each wanted to ensure that the new registering body would be constituted in such a way as to consolidate its position. There were personal overtones, too. Most people who came into contact with Mrs Bedford Fenwick either fell completely under her spell or found her quite intolerable.

The Nurses Registration Act set up a General Nursing Council for England and Wales which consisted in the first instance of nine lay members and sixteen nurses. Two of the lay members were appointed by the Privy Council, two by the Board of Education, and five by the Minister of Health, who also appointed the nursing members of the first Council. Later, when the Register was established, these were to be elected by the profession. A stormy future for the new Council was ensured by the inclusion among the nurse members of Mrs Bedford Fenwick. The first chairman of the GNC was a barrister, J. C. Priestley KC, but Mrs Bedford Fenwick secured the vital chairmanship of the Registration Committee. The GNC were to set up examinations, success in which would ensure admission to the register, but meanwhile 'existing nurses' would be entitled to registration on the basis of criteria to be decided by the GNC. Mrs Bedford Fenwick was anxious both to set a high standard for registration and to ensure that the electorate which would vote for the members of the next Council would be likely to support her policies. She and her allies were particularly keen to deny registration to ex-VADs (Voluntary Aid Detachment), women who had enrolled to nurse the troops during the 1914–18 War and who had for the most part no formal training. Each application for registration as an 'existing nurse' was scrutinized personally by the chairman of the Registration Committee, and progress was so slow that the chairman and sixteen members of the Council resigned in protest, leaving Mrs Bedford Fenwick and her five friends unable to form a quorum.

This was at the end of 1921. Early in 1922 the Minister of Health was able to persuade the sixteen members to withdraw their resignations and the Council met again, with a new chairman, Sir Wilmot Herringham, a consultant physician at St Bartholomew's Hospital, where Mrs Bedford Fenwick had formerly been matron. Controversy continued to surround the work of the Council over the next few years and on several occasions the Minister of Health had to intervene to ensure that the intentions of Parliament—i.e that 'existing nurses' should be registered on a reasonably generous basis and that criteria for recognition as training schools should be realistic—were not overruled by the professional aspirations of the nurses on the Council.

The first examinations, to be conducted by the Council were held in 1925 and from then onwards the examinations were held three times a year. In 1924 the GNC Disciplinary and Penal Committee heard their first case, and ordered the removal from the Register of a nurse who had been sentenced in the courts to six months' imprisonment. Over the years there were a number of cases where hospitals which the Council had refused to approve as training schools appealed to the Minister under Section 7 of the Act. In some instances the Minister upheld the Council's decision, but there were a number of cases where he allowed the appeal. Generally the stance of the Ministry was that the public interest required that the supply of nurses should be sufficient to staff the hospitals; the GNC put the emphasis on quality —how hospitals staffed their wards was their affair, not the concern of the Council.

The Council did not appoint the first inspector of training schools until 1936. Up until that time a limited amount of inspection had been carried out by members, but after 1936 it became the policy of the Council to ensure that each training school would be visited once in five years.

The Act had nine sections. Section 1 set up the GNC as a body corporate and Section 2 laid down that a register of nurses was to be formed and should comprise five parts: (1) a general part; (2) a supplementary part for male nurses; (3) a supplementary part for mental nurses; (4) a supplementary part for sick children's nurses; (5) any other prescribed part. The power given under (5) was used to establish a part for fever nurses. Because of the dramatic decline in infectious diseases this part of the register was closed in 1967. A separate part of the register for nurses of the mentally defective (later known as the mentally subnormal) was created by splitting the supplementary register for mental nurses. The supplementary register for male nurses was amalgamated with the general register under the Nurses Act, 1949.

Section 3 empowered the Council to make rules, subject to the approval of the Minister, governing admission to the register, professional discipline, examinations, uniform, schemes of training, and the conduct of business. Section 4 authorized the Council to employ staff and Section 5 to charge fees. Section 6 was concerned with the registration of nurses trained outside the UK, and Section 7 with appeals against decisions to remove a nurse's name from the register or not to approve a hospital for training.

Section 8 gave legal protection to the title of registered nurse and laid down penalties for persons who falsely represented themselves to be registered nurses. Section 9 confined the operation of the Act to England and Wales.

7.3 Report of the Lancet Commission on Nursing

Published: 1932

Chairman: *The Earl of Crawford and Balcarres PC, KT, FRS*

Members: *Miss M. D. Brock, OBE, MA, DLitt; Miss L. Clark MBE, RRC; Professor Henry Clay MA, DSc; Miss R. E. Darbyshire RRC; Professor F. R. Fraser MD, FRCP; A. Lister Harrison JP; Robert Hutchison FRCP; Mrs Oliver Strachey; Miss Edith Thompson CBE; Sir Squire Sprigge MD, FRCP; Dr M. H. Kettle (hon. secretary)*

Terms of Reference (1930): *To inquire into the reasons for the shortage of candidates, trained and untrained, for nursing the sick in general and special hospitals throughout the country, and to offer suggestions for making the service more attractive to women suitable for this necessary work.*

The action of the proprietors of the *Lancet* in setting up and financing an inquiry into the shortage of nurses was perhaps an example of enlightened paternalism more acceptable to the nursing profession in 1930 than it would be today. For a medical journal to take such a step, and to include on the Commission only two nursing members, would probably now produce an outcry from the nursing organizations, but in the 1930s they were willing to give evidence and to assist the Commission in every way possible. In fairness, too, it must be stated that there were only three doctors—four if we count the hon. secretary—on the Commission, and they were balanced by two women educationists, a professor of social economics, the chairman of the committee of management of the Metropolitan Hospital, and the chairman of the employment committee of the London and National Society for Women's Service. Of the twelve members of the Commission five, including the hon. secretary, were women.

On page 10 of the report it was stated that 'the establishment of this Commission was due to the initiative of one of our members. On her the work of collating evidence and of preparing drafts has chiefly fallen. It is at her express wish that no further acknowledgment is made of her signal services to the Commission'. The member referred to was Dr M. H. Kettle, hon. secretary to the Commission, wife of Professor E. H. Kettle FRS, and later an assistant editor of the *Lancet*. As a result of her work with the Commission, the Ministry of Health nominated her in 1933 as a member of the General Nursing Council.

The Commission worked quickly. The first meeting was held on 8 December 1930 and an interim report was published in the *Lancet* of 28 February 1931. This included a preliminary analysis of the responses to a questionnaire sent to more than 1,000 hospitals and returned completed by 686 of them (67 per cent). A second interim report, with Dr Bradford Hill's final analysis of the questionnaire responses, was published as a special supplement to the *Lancet* of 15 August 1931. Both interim reports were reprinted as appendices to the final report, published in January 1932, and the second in particular contained a wealth of information about nursing conditions at the time.

The first task of the Commission was to establish the extent of the shortage and to gather data about nurses' working conditions which might have a bearing on this shortage. They were fortunate enough to have the services of Dr A. (later Sir Austin) Bradford Hill as statistician. His analysis of the questionnaires showed that the shortage was both quantitative and qualitative. In quantitative terms it was not very great, most hospitals having about 90 per cent or more of their full establishment, but there was evidence that untrained staff were sometimes employed because trained staff could not be had, and many hospitals felt they were unable to secure staff of the standard they required. The report accepted the establishments at more or less their face value, but the evidence on the ratio of beds to numbers of nursing staff suggested that many of the establishments were themselves on the low side. It was probably the case that approved establishments were related rather to the numbers of nurses it was thought possible to obtain, and the numbers the hospitals could afford to employ, than to any measurement of the work that required to be done.

The survey showed that there was appreciable 'wastage' of probationers (the term 'student nurse' had not then come into general use) who failed to complete their training, and by far the greater proportion of these left during the first year of the three or four year course. 'This', Dr Bradford Hill commented, 'suggests that these hospitals are recruiting a considerable number of candidates who are never likely to become efficient nurses, and are eliminated after a few months' trial period. One hospital, in fact, reports "we have to engage all who apply and weed out later".' Wastage was particularly high in fever and mental hospitals, but was lower in the municipal hospitals than in the London and provincial voluntary hospitals. On the other hand, the voluntary hospitals had a higher proportion of trained to untrained staff than the municipal hospitals and a higher ratio of staff to beds.

The statistical evidence of shortage was echoed by the testimony of such bodies as the College of Nursing, the Association of Hospital Matrons, and the British Hospitals Association, but the emphasis was on a shortage of 'suitable' candidates rather than lack of applicants. London County Council stated that of 8,000 applicants for training, 6,000 were rejected, mainly on grounds of lack of education, although a secondary education was not demanded. Some hospitals declared themselves ready to accept any candidate who could read, write and spell, but those that were more particular experienced difficulty.

The *Lancet* Commission were therefore concerned to make nursing more attractive to the well-educated girl, particularly the girl who stayed at school until she was 18; and also that there should be experiments with ways of 'bridging the gap' between leaving school at 14, 15 or 16 and starting nursing at 18. The Commission suggested there might be scholarships to enable girls either to take a full-time pre-nursing course or to attend evening classes leading to Part I of the Preliminary State Examination in Nursing.

There was ample evidence in the report as to why nursing was not popular with educated girls. Senior nurses were out of touch with conditions outside the hospitals and regarded as tolerable conditions and practices which were no longer acceptable in other walks of life. Conditions in nursing had improved since the turn of the century, but they needed to improve much more if nursing was not to be regarded by many as over-regimented drudgery. The hours of work were excessive and they were so arranged that the nurse's free time was often of little use to her. Only 17 per cent of the hospitals in the survey had adopted a system to give the nurse reasonable notice of her off-duty hours. A letter from a nurse described how she made an appointment with a friend: 'If I don't come by 10 o'clock I will come by 2; if I don't come at 2 I will come at 5.' Lectures took place in off-duty hours, perhaps after a night's work on the wards. Hardly any hospitals employed enough cleaners, and nurses, especially probationer nurses, spent a good deal of their time in domestic work.

Discipline on the wards was not objected to, but the lack of privacy in the nurses' home, and rules requiring, for instance, that the nurse should be in bed by 10 p.m. and switch her light out by 10.30, were bitterly resented. The quality of the accommodation and food provided for nursing staff in those days, when residence was the general rule, varied widely. The Commission felt it necessary to recommend that 'A separate bedroom should be provided for each nurse.' In the letters received by the Commission, complaints of poor pay were nearly as numerous as those referring to long hours of duty. Within the profession, as well as among parents, it was the pay and prospects of the trained nurse that caused concern rather than the low pay of the probationer, and the Commission agreed that the policy most likely to attract suitable candidates was that of offering low salaries to probationers and increasing the pay of trained staff. They even suggested that as an experiment certain hospitals known to give good training should advertise for probationers without offering any pay, but offering six weeks' holiday a year and two short periods of study leave during the period of training. It was felt that such a scheme might attract to nursing a certain proportion of the girls who would otherwise take a university or other comparable course. Scholarships could be given to ensure the supply of sufficient candidates until the scheme became well known.

The Commission took a careful look at the question of who paid for the nurse's training. It was generally assumed that the nurse got her training free and was indeed unique among students for a profession in receiving a salary as well as board and lodgings while under training. This was often used to justify the low salaries offered to trained nurses. However, it was evident that hospitals would not spend money on training nurses if they did not effect some economy by doing so, as their funds were subscribed, or provided from the rates, for the care of the sick and not for the training of nurses. The Commission calculated that when the cost of training was offset against the savings effected by employing probationers instead of other grades of staff to do the work which they undertook, hospitals were decidedly in pocket, and so it was in fact the case that the probationer paid for her training by virtue of being underpaid for the work she did.

The Commission found that sisters were generally paid between £70 and £85 a year (approximately £290–£350 in 1970 values) in addition to their board and lodging, although the initial salary might be as low as £60 and the maximum after many years' service might rise as high as £150 (£620 in 1970 values). They recommended that the minimum salary for ward sisters in hospitals not approved as training schools should be £80, rising to £120 (£330–£500). In hospitals approved as complete training schools the scale should be £100 rising after eight years to £160 (£415–£665). All these salaries were in addition to board and lodging. Where a sister was non-resident the Commission recommended she should be paid not less than £250 a year (£1,040). For other grades the Commission were content to recommend for the most part that hospitals should adopt the scales suggested by the Royal College of Nursing.

In addition to improvements in the pay of trained staff, the Commission recommended that those voluntary hospitals which did not participate in a pension scheme for their nurses should do so. The span of work on day duty should not normally exceed thirteen hours, and at least three clear hours off-duty, in addition to meal times, should be allowed during this span. One free day each week should be allowed. The hours of night duty should not exceed fifty-seven in any week and the span of night duty should normally not exceed eleven hours. No nurse should be kept on night duty for more than three months in any year. Not less than three weeks' annual holiday should be allowed. Living conditions for trained staff should be much improved, and the possibility of giving some trained nurses the alternative of living out by the offer of non-resident allowances should be explored.

The Commission suggested some curbs on the powers of the matron; she should be entitled to suspend a nurse from duty pending a report to the board of management, but not to dismiss her. The application forms sent out by hospitals and the way in which hospital rules were worded should be examined to avoid giving a disagreeable impression. Some of the rules held threats of fines and dismissal over the nurse's head, and the report quoted examples to show that there were better ways of bringing a nurse's responsibilities home to her than this.

The report also included recommendations affecting the structure of nurse training and the rules of the General Nursing Council. The GNC's Preliminary Examination should be divided into two parts, of which Part I, consisting of papers in anatomy, physiology and hygiene, could be taken before the nurse entered the wards. This would enable secondary schools to prepare girls for this examination, and to be recognized by the GNC for the purpose. The Preliminary Examination was split in the way suggested in 1939 after a long and at times acrimonious controversy and the election in 1937 of a GNC the majority of whose members were in favour of the split.

Separate sections of the report were devoted to the problems of tuberculosis hospitals and mental hospitals, and in a final section on 'Some Questions of Policy' the Commission stepped largely outside their terms of reference to give their views on the establishment of university schools of nursing; the replacement of the five registers maintained by the GNC by one; the proposal to shorten the course of training to two years and four months; the recognition of a second grade of nurse; and publicity for nursing (the Commission actually used the term 'propaganda'—it had not then been discredited by Dr Goebbels). They were doubtful about university schools of nursing, but felt there would be an increasing need for university diplomas in special branches of nursing, in teaching and in administration. They were cautious about recommending the abolition of any of the existing registers, and felt they could never in any case be reduced below three—for general nurses, male nurses and mental nurses. The proposal to shorten the training, whatever its merits, would not, it was thought, be acceptable to the profession, and as far as the second grade of nurse was concerned the Commission sat firmly on the fence.

Lancet Report, 1932

NURSING CONDITIONS BETWEEN THE WARS

The element of apprenticeship is regarded by most of the leaders of the nursing profession, at least in this country, as a far more important part of a nurse's training than her theoretical studies. Some senior nurses, notably ward sisters, may still be heard to protest that the vocational spirit which inspired former generations of nurses has been dimmed by the introduction of a standard curriculum. Although most of them are now beginning to realise that their early fears in this respect were unfounded, they attribute the preservation of the vocational spirit to the retention of a factor in hospital life which has been severely criticised from outside the profession, and is stated to have prevented many girls from entering hospitals. This factor is the routine work of the probationer, occupying nine to ten hours a day. It has not been modified to give her more time and leisure for study; and though the passing of State examinations is now essential to her career, she must fit in her theoretical work and at least some of her lectures during her official off-duty time.

Women in other professions are apt to regard such long hours of routine work, the restrictions on liberty when off duty, in short, the scanty opportunity given to the nurse in training to lead a normal social life and to cultivate interests apart from her work, as being associated mainly with the desire of the hospitals to economise at the expense of their staff. They criticise senior nurses for acquiescing without protest in a system which admits of the exploitation of student labour. But they fail to recognise that a large section of the nursing profession, especially ward sisters, remain convinced of the value of a strict discipline, which is designed to plant and foster in the probationer certain qualities and habits. Among these are uncritical obedience; punctuality; loyalty to superiors and to the institution served; together with a sense of responsibility and of vocation which, in the opinion of many, is incompatible with the cultivation and maintenance of wide interests outside the hospital community.

It is this attitude which underlies the disregard of the mental conflict that may trouble a probationer who comes from a good secondary school; there her duty has been primarily to learn, her critical faculty has been stimulated, and her practical work has been assessed for precision and neatness and a grasp of principle, rather than for a speed of execution which to a beginner is incompatible with a high standard of efficiency. She soon learns in hospital that her first duty is to help to get the work done, and in some hospitals she must also learn to subdue her critical impulses and even her curiosity. It is assumed that she will never make a good nurse unless she regards her time as the hospital's and not her own, and her training as incidental to the work she does as employee. A receptive young nurse soon absorbs this spirit, and is in her turn shocked at the solecisms and breaches of etiquette committed by newcomers. But in the process of acclimatisation she is liable to adopt blindly the traditions of her seniors—the reaction has been aptly described as 'putting on the blinkers'—and to become as impervious as they are to the fact that the educational methods practised in hospitals have been largely superseded elsewhere by methods which rely on arousing, instead of damping, curiosity and initiative, and which insist on the importance of developing a student's personality and tastes outside the range of daily work.

paras. 34–6

The long hours of work demanded are criticised freely by matrons, nurses, prospective nurses, parents, headmistresses, women's organisations, the general public, and hospital authorities themselves. Among the replies to the questionnaires sent out by the Commission to probationers and trained nurses, such phrases as the following occur:—

'The hours of duty are usually too long.'—'Shorten the hours to the equivalent of an eight-hour day.'—'Better off-duty time for the trained staff.'—'Longer rest in the middle of the day.'—'On a lecture day we only get one hour of freedom instead of two.'—'Night duty 8.40 P.M. to 9.0 A.M. . . . . Lectures sometimes *after this* from 10 A.M. to 11 A.M.'—'I dislike working at night, especially on account of the length of the hours (i.e., 10½ really without a break).'—'Long hours—7 A.M. to 9 P.M. with three hours off duty.'—'The necessity for remaining on one's feet, often for 12 hours at a stretch with a mere half an hour for meals. —'The long hours, making it impossible not to be tired, a condition which indirectly reflects on the patients.'

Several experienced nurses, in a joint letter, say:—

'The hours are too long. The nurse in . . . rises at 6 A.M., makes her bed, then goes straight to breakfast and on duty, and finishes at 8.5 P.M., goes to supper and is literally not free till 9 P.M. What modern girl will tolerate this when other careers offer so much more freedom?'

This letter omits to mention the off-duty hours which break the day's routine, but we find that the prospect of two or three hours' freedom during the morning or afternoon means little to the girl contemplating nursing as a profession. Her thoughts evidently focus themselves on the long daily span, and she constantly compares nursing unfavourably with other occupations where her duties would end at 5 or 6 P.M. and her hours of liberty coincide with those of the majority of her friends. Attention is frequently drawn to the fact that in most other occupations women are free at the week-ends; as nursing is as necessary on one day as on another the nurse's off-duty day, as arranged by rota, must often fall on a week-day when other people are at work.

A grievance among probationers which undoubtedly antagonises their friends against nursing as a profession is inadequate notice of off-duty time. As one of them writes:—

'The fact that one seldom knows definitely one's off-duty time even for the following day makes it almost impossible to make any but tentative outside arrangements.'

The following typical letter emphasises the same point:—

'A young friend of mine has now been at one of the most noted county hospitals for a year. She is doing extremely well and they are most anxious to keep her. She had a night off just before I saw her, and did not know until just before the train started that she could go. I wished to make plans for the day I was there, but she said: "If I don't come by 10 o'clock I will come by 2; if I don't come at 2 I will come at 5." She never knew when it would be, though there was no special stress of work, and it was quite impossible even to telephone to friends to say when she was coming.'

Long hours of work are discussed in paras. 150 to 178, advance knowledge of off-duty time in para. 208, the use of the telephone in para. 210.

The majority of probationers say that they find the double burden of ward work and study for examinations a great strain; one describes the effort of keeping abreast of preparation for classes after an arduous day in the wards as almost a nightmare. That this difficulty is a serious one is implied in the evidence from the Association of Hospital Matrons, who draw attention to the possibilities of affording some relief from the pressure of work in the first and second years of training. A physician on the staff of a hospital, who lectures to nurses on anatomy and has for years been in medical charge of the nurses in his hospital, writes:—

'They are overworked and are compelled to use their leisure for rest, not recreation. First-year probationers should be learning the elements of nursing. Now their thoughts are distracted by the lectures and lecturettes, note-keeping and book-cramming, and by the growing dread of hospital and State examinations. . . . Physiology and anatomy are both taught and examined at too detailed a standard.'

The possible mitigation of some of the burdens related to examinations are discussed in paras. 215 to 242.

It is generally believed that a nurse is often tired because energy which should be devoted to the care of the sick is dissipated in the performance of unskilled domestic work. The Association of Hospital Matrons attach considerable importance to a reduction of the domestic duties of nurses. They state:—

'Some hospitals have already taken action in this direction, and much of the ward cleaning has been taken from the probationers in training and allocated to domestic workers, but this only applies to some hospitals. . . . Sweeping, brass-cleaning, polishing of furniture, and all similar purely domestic duties should be taken from the nursing staff, thus giving the probationer more adequate time to study her practical work by the bedside of the patient, without the jading atmosphere of rush which she now lives in, often throughout her whole period of training.'

The London and National Society for Women's Service also believe that with the elimination of domestic work one of the substantial objections to the nursing profession would be removed, and the same opinion has reached us from the College of Nursing, from many nurses in training, and from the groups of girls questioned, who appear to believe that a large part of a nurse's life is devoted to scrubbing floors. A teaching sister at a large London hospital summarises well the attitude of the educated girl:—

'The cleaning required is excessive: I objected to this, not because I dislike cleaning, but on the grounds that it was sheer waste to clean laboriously and in an amateur fashion what a professional with proper equipment could do with half the effort; and secondly, that we cleaned when we might have been looking after patients or studying.'

Anticipation of hard physical work in the wards evidently has an unfavourable influence on recruiting. There seems to be a general opinion that physical strain is aggravated by the speed at which the nurse is required to perform her work. The physical strain of nursing was criticised emphatically by the groups of girls questioned, and it is also an argument frequently used by parents who wish to dissuade their daughters from the choice of a profession which they believe makes an exceptionally high demand on the stamina of the worker. The girl who allows herself to be diverted from nursing as a profession by the fear of physical breakdown is not necessarily swayed by selfish motives; we have evidence that the dread of becoming a burden upon relatives is a real deterrent among those who have a sense of vocation, but whose parents do not consider them strong enough for the work.

Domestic work in hospitals is discussed in paras. 254 to 258. Considerable relief of the physical strain on nurses would follow the adoption of many of the recommendations made in this Report.

While we have received from no responsible quarter the suggestion that discipline in the wards should be relaxed, we have been informed repeatedly by nurses in training and by qualified nurses that the enforcement of the same rigid discipline in the Nurses' Home is resented by women accustomed to modern standards of liberty in their own homes. Regulations which prevent a nurse, though nominally off duty, from leaving the Nurses' Home without permission between 8 and 10 o'clock in the evening obtain in the large majority of hospitals and often apply to the qualified nurse equally with the probationer in training. One nurse writes: 'What girl nowadays wants to feel she can't go out unless she shows a pink slip to about six people, on her way probably to buy a stamp or post a letter?' In no other occupation, we are told, is the same degree of supervision found to be necessary. In the Nurses' Home, it is constantly urged, the nurse now has to conform to restrictions based less on the convenience of the community than on a traditional theory of discipline. Inspection of bedrooms and of personal cupboards and drawers is regarded as an intrusion. The Red Cross Scholarship Group* note that 'the living-in system as applied to nurses involves a lack of independence to which the modern girl finds it difficult to accommodate herself.'

Mixed dances are rare occurrences, and in some places even these entertainments are subjected to the prevailing discipline, as the following illustrates: 'Even at Christmas the only dance of the year in some hospitals is held in uniform. Can you imagine dancing, say from 8 to 12 P.M., in a stiff, starched frock with belt, collar, cuffs, cap, and strings complete?'

Conditions of social life are discussed in paras. 180 to 214.

Apart from the question of the suitability of uniform for social gatherings, we are informed by many writers of the inconvenience occasioned by some

---

*A group of British nurses who have followed the International Courses organised by the League of Red Cross Societies (at Bedford College and the College of Nursing) and certain others who are, or have been, connected with these courses.

patterns of dress, cuffs, and collars to nurses, even while at work in the wards. A mother of a nurse writes:—

'At one good London hospital a probationer's dress, apart from the putting on of cap and apron, needs 18 buttons, 6 hooks, and 5 studs to be done up. If she wishes to change, this seriously shortens her off-duty time and increases the mending of buttons and hooks crushed by the laundry.'

Poor food, or the spoiling of good food by careless cookery and service, is a discouraging factor in some cases.

Actually it is rare for the quantity of the food supplied to nurses to be criticised, but objections to the cooking and service occurred repeatedly in the answers to the questionnaire sent to nurses in training, and this was a favourite source of comment among the girls outside the nursing profession who were questioned. The food provided for nurses engaged in night duty is often criticised. In some hospitals the night nurse is given a portion of the dish served at the midday meal of the day nurses, and has to warm it up for herself. The time usually allotted to meals in hospitals is regarded by many as too short; from the replies to the questionnaire sent to hospitals it appeared that at 66 per cent. of hospitals only half an hour is allowed for the midday meal.

Accommodation appears to be unsatisfactory in many hospitals; the Association of Hospital Matrons regard this as exercising an unfavourable influence on recruitment. Not many criticisms of hospital accommodation have reached us from nurses; three writers of spontaneous letters mention it, and two of the probationers in training. It does not seem to figure largely in the minds of girls eligible for the profession as a reason against adopting it, but it may well cause leakage.

paras. 54–60

7.4 Interim Report of the Inter-Departmental Committee on Nursing Services (Athlone Report)

Published: 1939

Chairman: *The Earl of Athlone KG, GCB, GCMG, GCVO, DSO*

Members: *H. S. Souttar CBE, DM, MCh, FRCS; Miss M. Dorothy Brock OBE, DLitt; E. W. Cemlyn-Jones; Miss Gertrude Cowlin SRN; Rhys J. Davies MP; H. A. de Montmorency OBE; Sir Francis Fremantle OBE, MA, MD, MCh, FRCP, DPH, MP; Sir Arthur J. Hall MA, MD, DSc (Hon.), FRCP; Alderman Mrs F. A. Keynes JP; Miss Megan Lloyd George MP; C. W. Maudslay CB; Sir Frederick Menzies KBE, MD, LLD, FRCP, KHP; Miss E. M. Musson CBE, RRC, LLD, SRN; R. H. P. Orde BA; Gilbert E. Orme MA, MB, ChB, MRCS, LRCP; Professor R. M. F. Picken BSc, MB, ChB, DPH; Miss D. M. Smith SRN; W. Rees Thomas MD, BS, FRCP, DPM; Miss Frances Wakeford SRN, SCM; H. M. Walton MA; Sir Weldon Dalrymple-Champneys Bt. MA, DM, BCh, DPH, FRCP and W. A. B. Hamilton (joint secretaries)*

Terms of Reference (1937): *To inquire into the arrangements at present in operation with regard to the recruitment, training, registration, and terms and conditions of service of persons engaged in nursing the sick and to report whether any changes in those arrangements or any other measures are expedient for the purpose of maintaining an adequate service both for institutional and for domiciliary nursing.*

The Athlone Committee, appointed at a time when unprecedented militancy among nurses was bringing their demands for a 96-hour fortnight and better pay before the public and winning increasing support in Parliament, produced only an interim report before the outbreak of war brought an end to their deliberations. One of the first points which came to the notice of the committee as they set about their task was the paucity of reliable statistical material relating to nursing, material such as the numbers of nurses of various grades employed in hospitals, the rates of pay, and the hours worked. They therefore issued a questionnaire to all hospitals asking for information of this kind, and one of the matters outstanding at the time when they published their interim report was the results of this questionnaire. However, although a final report incorporating these results was never published, the statistical material was eventually published in 1960 as an appendix, 'Hospital Nurses in 1937', to Brian Abel-Smith's *A History of the Nursing Profession.*

The Athlone Committee had the unusual satisfaction of seeing nearly all their main recommendations implemented within a relatively short space of time, by the end of 1943 in fact. No doubt this was partly because war made steps to maintain an adequate nursing service all the more urgent. The report called for higher pay for nurses and a national negotiating body to establish national rates of pay. At that time each voluntary hospital and each local authority was free to offer what rates of pay it chose, and hospitals were forced to compete against each other to get nurses. The Athlone Committee felt that this was good neither for the employer nor the nurse, who was encouraged to move from one hospital to another at frequent intervals. On the other hand, if national negotiations resulted in the award of substantially increased salaries, would the voluntary hospitals be able to pay them? It appeared they would not be able to afford to pay their nurses more without grants in aid from public funds, and this the majority, of the Athlone Committee were prepared to recommend—a note of reservation signed by four members of the committee asked that similar help from the national Exchequer should also be extended to local authority hospitals. The report also suggested that grants should be paid to hospitals in respect of the work done in training nurses—again three members of the committee dissented.

The immediate decision of the Government was that it was 'neither sound nor proper for the Government to make itself responsible for the payment of salaries to members of a particular profession', but in 1941, fearing that the progress of the war would impose demands on the nursing service that it would not be able to meet if salaries were not improved, the Ministry of Health guaranteed starting salaries of £40 a year for probationers, £95 a year for trained nurses and £60 a year for assistant nurses (all these salaries were in addition to bed, board and uniform), and promised financial help through the emergency medical service to enable hospitals to meet the cost. In real terms these salaries did not represent an improvement on those paid in the majority of local authority hospitals before the war, but they did represent some levelling up for nurses in the voluntary sector. In October 1941 a salaries committee for nurses in England and Wales was constituted under the chairmanship of Lord Rushcliffe. The committee had a staff side consisting of representatives from the main professional associations and trade unions with nursing members, and an employers' side with six voluntary hospital representatives, one representative of the Queen's Institute of District Nursing, and thirteen local authority representatives. The Rushcliffe Committee negotiated salaries and later also conditions of service for nurses in England and Wales, until they were superseded by the Whitley machinery set up under the National Health Service in 1948.

An interesting light on attitudes in the nursing profession over many years was that when the Ministry of Health announced the new guaranteed salaries the Royal College of Nursing objected that the salary offered to probationer nurses was too much; £30 a year would have been sufficient. The Athlone Committee had argued that

> It is fundamentally wrong to attempt to attract recruits of the proper type by offering initial salaries which are high by comparison with those offered to the trained nurse. The entrant to the profession who intends to make a success of her work and remain a nurse is naturally more interested in her prospects than in the immediate reward.

The College took the same attitude, then and much later, and was always greatly concerned that better rates of pay for student nurses might on the one hand reinforce the view of the student as an employee at the expense of her status as a student, and on the other attract into nursing the 'wrong type' of girl, the one who was interested in financial reward rather than vocational satisfaction and service.

Another Athlone recommendation that was accepted only reluctantly and with reservation by the nursing establishment was that a second grade of nurse should be trained and recognized. The nurse members of the committee did not want them to be called nurses at all, and they signed a reservation suggesting that they should be called 'Registered Invalid Attendants'. However, there was a clear case for regularizing a situation in which there were certainly not enough registered nurses to staff the hospitals of the country and large numbers of unqualified women were being recruited, and in some instances given some training, to fill the gaps. After the subject had been further explored by the Horder Committee, set up by the Royal College of Nursing to prepare plans for nursing after the war, the Nurses Act, 1943, made the General Nursing Council responsible for establishing a roll of assistant nurses and for regulating their training.

Athlone Report, 1939

THE ASSISTANT NURSE

The evidence placed before us shows that a large body of women, varying greatly in age, skill and experience, who are not trained nurses or training for admission to the Register, are engaged in nursing the sick, and, in so far as they are employed in hospitals or institutions, are usually known as 'Assistant Nurses.' In many instances these women render very useful services and it appears certain that however rapidly recruitment to the nursing profession may improve in the near future, as the result of the reforms now being carried out or those suggested by this Committee, it will not be possible for at least some years to come, or perhaps ever, to carry on the nursing services of the country without the aid of assistant nurses. We are satisfied that if these assistant nurses always worked in hospitals and other institutions under trained supervision their employment would be of great help to the community, but we are equally convinced that their uncontrolled employment constitutes a definite danger to the patients under their care and tends to lower the status of the whole nursing profession.

At the present time many of these women are doing excellent work in hospitals and institutions, especially in caring for the chronic sick. Others, however, leave the hospitals or institutions where they have been employed in this work, or the training schools in which they have started but failed to complete their training for the State Examinations of the General Nursing Council, or other hospitals for the acute sick which are not recognised as training schools, and either find employment in private nursing homes or join nurses' co-operations from which they are sent to nurse patients in their homes or are supplied to hospitals for temporary work during a shortage of nurses. We have been told of many cases where a probationer who has not completed her training or who has failed to pass her examinations has later been sent by a co-operation to the hospital which first employed her at a much higher salary than she was formerly receiving in the hospital, though no better qualified than when she left, and we understand that such an event is frequently followed by a crop of resignations of probationers who prefer to follow her example and earn a good salary rather than make the effort necessary to complete their training and become State Registered Nurses.

It is therefore obvious to us that a proper control of these assistant nurses is urgently required and that their position in the nursing profession should be regularised. Some of our witnesses have represented to us that any action to give assistant nurses a recognised status would react adversely on the status of the State Registered Nurse and that, particularly in the sphere of domestic nursing, the State Registered Nurse would experience unfair competition from the assistant nurse. We are unable to accept this view. At the present moment State Registered Nurses do experience competition from assistant nurses and the patient has no means, except by asking the nurse to state her qualifications, of distinguishing between the trained and the untrained nurse. However prudent it may be to make such an inquiry in all cases where the services of a nurse are required in the home, it is not a step which is usually taken and it appears to us that, far from imperilling the status or economic position of the State Registered Nurse, her position will be much more assured if the assistant nurse is recognised and her status defined, and if at the same time legislative measures are taken to protect nurses of both categories.

It follows that for the assistant nurse a measure of State control is essential and we recommend that this should be done by placing these nurses on some form of register or roll. The most suitable body to keep such a Roll of Assistant Nurses would seem to be the General Nursing Council and if it should be found that the powers conferred upon the Council by the Nurses' Registration Act,

1919, are too limited for this purpose, then these powers should be extended by suitable legislation.

It will of course be necessary to determine what qualifications should be required for admission to this Roll and what training in future the assistant nurse should receive.

We have received evidence of a scheme for the training of assistant nurses inaugurated by the Public Assistance Committee of the Essex County Council. The object of the scheme is to provide a training in the care of chronic and senile patients in Public Assistance Institutions and the training course lasts for two years. A simple test examination is given at the end of the first two months' preliminary training and there is a final examination at the end of the course. Trainees are recruited normally from persons of 18 years of age or over and the syllabus covers lectures and practical demonstrations on the theory of nursing, practical nursing, elementary anatomy and physiology, first aid, dietetics and hygiene. Many of our witnesses have spoken highly of this scheme and of the product, and it is clear that there is no insuperable difficulty in constructing a scheme of training suitable for girls with a practical bent for nursing but without the intellectual equipment necessary to pass all the examinations for State Registration.

We are not in a position to lay down the details of a general scheme for the training of assistant nurses but we would suggest the following as points for consideration when the conditions of admission to the Roll we have recommended are being framed.

Admission to the Roll should be open to women over the age of 21 years who have passed a medical examination, have produced satisfactory evidence of character and general suitability and have completed two years' training in an approved institution. We would stress that we attach much importance to the approval of an institution for training purposes, since careful inspection before approval, with subsequent inspections at reasonable intervals, will give a *prima facie* guarantee that the assistant nurse trained in that institution is a suitable person for admission to the Roll. Institutions approved for the training of assistant nurses will not normally be training schools approved by the General Nursing Council for the training of nurses for the State Examinations and the standard of approval must obviously be lower in the former case than in the latter. It is essential, however, that there should be adequate opportunities for obtaining the qualifications of an assistant nurse. It may, therefore, become necessary, in certain circumstances, to approve as an institution for the training of assistant nurses a hospital already recognised as a training school for State Registration, in spite of the objections which may be felt to the concurrent training of two types of nurse in the same institution.

As a considerable number of women who are suited for the type of work now carried out by assistant nurses might have great difficulty in passing a written examination of a uniform national standard, we are of the opinion that such an examination should not be a condition of admission to the Roll. The conditions for admission to the Roll should include a test in practical nursing and we have in mind that assessors, who would be senior State Registered Nurses, should inspect the candidates at work on behalf of the enrolling body. The assistant nurse would then be seen at work in her normal environment and not in the atmosphere of an external examination. The more informal the assessor's visit could be made, the more satisfactory the results would be, and the assessor's opinion of the candidate's suitability should carry equal weight to that of the matron of the institution. In our view, therefore, admission to the Roll should be granted on the production of a certificate from the managing body of the hospital or institution, endorsed by the medical officer, the matron and the assessor, which would state that the candidate had received a continuous period of training in an approved institution, or associated group of institutions, for a period of two years, that she was competent in her work and that she was in all other respects a suitable person to be admitted to the Roll.

The expenses involved by the establishing of the Roll, inspection of institutions, and the payment of the assessors' fees would be met by the fee charged for admission to the Roll. This fee should, of course, be as reasonable as possible and we doubt whether it would be necessary for the enrolling body to incur the heavy cost of publishing the Roll in full each year. Publication in full every five years, with annual supplements, might prove sufficient.

It is, of course, obvious that there must be a transition period and that, since a very large number of assistant nurses are now in employment in this country, some means must be found of admitting them to the Roll. It appears to us that a certificate from the matron of the hospital where they are now employed or from the co-operation or agency through which they are engaged is the only practical way of achieving this. Evidence should be required that such women have practised nursing of the sick for at least two years and are of good character.

In hospitals and other institutions we are satisfied that assistant nurses should only be employed under the supervision of a trained nurse. It is clearly impossible to attach a similar restriction to the employment of an assistant nurse in domiciliary nursing, but what we are concerned to ensure is that the patient is aware whether or not the services received are those of a trained State Registered Nurse or an assistant nurse. We would emphasise that our recommendation that a Roll should be established for assistant nurses is contingent upon the enactment of the safeguards for the public which we discuss in paragraph 165.

We believe that the institution of a Roll of Assistant Nurses would not only help to remove existing abuses but would do something to remedy the shortage of nurses. This special work would attract older women who may find their present occupation lacking in interest or who have been detained by home duties until too late to enter any other profession, but whose qualities and experience would make them particularly suitable for the work of an assistant nurse. Thus many State Registered Nurses would be released for work which cannot be done by assistant nurses and for which State Registered Nurses are so badly needed. Needless to say the conditions of service for assistant nurses should be such as to make this career attractive to the right sort of woman and we recommend that their rates of salary should be regulated by the Salaries Committees and that they should be eligible for pension. . . .

paras. 158–64

It has been suggested to us that the term 'nurse' should be legally defined as connoting a State Registered Nurse and that the same should be done for whatever appellation might be adopted for the assistant nurse, and that persons using these names who are not entitled to them should be liable to legal prosecution.

Some of our witnesses and individual members of the Committee have suggested that the assistant nurse might be known as 'nursing aid,' 'invalid aid,' 'hospital aid,' 'nursing assistant,' etc., but on the whole it appears to us that titles of this kind would never win popular acceptance. The word 'nurse' is embedded in the structure of the language and it is impossible to expect that the assistant nurse, whatever her official title, would be known to the public other than as 'nurse.' It follows that it is not practicable, either, to limit the use of the term 'nurse' to the State Registered Nurse. It is every day practice to designate those who take care of healthy children 'nurses' whether they are qualified or not. It is, moreover, imperative that any name adopted for the assistant nurse on the Roll should be indicative of her function and should not be such as to lower in any way the status of the assistant nurse who has rendered and is rendering a valuable service to the community.

After very careful consideration we have come to the conclusion that we should recommend that the term 'Assistant Nurse' should be retained, and that it should be given legal recognition and protection.

We recognise that in the public mind some confusion may be caused between the Assistant Nurse and the State Registered Nurse if both are in practice known as 'nurse'. We hope that the recommendation we have made in paragraph 165 with regard to the declaration of the nurse's qualifications will go some way to obviate this. The problem of easy differentiation between the two grades assumes real importance only in domiciliary nursing, and we would suggest that a development of the practice, which already exists to some extent in private nursing, of knowing all State Registered Nurses as 'sisters' would prove of value in making clear to private patients the difference between a State Registered and an Assistant Nurse. General use of the term 'Sister' as a title by State Registered Nurses who practise privately would soon establish the distinction.

paras. 167–8

7.5 Report of the Working Party on the Recruitment and Training of Nurses (Wood Report)

Published: 1947

Chairman: *Sir Robert Wood KBE, CB*

Members: *Miss D. C. Bridges RRC, SRN, SCM; Miss E. Cockayne SRN, SCM; J. Cohen MA, PhD, FBPsS; T. Inch CBE, MC, MD, FRCP (Edin.), DPH; J. McCree (secretary); D. Somerville (assistant secretary)*

Terms of Reference (1946): *To review the position of the nursing profession [and to] survey the whole field of the recruitment and training of nurses of all types, including an examination of such questions as: (a) what is the proper task of the nurse? (b) what training is required to equip her for that task? (c) what annual intake is needed and how can it be obtained? (d) from what groups of the population recruitment should be made? (e) how can wastage during training be minimized?*

The Wood Report was perhaps twenty-five years ahead of its time in its recommendations for the reform of nurse training and it still makes stimulating reading. It was published in two parts, a majority report and a minority report by Dr John Cohen. In preparation for the establishment of the National Health Service the working party gathered a good deal of information on the country's nursing resources, on the structure of the nursing profession, and on such topics as selection and wastage during training. This information appeared either in the body of the report or in a number of useful appendices which also included papers on selection for senior posts in hospitals, post-registration nursing courses, the supervision of nurses' health, the nursing of the chronic sick, and mental nursing.

The working party identified as the principal problem the fact that 54 per cent of student nurses failed to complete their training. The answer to this high level of wastage was to be found partly in initial selection, partly in the conditions of training, and partly in the training itself. Nurses in training should no longer be regarded as junior employees, subject to an outworn system of discipline. They must be accorded full student status with the conditions of work that this status implied, so far as the intrinsic requirements of nurse training permitted. There should be more careful selection of students, including the use of psychological tests, and there should also be more careful selection procedures for appointment to senior posts, which would help to ensure that those who were appointed possessed the capacity to develop satisfactory human relationships. Nurses' food, accommodation and amenities should be improved, and a three-shift system of working introduced.

It was estimated that if student nurses were relieved of domestic work and of nursing duties which contributed little to their training but which were dictated solely by the staffing needs of the hospital, a period of two years would suffice for general nursing training. Within these two years it would be possible to provide a training at once more comprehensive and more effective than the existing three-year course, and to allow student nurses to work a five-day, forty-hour week, with six weeks' annual holiday. The normal working week for student nurses in 1947 was forty-eight or more hours a week with four weeks' holiday. It was proposed that the first eighteen months of the two-year course should be devoted to fundamentals common to all fields of nursing, and the remaining six months to concentrated study and training in a chosen field, such as public health, paediatrics or psychiatry. It was thought that the common qualification of SRN at the end of the two-year course, and the common basic training, would bring the various fields of nursing closer together and enhance the status of the less popular branches, such as mental nursing.

After completing her two-year course and passing the necessary examinations—one at the end of the eighteen months' basic training and one at the end of the specialist training period—the nurse would be given the pay and status of a SRN but would be required to work a further year under supervision before being licensed to practise. The working party suggested that the application of this scheme of training to midwifery should be considered, and this suggestion was taken up in the Stocks Report, published in 1949.

The working party recommended there should be one General Nursing Council for Great Britain, in place of the separate councils for England and Wales, Scotland and Northern Ireland, and if the suggestion regarding midwifery were accepted, the General Nursing Council and Central Midwives' Board should merge. As a consequence of the training recommendations there would of course be a common register, replacing the existing general register and the supplementary registers for mental nurses, male nurses, fever nurses and sick children's nurses. In each region there should be a regional nurse training board with wide representation to plan and co-ordinate training facilities, to co-ordinate standards of admission and to allocate students to training units, as well as to approve practical supervisors and assist with recruitment. Within each region selected hospitals and public health agencies should be grouped together to form training units covering all fields of nursing. Students would be students of the unit, passing from one institution to another in the course of their training.

The Wood Report recommended that while for some time it would be essential to use the services of assistant nurses then employed in hospitals, such a grade with a two-year training should not be perpetuated. The Roll should be closed at a given date and the duties undertaken by assistant nurses should be allocated partly to trained staff and partly to nursing orderlies, who would replace assistant nurses. Implementing student status and the three-shift system would require the trained nursing force to be raised from the 88,000 employed in 1945 to 112,000. The working party thought this could be achieved in five years by reduction of wastage during training, but there would also be a need for more staff to expand the service. All restrictions on the employment of married nurses—it was then unusual for married nurses to be employed in hospitals—should be removed, part-time service should be encouraged, and the use of male nurses should be extended.

Dr Cohen's Minority Report was a prolonged plea for more research to provide a sound basis for action. His thinking had been influenced by close association with Geoffrey Pyke, who at the time of his death was engaged on a study of the economic and sociological problems of health planning which Dr Cohen had hoped to publish as an appendix to his report. How could we plan a future nursing service, Dr Cohen asked, if we did not know how many nurses we required, and how could we say how many nurses we needed if we had no reliable indications of how many hospital beds should be provided? He quoted a large number of examples to drive home his point that opinion was no substitute for knowledge of the facts, and that statistical and other techniques were now available to measure things that in the past had not been thought susceptible of measurement. He pleaded for experiment. He was not opposed to the majority's two-year training scheme as such, but he was opposed to its adoption as a permanent solution without further research. The merits of courses of different length should be scientifically investigated.

The Wood Report was not well received by the nursing profession. Senior members of the profession were affronted by the outspoken criticisms of nursing administration and discipline, and by the generous selection of extracts from letters by former student nurses which Dr Cohen printed as an appendix to his Minority Report. The General Nursing Council opposed the recommendation to reduce the length of training to two years. Matrons everywhere were opposed to the suggestion that training schools should be administered separately from the hospitals and that students should be allocated for practical experience by the schools. Hospital authorities wondered how patients would be nursed if the contribution to staffing needs made by students was withdrawn.

On the main recommendations no immediate action ensued. The area nurse training committees set up under the 1949 Nurses Act were a pale reflection of the Wood Report's powerful regional nurse training boards. Schools of nursing remained hospital based and the tutors continued to be responsible to the matrons. The training of assistant nurses continued, although certain modifications were made which may have represented some response to the reasoning in the Wood Report. In 1950 the training period was reduced from two years to one year, followed by a further year of work under supervision to qualify for admission to the Roll. At the same time it was made possible for any type of hospital to apply for approval as an assistant nurse training school and pupil assistant nurses no longer had to spend a minimum of a year nursing the chronic sick.

Progress in the improvement of nursing conditions and the reduction of wastage during training proved slow, and reflected the normal process of negotiation at national level and the impact of more general social changes at the periphery, rather than the determination to take prompt and effective action which Dr Cohen had called for. Equally gradual was the movement to close the smaller training schools. Only after 1962 did it become necessary for a hospital to have a minimum of 300 beds to be recognized as a training school.

Wood Report, 1947

WASTAGE DURING TRAINING

Any impartial investigator entering many nurse training schools encounters an atmosphere of dissatisfaction or even discontent. Generally speaking, there is a considerable sense of frustration, and discipline is felt to be harsh and cramping and quite out of accord with modern notions of personal freedom. We are not referring so much to disciplinary requirements in periods of duty, but more to the restraints imposed upon a nurse's freedom in her personal life when she is not on duty. The very contract most student nurses are compelled to sign at the outset of their training, with all its vague but ominous legal implications, must prejudice them against their future career. The term 'abscond', which some hospitals use to describe a nurse's sudden departure, is consistent with the spirit of the contract.

The impression is sometimes left that senior members of staff are not really aware of, or fail fully to appreciate, the outlook of the younger generation. An interview first with the medical superintendent or matron or with ward sisters, followed up by confidential interviews with student nurses generally leaves the investigator with two contrasting pictures of hospital life as far as the students are concerned.

The opinion studies which we have made of student nurses who are still in training, as well as of qualified nurses, suggest strongly that the difference in attitude between a nurse who gives up training and one who does not is a difference in degree not in kind. Under the present system, a point is reached during the training period when many students 'waste'. They are not necessarily altogether different in kind from their fellow-students who remain. Many of those who stay on, if what they say is true, would almost certainly leave were it not for the direct or indirect pressure exerted on them by their parents or their own sense of vocation. In many cases they would leave not because they dislike nursing but because the conditions of training are to them all but intolerable. Similarly many, perhaps most, of those who leave do not do so necessarily because they dislike nursing, but because they have reached breaking point. In other words, the 'wasters' and 'non-wasters' are, generally speaking, a homogeneous group so far as their general attitude to nursing life and training is concerned.

paras. 91–2

Special study of causes of wastage. In order to examine more closely the causes of wastage, we have carried out a special analysis of 400 statements or letters submitted by 400 ex-student nurses, explaining why they gave up training. These were students whose names were submitted by the sample hospitals as having left in 1945 and who were not visited at their homes.

The results of the analysis indicate that the reasons given in the 400 statements are due to a general factor underlying all causes of wastage: this factor is composite and appears to exert a pressure on student nurses to abandon training. It manifests itself as the combined effect of all the various reasons for leaving— hospital discipline, food, pay, and so on, and is not to be identified with any single facet or feature of hospital life. The individual reasons themselves interact with one another. Thus, unsatisfactory food or poor accommodation might be tolerated if the discipline were less severe.

But the reasons which enter into this composite factor are far from being equally important. The first in significance is hospital discipline; the second, the attitude of senior staff; the third and fourth, food, and hours and pressure of work.

The conclusion emerges clearly from this analysis that the type of discipline which pervades the training schools today is unquestionably the most important cause of wastage. This code of discipline is intelligible historically inasmuch as it was originally inspired by a conventual tradition. Self-abnegation was the keynote of this tradition which the insularity of institutional life has preserved more or less unaltered by the profound changes in social outlook which have affected the community as a whole. Nursing titles are survivals of this regime. During the inter-war years a generation has grown up nurtured on modern ideas of personal freedom and relationship between the sexes and, inevitably, a gulf has separated the representatives of the old order from the newcomers to nursing. Potential student nurses today for the most part regard nursing as a profession with no more justification than any other for encroaching unduly upon the personal life. In these circumstances it is not surprising that friction should occur between the older and younger generations of nurses. Feelings tend to be exacerbated by the psychological deprivations which the older generations had perforce to suffer and from which the emancipated younger nurse is free.

Inadequacy of food, both in quantity and quality and the span and pressure of working hours, come next in that order. Following on these are poor accommodation, insufficient pay, poor social and recreational facilities, and the domestic work which student nurses have to carry out. Dissatisfaction either with training methods or examinations is apparently unimportant in its effect upon attitudes towards nurse training. Dissatisfaction with arrangements for the care of nurses' health is in rather a different category: it does not tend to provoke discontent with other features of hospital life, as do hospital discipline and attitude of senior staff. Private reasons and marriage exert a kind of 'negative' effect. In other words, a nurse who leaves training for private reasons, or because she intends to get married, will tend to overlook the reasons for leaving frequently mentioned by other nurses.

It follows that in order to reduce wastage to reasonable proportions steps must be taken to eliminate the main causes which would appear to operate. Experience teaches that, as far as the first two causes are concerned, it is of little use merely *appealing* to hospital authorities to modify discipline or to adopt more understanding attitudes. The introduction of *structural* changes in the organisation and staffing of training schools is certainly needed. The same applies to the changes required to lessen the 'wastage' effect of long hours and undue pressure of work. The elimination of 'food' as a contributory cause of wastage should be, administratively, the easiest to achieve.

The foregoing paragraphs are concerned with the evidence obtained from ex-students. In the course of our visits to hospitals we sought the views of random groups of nurses of all grades, and we also obtained a number of written statements from nurses. The views so expressed fully confirmed those of the ex-students.

A number of important conclusions follow directly from this inquiry. If the wastage of student nurses is to be reduced from the present rate of about 50 per cent. of the intake to reasonable proportions, the following changes must in our view be introduced:—

(i) Nurses in training must no longer be regarded as junior employees subject to an outworn system of discipline. They must be accorded full student status with the conditions such status implies, so far as the intrinsic requirements of nurse training permit.

(ii) A new selection procedure for student nurses.

(iii) A method of selection for appointment to senior posts which will help to secure that only those are appointed who possess the capacity for developing satisfactory human relationships.

(iv) Steps must be taken to improve the quantity and quality of diet and to provide suitable accommodation and other amenities.

(v) The training day must be reduced in span so that it approximates as closely as is practicable to that of a 'normal' working day. This involves the introduction of a three-shift system.

paras. 103–8

IMPLICATIONS OF THE NEW SCHEME OF TRAINING

If student nurses are to be treated as students, and the new training scheme successfully implemented, certain requirements must be met as indicated in the following paragraphs.

Basic Conditions. Conditions must be such as to permit the planning and conduct of training courses unhampered by the staffing requirements of particular hospitals. It follows that there must be an adequate and stable domestic and nursing staff in whatever hospitals, wards or departments are used for training purposes, to perform the domestic duties now falling on the student, and to fill the gap created in the ward services by eliminating unnecessarily repetitive work.

The rotation through hospital wards and departments, or through other branches of nursing, must be dictated by the nurse's needs as a student. A complete course of training must be laid down and adhered to, with teaching planned and continuous in all essential subjects and aspects of nursing, including systematised practice in techniques.

The dissociation of training from staffing needs, which follows from the above, will place the student under the control of the training authority . . . and not under that of the hospital. Senior nursing staff will exert authority over the student only in so far as this is necessary in the exercise of teaching functions or for the care of patients.

The cost of training should be dealt with entirely separately from the general maintenance expenditure of the hospitals in which training is given. Without question the present financial dependence of nursing schools upon the finances of the hospitals to which they are attached nullifies any serious attempt to improve the training of nurses. Student nurses would cease to be employees of the hospital and would not be bound by contract to an employing authority.

If the nurse in training is to be a student in the full sense of the word, the notion of 'recruitment', implying recruitment to employment, will no longer apply to her, though the machinery of the Ministry of Labour and National Service would continue to function in so far as it deals with choice of careers and is in touch with the training authorities. Just as in the educational sphere a responsibility rests upon the Minister of Education and the Secretary of State for Scotland for ensuring, so far as lies in their power, that sufficient teachers are available for the education services under their charge, so, we conceive, should a responsibility rest upon the Minister of Health and the Secretary of State to ensure that the nursing personnel required for the public health services are secured. It will be their concern to watch demand and supply and to take steps as necessary to stimulate the flow of students so as to ensure that supply meets demand.

Span of training day. We have concluded from our study of wastage that the training day must be reduced in span so that it approximates as closely as is practicable to that of a 'normal' working day, and that this involves the introduction of a three-shift system. Such a system is no less necessary to provide a normal working day for qualified staff than it is for students. Given the necessary staff it would be quite practicable to arrange this in spite of the fact that hospital routine requires a 24-hour working day. We have discussed the question with large numbers of nurses of all grades and, generally speaking, they declare their wholehearted preference for a shift system.

We have not met any evidence that the shift system is unpopular with patients or is bad for them. It is desirable that a patient should know which nurses he can turn to for nursing care, but this is no more difficult with the shift system than with the 'split duty' day. Moreover, the case assignment method is easier to work under this system. The present arrangement in training hospitals is, in fact, so confusing that few patients can know which of the ward nurses are really available. A patient in a ward of 25 to 30 beds is probably treated by six or eight different nurses during a day of 24 hours. The need for continuity of supervision in the ward may be met by a system of overlapping during the change-over period, ensuring that a qualified nurse will always be immediately available. A nurse's care and supervision of her patient are likely to be more efficient in an eight-hour span than in one of 12 or 13 hours. The rest period introduced under the split duty system is a poor compensation for the long stretch of duty.

As far as student nurses are concerned, the day is now broken up into periods in the wards, in lecture rooms, or off-duty, and is more fragmented than it would be under a shift system which would make it easier to systematise training. Among its many advantages may be counted the opportunities of non-residence, of having free time at the same hours as persons in other occupations, and avoidance of the insular and cloistered life of an institution.

The time for starting the day shift in the wards in most hospitals seems to us to be earlier than it need be; indeed, the present system would appear to rest in part on the inertia of tradition. The doctor's morning round all too often dominates the picture and, in preparation, patients are awakened at an hour they would not tolerate if they were at home. The aim should be to depart as little as possible from normal home routine for patients and, so far as student nurses are concerned, we consider that the span of daily duty should not begin before 8 a.m.

Teaching needs. The success of a scheme on the lines we have propounded will depend on the sufficiency and quality of the teaching staff provided. There were in August, 1943, 834 sister tutors in hospitals, but not all of these were qualified. In 1944 there were 417 qualified and 267 unqualified sister tutors training students for the General part of the Register. The number at that time teaching for the Supplementary Registers is unknown. It seems probable that by the end of 1946 there were some 1,000 sister tutors (qualified and unqualified) in all the hospitals of Great Britain. According to an estimate made in 1943, 900 qualified sister tutors would be needed by 1947 for training State Registered Nurses. This estimate must certainly be revised in the light of the new tasks that will fall to those responsible for instruction.

It will also be necessary to review the training of nurse instructors to bring it into line with their new functions. The main part of the training course for sister tutors or nurse instructors would need to be devoted to the study of modern educational methods. Nurse training calls for all the devices—classroom technique, visual aids, practical demonstration, experiments, case history study—which the well-equipped teacher would employ.

Particular consideration will need to be given at an early stage to the provision of adequate facilities for teaching in the various branches of public health. This is necessary because in the proposed scheme a period of public health experience is included in the training of every student, apart from the optional six months which some may devote to public health. Similar measures will need to be taken in certain hospital fields now lacking organised teaching facilities.

Nurse training has much to learn from developments in other training fields. The potential value for nursing of applying principles of work simplification, long established in industrial psychology, is all but unexplored. Such principles have a direct bearing both on methods of nurse training and on the performance of many duties falling to the lot of the trained nurse. Work simplification leads to economies of time and effort and to reduced fatigue. No less important an item in the smooth and efficient running of a training or working unit is the human factor in staff relations. In nursing, as elsewhere, incentives must be kept alive, interests must be sustained, and team-work must be inspired. To achieve these ends, suitably selected teachers and other senior staff must be trained to acquire the necessary skill in handling people and in understanding their needs.

Remuneration—Training Grants. Under present arrangements student nurses, in addition to receiving free tuition, board residence, uniforms and laundry, are paid small salaries under the Rushcliffe scales. These salaries are payable to them in virtue of their position as employees of the training hospitals and essential members of the nursing staffs. If in the future student nurses are to be treated as students and, instead of training being incidental to their work in the wards, the service they render to the hospitals becomes incidental to their training, the basis of their remuneration will call for reconsideration.

Methods of dealing with this question vary from country to country, in some cases taking the form of payment during training to all students as is the practice here now, and in others providing for payment only during the final period of studentship, or actually for the payment of fees *by* students to the training hospital.

An analogy is sometimes drawn between the financial terms offered to young women to train as nurses with those available for would-be entrants to the teaching profession. The intending teacher is assisted by the provision of free tuition in a Training College and also, subject to a parental contribution on an approved income scale, with board and residence in College or Hostel during term, or equivalent subsistence allowance. Actually, as will be seen, student nurses are offered much more favourable financial terms. But such an analogy is irrelevant if it is confined only to this aspect of the problem and does not take into account the type, hours and conditions of work and the future prospects of promotion in the two professions.

It is, however, sometimes suggested that student nurses training for the public health services should be regarded as in much the same position as intending teachers training to serve in the public system of education, and that there is no case for continuing any payment to student nurses when they cease to be employees of the hospitals. Indeed, the Horder Committee supports the principle that, when possible, the student should pay for her training; but with the proviso that no good potential nurse should be debarred from training through lack of money.

In our opinion the case for providing a grant to student nurses stands on its own merits. The fact is that we are faced with the practical and pressing problem of providing an adequate number of nurses of the type required by the community. In principle the case for the provision of training grants to student nurses rests, in part, on the services they will render during the course of their training, but, in the main, on what it is worth to the community to get nurses at all.

We are led to the view that the nursing needs of the community will not be met unless the training grant given to a student nurse is adequate to cover reasonable personal expenses (including on vacation), in addition to board residence or an allowance in lieu, and free tuition. The grant would be paid by the training authority. What modification, if any, in the present scale of payment might thus result we have not attempted to determine.

Finally, we would add a further observation to which we attach considerable importance and which is supported by views we have elicited from large numbers of nurses. What the nursing profession requires is, not so much slight changes in the size of grants paid during the relatively brief phase of training, but better training and wider career prospects with enhanced status and opportunities. Only by offering such a career is the profession likely to attract the candidates it needs.

paras. 146–61

7.6 The Work of Nurses in Hospital Wards

Report of a Job-Analysis by the Nuffield Provincial Hospitals Trust

Published: 1953

Director of the Job-Analysis Team: *H. A. Goddard*

Nursing Adviser: *Miss C. M. Grant Glass SRN, SCM, HV*

Advisory Panel: *Sir Ernest Rock Carling FRCS, FRCP, HonLLD; Miss C. F. S. Bell SRN, SCM; Miss E. Cockayne SRN, SCM; Donald Court MD, MRCP, DCH; J. W. B. Douglas BA, BSc, MB, BS; Miss A. M. D. Leslie SRN, SCM, DN (Lond.),; S. C. Merivale MA, FHA*

Terms of Reference (1948): *To carry out a complete job-analysis of the work of the nurse and other members of the health team in order to obtain the necessary data so that an answer can be given to the fundamental question 'What is the proper task of a nurse?'*

When the Wood Report on the Recruitment and Training of Nurses was published in 1947, the Ministry of Health invited various interested bodies to comment. The Nuffield Provincial Hospitals Trust pointed out that the principal shortcoming of the report was the absence of objective research findings to throw light on the first of the main questions which the working party were asked to examine, namely 'What is the proper task of the nurse?' The Trust went on to recommend a study, using the technique of job-analysis, to provide 'an essential foundation of long-term policy'. The study should analyse the work of 'the whole health team', but the study that the Trust itself mounted, as 'a practical demonstration of the earnest desire of the Trust to make a worthwhile contribution to the solution of the many problems which beset the nursing profession', was limited to general hospital nurses working in wards, together with the ward orderlies and ward maids who assisted them. The Trust recognized that although ward work occupied some 70 per cent of the nursing staff of a hospital, such a study was only a starting point, and expressed the hope that it would be followed by others.

Job-analysis is a technique defined as 'the scientific study and statement of all the facts about a job which reveal its content and the modifying factors which surround it'. In this context the word 'job' refers to an occupation, the whole group of duties, responsibilities and activities assigned to an individual, and not to an individual activity, such as typing a letter or changing a dressing. The Nuffield study involved a team of observers who recorded, minute by minute, the activities of staff in selected wards in twelve general hospitals in different parts of the country for a week at a time over a period of eighteen months between January 1949 and July 1950. In all, some 15,729 hours' work was observed.

The report included the findings of the study; observations on these findings by the director, H. A. Goddard, and his team; and observations by the advisory panel. The findings continued to be discussed and to influence policy proposals for many years. Some of the most important were as follows.

(1) Student nurses contributed 74 per cent of the time recorded as spent on nursing duties.

(2) Ward sisters spent nearly half their time on ward organization, and staff nurses (state registered nurses other than the ward sister) spent just over one-third of their time on ward organization.

(3) Ward sisters spent, on average, only five minutes a day specifically giving tuition to student nurses.

(4) In most cases, student nurses spent relatively little time (an average of thirty-five, thirty and twenty minutes a day in their first, second and third years respectively) on domestic work.

(5) Student nurses spent more time on technical nursing and less on basic nursing as they progressed through their training.

(6) The average length of the patient's day was from 5 am to 10 pm, with little opportunity for undisturbed rest within that period. There was a peak of activity between 5 am and 9 am in order to get wards 'open' for doctors' rounds by 9 am, which made it necessary in some cases to wake patients even earlier than 5 am.

The heavy contribution made by student nurses to the work of the ward was inevitable, as they comprised 60·8 per cent of the ward staffs, and whatever the size of the ward the trained staff normally consisted of one ward sister and one staff nurse, each of whom spent a substantial part of her time in ward organization (including clerical duties). This finding set in perspective the Wood Report's recommendation of 'student status' for student nurses.

If students' educational needs were to take priority over service demands, who would take over this substantial chunk of work? One possibility was the employment of more auxiliary help on the wards and in fact the numbers of 'other nursing staff', as they were referred to in the Ministry statistics, grew steadily in the later 1950s and the 1960s—not without agonized cries of 'dilution' from some sections of the nursing profession. It was an interesting reflection of the failure, at this stage, of the enrolled assistant nurse to secure acceptance within acute general hospitals, that the staffs of the wards studied included only one assistant nurse; it was therefore not possible to offer any conclusions on the work of this grade. Enrolled assistant nurses (the word 'assistant' was later dropped) were still working almost exclusively in long-stay hospitals, which did not come within the scope of this study.

It had been traditionally assumed that the student nurse received her theoretical training in the classroom, from medical lecturers and the sister tutors, and her practical training in the wards and departments, at the hands of ward and departmental sisters and other trained staff. The Nuffield finding that ward sisters spent very little time on their teaching duties was hotly disputed by the nursing profession. Goddard and his team were accused of adopting an unduly rigorous definition of 'tuition' and of ignoring the sisters' contribution to the training of student nurses through teaching by example. The Royal College of Nursing persuaded a group of ward sisters to keep diaries, and these purported to show that sisters spent 5·9 per cent of their working time in tuition, compared with the Nuffield figure of 1·1 per cent. Subsequent studies, both of ward activities and of student nurses' perceptions of the teaching they received, tended to confirm, however, that ward teaching was largely neglected, a situation which only started to be remedied with the introduction in the early 1960s of clinical instructors, trained nurses working in the wards with a specific responsibility for teaching student nurses and no administrative load to carry. Interestingly, where clinical instructors were employed the student nurses got more teaching from the ward sisters too.

Goddard's suggestion that his findings showed the end result of nurse training to be not the nursing of patients but ward administration provoked a reaction among nurses that this was an unhealthy situation, that the proper task of the nurse was to nurse patients, and that patients were entitled to the skills of a trained nurse. The finding that the time spent on ward organization did not vary with the size of ward led to experiments with larger wards when it was fed into the parallel Nuffield study of the design of hospital wards. Various experiments with 'team nursing', in which patients on a ward were divided into groups and total responsibility for the care of each group was assigned to a team of varying grades, led by a trained nurse or senior student nurse, also stemmed from this finding.

The Nuffield study showed that some of the claims that nurses were overburdened with domestic duties over-stated the situation, but there was plainly room for further improvement. The inhumanity of a system which exposed the patient to being wakened at 5 am or earlier and which gave sick people little chance to rest during a 17-hour day (and presumably a rest was, at least in part, what some of them were in hospital for!) was highlighted in this report and was to continue to cause concern for a number of years. The report also spelled out what every nurse knew, but those responsible for the administration of hospitals chose to ignore, that the work required of the night nurses between 5 am and going off duty was quite beyond the capabilities of the numbers of staff available.

7.7 Report of the Committee on Senior Nursing Staff Structure (Salmon Report)

Published: 1966

Chairman: *Brian Salmon*

Members: *J. Greene SRN, RMN, RMPA; Miss J. T. Locke OBE, RGN, SCM, RNT; T. T. Paterson BSc, MA, PhD; Miss M. B. Powell CBE, SRN, SCM, RNT; Miss E. M. Rees SRN, SCM, RNT; John Revans MBE, MRCP; Miss G. M. Westbrook SRN, SCM, RNT; G. H. Weston FHA; S. R. F. Whittaker MA, MD, FRCP, DL; F. D. K. Williams (secretary)*

Terms of Reference (1963): *To advise on the senior nursing staff structure in the hospital service (ward sister and above), the administrative functions of the respective grades and the methods of preparing staff to occupy them.*

In 1948 hospitals had been grouped under hospital management committees and on the lay administrative side a chain of command had been established between administrators of the hospitals comprising the group and the new post of group secretary. No comparable development took place on the nursing side until the early 1960s, when a few 'group matrons' were appointed in scattered parts of the country. This pattern was, however, not at all widespread by the time the Salmon Committee reported, and in most groups the matrons of individual hospitals jealously guarded their own autonomy and their right to be considered directly responsible to the HMC.

The fact that most groups comprised a number of hospitals, each with its own matron (or in the case of a mental hospital with a matron *and* a chief male nurse) made it difficult, if not impossible, for HMCs to continue the practice that had been general among voluntary hospital boards of having the matron in attendance at meetings of the hospital authority, to give her advice on nursing matters and take part in discussion of future policy. This exclusion from policy-making discussions was felt by matrons as a blow to their status. Already the position of the matron had changed with the appearance within the hospital of other, independent, professions open to women, such as physiotherapy and radiography; and with the appointment of specialists in catering, laundry management, cleaning etc. to take over many of the 'housekeeping' aspects of the matron's task. In most cases these new specialists were made responsible to the hospital secretary rather than the matron. While matrons had previously had much of the day-to-day control of the hospital in their hands, they now saw themselves becoming mere departmental heads.

A number of compromise arrangements were tried in order to meet the matrons' demands that they should have a voice in policy-making and should be allowed to put the nursing view at meetings of the hospital authority. In a few groups it was possible to continue previous arrangements virtually unchanged, because there was only one hospital of any size or significance; other groups established matrons' advisory committees and asked them to nominate a representative to attend meetings of the HMC. However in 1964, soon after the Salmon Committee were given their terms of reference, the Royal College of Nursing published a report entitled *Administering the Hospital Nursing Service* and suggesting that:

> For each group of hospitals there should be one top level nursing administrator, who for the purposes of this report will be described as 'Group Nursing Officer'; her span of control would equate with that of the group secretary. . . . At hospital level there should be a senior nurse administrator who, in turn, would equate with the hospital secretary. . . . This officer could appropriately be described as a 'Hospital Nursing Officer'.

These and other recommendations anticipated many of the points made in the Salmon Report—even if only approximately—which is hardly surprising, since several members of the Salmon Committee were leading members of the College. Yet it was only a few years since the suggestion that each group should have a matron-in-chief and that other matrons in the group should be subordinated to her would have been inconceivable to any right-thinking matron.

Another aspect of nursing administration that had given rise to unease within the profession was the role and function of assistant and deputy matrons. There were many ironical comments in the nursing journals of the 1950s about assistant matrons whose main jobs appeared to be to fill matron's ink-well, put out her blotting paper, and rule lines in books. As the Salmon Report explained, 'the Assistant Matron is often treated exactly like an assistant, not as a person between the Matron and the Ward Sister, and to whom the right to command the Ward Sister . . . is delegated by the Matron'. A few hospitals broke away from this pattern with the appointment of 'clinical assistant matrons' who were each made responsible for a block or group of wards, and it was no doubt this development that was responsible for the recommendations regarding Grade 7' in the Salmon Report.

The Salmon Report introduced to nursing a new language, the language of management. It was therefore found necessary to print as an appendix a four-page glossary, distinguishing between such terms as *structural authority* and *sapiential authority*; *full control, actual control* and *direction; line* and *staff*; *job description, job grading* and *job specification*. In the body of the report, equally careful distinctions were drawn between *directive* and *executive committees*, and *informative* and *conclusive conferences*. The report met with some criticism for its rigidly structuralist approach but there is no doubt that it taught many nurses to think systematically about management for the first time.

The main recommendations were quickly accepted in principle by the Minister of Health, Kenneth Robinson, but it was decided to proceed cautiously by means of a limited number of pilot schemes which would test out the new structure before it was generally adopted. The pilot groups were selected so as to be reasonably representative of the different types of group to be found in the country as a whole—teaching and non-teaching, mental, general and mixed, large, medium and small etc.—and so as to give the new structure a fair chance; for it was realized that it would have considerable repercussions throughout the hospitals of the group and that if the medical staff, the committee and the hospital administration did not clearly understand and support it, it could not work. An end was put to this careful approach when the Prices and Incomes Board published their Report No. 60, on the pay of nurses and midwives, in March 1968. This report called for complete implementation of the Salmon proposals at an early date, and so from 1969 onwards reorganization was set in motion in the majority of groups in the country without waiting for the experience of the pilot schemes to become available.

It was decided not to set up regional nursing staff committees, as recommended by the report, but a National Nursing Staff Committee for England and Wales was set up in 1967 to advise the Minister of Health on management training and selection and appointment procedures for senior posts. Close liaison with the National Staff Committee, the similar body for hospital administrators set up on the recommendation of the Lycett Green Report (q.v., p. 189), was ensured by the sharing of premises and, following the death in 1968 of Sir Albert Martin, by the appointment of the same chairman, Dame Isabel Graham Bryce, to both committees. The National Nursing Staff Committee devoted most attention during their first few years to the launching of a massive programme of management training for all grades of nurse from ward sister upwards, to the establishment of standardized procedures for appointments to senior posts, and to the introduction of a scheme of staff appraisal and counselling.

The implementation of the Salmon Report at hospital group level was found to require much thought, preparation and planning. More money was required, not only to pay for additional nursing administrators (in fact very often fewer nursing administrators were required in the new structure than the old), but also to pay other staff to relieve senior nurses of the supervision of non-nursing services such as housekeeping and staff residences. Additional office space and secretarial staff also had to be provided. Of course, it was hoped that this would be justified by the improvement in the standard of management of nursing services and ultimately by an improvement in the care received by patients. Staff throughout the group had to learn new channels through which to communicate and to co-ordinate their activities with the nursing staff. Much obviously depended on the calibre of nurses available to fill the new posts. In the early days, some groups were obviously much more fortunate in this respect than others.

Salmon Report, 1966

Despite the Bradbeer Committee's remarks on the partnership of nursing with medical and lay administration, nursing appears to occupy a secondary position. This stems from the incoherence of the nursing administration itself and a seeming inability on the part of nurses to assert the rights of their emergent profession. The profession is not represented officially and with the same status at meetings of all governing bodies as are the medical staff and the hospital administration. It seems to us that the assertion of the professional status of nurses could best be achieved by assuming the right of the profession to be heard (sapiential authority, as it is called) on all matters concerning nursing that are controlled by governing bodies; to present to those governing bodies the profession's concept of nursing policy; and, so far as possible (that is, where co-ordination with the other administrations is not involved) to decide the policy. This will require elevation of the status of the most senior nurse administrator in each hospital group.

STAFFING STRUCTURE AND GRADES

Confusion arises from the indiscriminate and imprecise use of the title 'Matron'. It is applied equally to the nursing heads of large hospitals of over a thousand beds and of small hospitals of as few as ten. The Matron of a small hospital is recognised as having the same duties and so the same rights as the Matron of a large hospital within the same group, rights such as attending the Management Committee or Board of Governors to which all matrons are directly responsible. The only recognition of difference lies in the Whitley salary grading which is based upon number of beds, not upon the importance of the decisions taken. The Assistant or Deputy Matron in a large hospital may well have as onerous tasks as the Matron of a small hospital but is accorded neither the status nor the prestige.

There is also confusion about the functions of nurse administrators in the hospital organisation, least for the Ward Sister, more for the Matron and most for nurses in the intermediate grades. As in industry and commerce where the belief survives that ability to manage is not learned but innate, nursing administration is still in the process of development. Matrons tend, for example, to hold on to tasks in which they are interested, tasks which could be carried out by other nurses or even a well-trained clerk. Few matrons appear to practise the technique of delegation. Nor do they seem to aim at decentralisation, that is, arranging that decisions of the appropriate level are taken as near as possible to the scene of the activities where these decisions are required. The Assistant Matron is often treated exactly like an assistant, not as a person between the Matron and the Ward Sister, and to whom the right to command the Ward Sister (structural authority) is delegated by the Matron. The Ward Sister feels she is responsible to the Matron, a remote person in a big hospital, and not to the Assistant or Deputy. The result is that Ward Sisters regard Assistant Matron and such 'administrative posts' as of no great importance or consequence and merely as tiresome stepping stones in advancement to the desirable post of Matron.

The confusion is further complicated by difficulties stemming from traditional and widely differing beliefs on the relative status of administrative nurses in general nursing and of those in teaching and midwifery, as well as a feeling that psychiatric nurses and midwives are of a nursing world apart.

We distinguish the decision to establish a nursing *policy* from the decision concerning the *programming* of the policy, that is setting the limits within which those who *execute* the policy, may decide to act. For example, a nursing policy decision may be the specification of a procedure for carrying out a nursing technique. The relevant programming decision may be concerned with the ordering of new equipment and the withdrawal from ward stocks of items no longer required, the communication of the new procedure to all concerned and the organisation of any necessary instruction for nursing staff and nurses in training. The executive decision, the act of bringing the new procedure into operation, will be undertaken by the ward staff under the control of the Ward Sister. Those who decide policy, the most senior officers, we propose to call *top management*, those who programme policy *middle management*, and those who control the execution *first-line management*.

At present, in a small hospital, the Matron may carry out both top and middle management functions, whereas in a larger hospital she may (or should) delegate to the Deputy and Assistant Matrons the tasks of middle management together with the right to give orders for the programme to be executed. If the small hospital is properly integrated within a group, or is satellite to a large hospital, the policy decisions should be made by the controlling or co-ordinating head nursing officer, and the Matron of the small hospital should be delegated only the tasks of middle management. She is then of status equivalent to that of the nurses in middle management in the large hospital. Status is established by the kinds of decision that are made not by numbers of beds controlled.

In large hospitals, and especially in the larger district general hospitals proposed in the Hospital Plans, the organisation of necessity becomes more complicated. The number of nurses executing the programme is large (the Staff

Nurses). Their tasks and they themselves are organised and co-ordinated by the Ward Sister or Charge Nurse who is then in control of what may be called a *section*. (This may be an operating theatre section, a teaching section or out-patient section with no beds as well as a ward.) A logical grouping of such sections (three to six) constitutes a *unit*, the sphere of authority of a nurse in middle management; and again, a grouping of units constitutes an *area*, co-ordinated by a more senior middle manager. (We use the term area since very often the units to be co-ordinated are in physical proximity.) Areas and units are brought together as a *division*, the sphere of authority of a nursing officer in top management.

There are three possible kinds of division—nursing, teaching and midwifery—for, wherever possible, a single school of nursing should be formed for the hospitals of a management group, and midwifery has peculiarities, statutory and otherwise, which distinguish it from general nursing. Where there is more than one division a more senior nursing officer in top management should co-ordinate the work of heads of divisions and be the nursing representative to present matters of nursing policy to the governing body of the hospital management group.

The organisation of nursing posts in a group can then be set out fairly simply and numbered in grades from 10, for the most senior nurse in top management, to 5 for the Staff Nurse who executes the programme (the lower numbers, 4 to 1, are applicable to grades below Staff Nurse).

Level	*Number and general title of grade*		*Local titles of posts*
Top management:	10 Chief Nursing Officer	C.N.O.	Chief Nursing Officer.
	9 Principal Nursing Officer	P.N.O.	Principal Matron, Principal Tutor.
Middle management:	8 Senior Nursing Officer	S.N.O.	Senior Matron, Senior Tutor, Senior Midwife Teacher.
	7 Nursing Officer	N.O.	Matron, Tutor, Midwife Teacher.
First-line management:	6 Charge Nurse	C.N.	Ward Sister, Section Sister, Midwifery Sister, Charge Nurse.
	5 Staff Nurse	S.N.	Staff Nurse, Staff Midwife.

The general titles can be used in any system for either sex, but they need not be applied rigidly in all hospital groups. Other local titles can be used, of which examples are given above, provided the grade is clearly specified. There is good reason for retaining the title of 'Matron' for women. It has a long and honoured tradition and has profound significance to the general public. In general we recommend the use of 'nursing officer' (which can be applied to male as well as female nurses) with appropriate adjectives to indicate the grade of management. We think the prefixes 'assistant' and 'deputy' should be abolished since they are confusing and do not indicate the nature of a job. An even number grade indicates a co-ordinating function in each of the three management levels, this co-ordination being exercised either by *full control* (the juniors being responsible to the superior) or by *actual control* (the juniors being responsible to a nurse in the level next above but reporting to the immediate superior). In the top-management level the Chief Nursing Officer (Grade 10) may have either full or actual control—the heads of divisions being responsible to the governing body in the latter case—or may co-ordinate by the use of her greater knowledge of the total nursing situation (sapiential authority), that is, by the use of *direction* as distinct from *control*.

This use of sapiential authority is also the essence of the process of *secondment* by which nurses can co-ordinate the activities of persons under the control of the hospital administrator, persons who can carry out many of the tasks now performed by nurses that are not properly nursing. We recommend that, wherever possible, nurses and nursing officers be relieved of all such tasks.

paras. 1.1–1.11

IMPLICATIONS FOR NURSING CAREERS

The proposed structure is diagrammatically, but not completely, represented in Figure 1. This shows the pyramidal nature of the structure which is of great concern in the matter of promotion. At present the pyramid is very narrow and insufficiently extended in the upper portions, that is to say there is limited scope for promotion. There is little incentive on this account for highly competent nurses to stay in the profession and it is disheartening for those who do. The addition at the top to the rungs in the promotion ladder, as well as the widening of the lower ones, will permit of more frequent, and evident, progression upwards in status—reward for work well done. The uniform grading, too, will remove many present anomalies in relative status and will reduce the discontent that is a consequence.

The recommended structure may also answer a need that was often expressed in evidence, a desire to remain 'close to the patient'. This attitude, wholly admirable and indicative of the professional sense of service, is also a contributory cause of some of the defects in the working of the present structure. Senior nurses tend to interfere in ward matters more than they ought to, and, however laudable it may seem for the administrative nurse to 'roll up her sleeves' in the wards, it is often really a satisfying of her own needs and not a service to patients or Ward Sisters. If the senior managerial positions are clearly seen to be of greater importance, in service to more patients rather than 'to the patient', these positions become desirable to the nurse with a developed sense of vocation.

Nevertheless many nurses do not wish to exchange practical nursing for managerial posts and it must be admitted that some highly skilled nurses do not have the managerial capacities that are necessary for the most senior positions. Their particular skills must be recognised and used to the full. There can be promotion to Nursing Officer (Grade 7) in control of a specialised *unit*, or *area* even in some cases. A Nursing Officer in such a post can use her accumulated specialised skill in developing her unit; and the title of Matron then becomes a mark of that nursing skill. Similarly, by the institution of teaching divisions, a promotional ladder is provided for nurses who have a proved aptitude for teaching and who wish to remain in that field. The structure we recommend is suitable for advancement of nurses in three different ways, according to the manner in which they wish to serve in their profession—in specialised nursing, in nursing administration and in teaching.

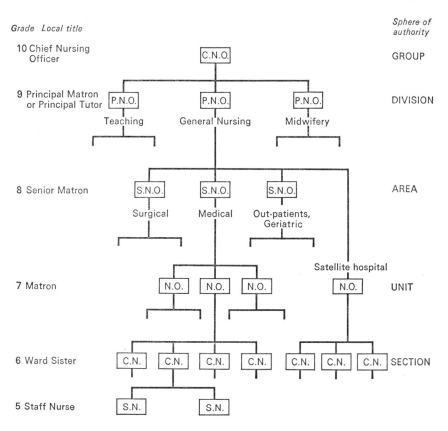

Nurses in top management need, most of all, well developed managerial skills. They should not be required to have a basic qualification in each kind of nursing represented within their sphere of authority. We see no reason at all why the head of a midwifery, or a psychiatric or a teaching division should not become a Chief Nursing Officer of a group of hospitals. Provided he or she has shown the proper managerial ability it does not matter the route taken to the top. The Chief Nursing Officer can adequately represent all divisions of nursing to the governing body and its committees by proper managerial consultation with the Principal Nursing Officers controlling the various divisions. Depending upon the composition of the group of hospitals the Chief Nursing Officer may have full control of all the hospitals, or may control only some and co-ordinate them with the others, either by actual control or direction. . . .

paras. 1.11–1.15

7.8 Report of the Committee on Nursing (Briggs Report)

Published: 1972

Chairman: *Professor Asa Briggs*

Members: *Ian M. Adam SRN, RMN, RNT;* Alan S. Anderton FHA;†
Miss Margaret G. Auld SRN, SCM, MTD, Cert. of Nurs. Admin. (Edin.);
Professor Ivor R. C. Batchelor MB, ChB, FRSE, FRCPE, FRCPsych,
DPM; Miss Sheila M. Collins SRN, RSCN, RNT; Mrs Susan Cooper
SRN;‡ Professor J. R. Crossley; D. W. Daly ChM, FRCS; Miss Winifred
Eustace SRN, SCM;§ Miss W. Frost OBE, SRN, SCM, HV, Queen's
Nurse; Dulcie Gooding MB, BS, MFCM, DPH; Vincent Gorman SRN,
RNMS; William L. Griffiths; Lady Howe JP; R. F. Kempster SRN,
RMN, RMPA;‖ Miss Susan Pembrey SRN, DSA; Robert E. Presswood
BSc, MEd; Professor Margaret Scott Wright MA (Hons.), PhD, DMSA,
SRN, SCM; Miss G. E. Watts Hon. LLD, SRN, SCM, RNT, Cert. of
Nurs. Admin., RCN*

**Appointed 29 July 1970; resigned to take up appointment at DHSS 31
August 1971*
†Appointed 4 September 1970
‡Resigned for personal reasons 26 October 1970
§ Appointed 9 February 1971
‖Appointed 28 June 1971

Advisers: *Nicholas Bosanquet BA, MA, MSc; Mrs Jillian MacGuire
BA, PhD*

Research Assistants: *Richard F. Clifton BA (Econ.), MA; Miss Christine
Hancock BSc, SRN; Ken Jarrold BA; Brian H. Merriman BSc, FRGS*

Terms of Reference (1970): *To review the role of the nurse and the midwife
in the hospital and the community and the education and training required for
that role, so that the best use is made of available manpower to meet present
needs and the needs of an integrated health service.*

On the eve of the reorganization of the National Health Service the Briggs Report proposed a major reform of nursing education designed to provide nursing with an appropriate structure of training and qualification to meet the needs of a unified health service. The committee examined many of the problems that had concerned, in turn, the Lancet Commission, the Athlone Committee, and the Wood Committee, but were careful to distinguish between myth and reality, between problems which were inherent in the nature of the profession and in its predominantly female composition and problems which ought to be susceptible of solution.

For instance, a balanced view was taken of wastage during training. It was calculated that on average one student nurse in three failed to complete her three-year training. 'These rates of wastage are higher than those for trainee teachers and for students in higher education. Yet they are somewhat lower than the turnover rates found among young women at work.' Although wastage could no doubt be reduced by better initial selection, by improving working conditions, and above all by raising the quality and quantity of training, much of it was explicable in terms of 'the highly demanding work and the often unpredictable stresses associated with it'.

Nor was turnover among trained staff as serious a matter as was sometimes thought. Table 28, 'Percentage of Employees in Various Categories Who Had Been Employed by their Current Employer for Twelve Months or Less at 1 April 1971' showed that, overall, nurses did not change their employment more frequently than other groups of women workers. There were, however, important variations between grades, and the statistics showed nursing to have a stable core of sisters, enrolled nurses, and older staff nurses and midwives. There was higher than average turnover among young staff nurses and among nursing auxiliaries, and the use of carefully compiled statistics to focus attention upon specific problems in this way was typical of the whole report.

In addition to drawing on data readily available from government and other sources the committee set up a small research team and commissioned a number of surveys from other bodies. Attention was paid to the collection not only of facts, a wealth of which appeared in the report's 50-odd tables, but also of opinions, which formed the basis of some of the discussion in Chapter II: 'Nurses and Midwives and the Public: Images and Realities'. The committee were adamant that while they did not necessarily agree with all the opinions expressed by nurses and others on current conditions in the profession, it was necessary to take into account opinions and attitudes as well as hard facts. The report was thus considerably more sophisticated than some of its predecessors in its use of the techniques and insights of the social scientist.

As far as nursing education was concerned the report pointed to six fundamental problems:

(1) the ambivalent position of the nurse in training both as learner and worker;

(2) determining the balance of theoretical and practical work in the learning process itself;

(3) the dual role of the hospital as the provider of nursing care for patients and the provider of education for nurses;

(4) the wide range of institutions providing education and the limited viability of many of them both as educational and social institutions;

(5) the mix of entrants of very different academic abilities;

(6) the timing of specialization and elucidating the relationship between basic nursing and specialized nursing.

All these problems were seen against the background of health service reorganization—and since nurses and midwives constituted the largest group of staff in the NHS the success of an integrated service Many depend largely on their ability to work in an integrated way. would previous discussions of the problems of the profession had been conditioned by a view which saw the nursing of patients in hospitals for the physically ill as the main focus of concern, with nursing in the community and in hospitals for the mentally ill and handicapped as well as for the chronically sick, as distinctly subsidiary branches of the profession. The Briggs Committee leaned over backwards to avoid giving this impression. They emphasized the need to plan nursing and midwifery requirements across the current dividing lines of hospital and community and to bear in mind current policies of treating patients whenever possible without admission to hospital and of discharging them from hospital as soon as possible.

The General Nursing Council for England and Wales had declared in their evidence to the Briggs Committee that 'the role of the nurse is constantly changing'. It must 'always be closely related to the needs of the patients' and these varied 'according to . . . medical and technical advances, and developments such as the possibility of a unified nursing service.' The Briggs Committee commented that there was growing recognition of the variety of jobs that existed within the nursing profession. They also drew attention to the range of abilities and qualifications to be found among those whom the public commonly regarded as belonging to the nursing profession—from the nursing auxiliaries and assistants with virtually no training and no formal qualifications at one end of the spectrum to graduate nurses holding senior positions at the other; (a member of the Committee was Dr Margaret Scott Wright, first professor of nursing in a British university.) There was obviously a place within the profession not only for many different skills and specialisms but also for many different levels of ability. The structure of the profession and its training arrangements should be so devised as to take advantage of recruitment from all sections of the community and to enable nurses to be deployed flexibly.

The solution that was reached owed a great deal to suggestions put forward by Dr Jillian MacGuire, who was employed by the committee as an adviser and whose early research into problems of wastage during nurse training had led her to publish in 1968 a scheme based on a common basic qualification, which could be obtained by following a variety of training pathways according to basic education and intelligence. The scheme outlined in the Briggs Report incorporated the idea of the common basic qualification—the Certificate in Nursing—but recommended that all recruits to nursing should be initiated to the profession through the medium of one basic course designed to produce at the end of eighteen months a competent and confident practical nurse, able to work as a basic member of the nursing team in any field of nursing.

Following basic training, those nurses who wished and had the ability to do so would proceed to a further eighteen months' training for registration possibly preparing at the same time for a Higher Certificate which would be recognized as an advanced qualification in a particular field of nursing. If taken after registration, the Higher Certificate course would last six months. A nurse might proceed from the basic certificate to registration and from registration to a Higher Certificate course at any time. Thus a nurse who had practised at the basic level and then married might after bringing up her family be accepted to train for registration without any loss of credit for her existing qualification.

The Briggs Committee built further flexibility into their scheme by constructing the courses for the basic certificate and for registration on modular principles, so that account was taken in the teaching and experience received of the student's own preferences and aptitudes, on the one hand, and on the other of what was seen as the necessity of providing a satisfactory balance of experience between various fields of nursing and between acute and long-term illness. The committee saw courses in universities and other institutions of higher education as an essential part of their long-term strategy for the profession, but did not feel called upon to outline possible university courses leading to degrees in nursing and midwifery. They merely expressed the hope that wherever practicable the Certificate in Nursing Practice and a shortened Higher Certificate course would be incorporated within a degree course for new entrants to nursing.

Apart from courses in universities and polytechnics, the design of which would be a matter for the educational institutions themselves, nursing education would be based on Colleges of Nursing and Midwifery, each with its own governing body, responsible in turn to an Area Committee for Nursing and Midwifery Education. The existing national statutory bodies, the General Nursing Councils and the Central Midwives' Board, would be replaced by a new statutory body, a Central Nursing and Midwifery Council for Great Britain. Separate Nursing and Midwifery Education Boards for England, Scotland and Wales would deal with matters specific to each country and would report direct to the Central Nursing and Midwifery Council. It was recommended that a statutory standing committee should be set up to deal with questions relating to midwifery.

The recommendation to abolish the separate statutory body for midwifery was not unexpected, but was regarded sadly by many midwives, who felt that the standards of inspection and general regulation of the profession set by the CMB were somewhat higher than those maintained by the GNC, whose surveillance of training schools and nursing practice was of a more general and less detailed nature. Midwives were, however, appreciative of the fact that the Briggs Committee recognized the midwife's 'unusual degree of clinical responsibility and independence, greater traditionally than that possessed by nurses'. This recognition was expressed in the recommendations for a statutory committee and separate registration for midwives—although the basic Certificate in Nursing Practice would be common to both nurses and midwives.

A number of bodies had urged the committee that nursing and midwifery education should be made the responsibility of the Department of Education and Science and that all nursing and midwifery students should be integrated into the higher education system. The report rejected these arguments and recommended that in order for educational policies to be properly related to long-term manpower needs overall responsibility should remain with the Health Departments.

The proposals for the setting up of some 200–300 Colleges of Nursing and Midwifery Education did not of course mean the Committee were suggesting a vast building programme. Most colleges would be based on mergers between existing schools of nursing and midwifery and would use both the existing buildings and existing opportunities for clinical experience. The establishment in each college of a post of Principal, responsible directly to the governing body, meant, however, that nurse tutors were at last scheduled to achieve full independence from the nursing administrators, under whose yoke they had chafed for so long.

Among the more controversial recommendations were the suggestion that the minimum age of entry to nurse training should be reduced to seventeen years, and that educational qualifications as such should not determine eligibility to train as a nurse.

Viewed in terms of the existing structure of the nursing profession and existing arrangements for training, the Briggs proposals were radical, but the report incorporated no new ideas that had not been common currency for some time. Like the Todd Report, it put the stamp of approval on what 'progressive' elements in the profession had been saying and thinking for several years. This is perhaps the British way of doing things. Reports that are too radical and visionary are quietly shelved.

To have broken new ground the committee would have had to adopt a more daring stance than that implied in their declaration (para. 141):

'Nurses and midwives must maintain a distinct professional identity.' And again (para 142): 'We believe that medicine and nursing and midwifery will remain distinct but related professions in the future.' The interesting thing is that the Briggs approach to professional structure and training puts in question the whole traditional concept of a 'profession' and it would not have required much more than a logical extension of this kind of thinking to have embraced the suggestion that medicine, nursing, midwifery and all the professions supplementary to medicine should see themselves as part of a 'greater medical profession', with the possibility of transferring, by means of appropriate training, from one to another. The Briggs Committee stated (para. 150) 'We do not consider . . . that the future of the nurse or midwife lies in her becoming a junior medical assistant. The image of the *Feldscher* does not in our view fit into the health pattern of this country. If the nursing and midwifery profession were to be expected to undertake a greater proportion of the more frequent, boring, inconvenient or time-consuming of the doctor's tasks . . . then the caring function, to which we attach such basic importance, could be jeopardised.'

But need it be like that? About this time the nursing profession was much occupied with the problem of providing an avenue of progression for the clinical nurse, to parallel the opportunities (in terms of salary, status and satisfaction) which existed in teaching and administration. The logical solution to this problem would seem to be the development of a pathway which would lead eventually to a full medical qualification for those nurses who wished to stay in the clinical field. As an alternative to using the emotive 'image of the *Feldscher*' the committee might have examined more closely the position of the midwife, who within certain limits treats patients and administers powerful drugs on her own responsibility.

This, however, is not the place for an extended discussion of these matters. In the last chapter of the report, the committee examined the costs of implementing their recommendations and the problems, particularly of availability of manpower, to which implementation would give rise. They took a fairly optimistic view of the manpower implications. The extra expenditure on nursing and midwifery education would, they admitted, be 'substantial' and they would have liked to be able to justify this by a detailed assessment of the benefits in terms of patient care and quicker recovery. This was not possible in the existing state of knowledge and the case for increased spending therefore had to rest, as in so many previous reports, on a general conviction that a more appropriately trained profession 'could make a substantially greater contribution to patient care'.

Briggs Report, 1972

THE BASIC NURSING COURSE
Once students have been accepted, we believe that there are great advantages
both from an educational and from a social point of view in initiating all of them
to the profession through the medium of one basic course. This course would
contain a common core of clinical experience but there would be scope for
limited options. Within the framework of the course students should be able to
develop their theoretical knowledge according to their ability. We have tried to
outline the shortest possible course which will produce a safe and confident
practical nurse. The basic qualification for all students at the end of such a
course, whatever their qualifications at entry, will be a Certificate in Nursing
Practice. The objectives of all courses leading up to the acquisition of this
Certificate should be:

(a) to provide experience and related teaching in the basic nursing skills;
(b) to provide experience and related teaching in the nursing of patients with
    physical, mental and behavioural disorders, in the nursing of patients of
    different age groups and levels of dependency and, of equal importance,
    in the nursing of patients in both hospital and community settings.

Basic nursing skills can be learnt thoroughly, we believe, only in clinical
practice. A considerable part of the necessary preparation for the Certificate
should be carried out, therefore, in a variety of clinical settings, including training in an acute general hospital (adult or children's), experience in a psychiatric
service, and work with old people. Theoretical instruction should be related
step by step to the relevant practical instruction. We recognise the complexities
inherent in balancing work in the clinical and other settings, but stress that basic
education should fit a nurse to work in any field at the basic level of membership
in a nursing team.

All students would spend time on the study of the problems of nursing in the
community, and visits, attachments and courses would be arranged. This
element in education is of the utmost importance in the strategy of integration.

We do not believe, however, that experience in intensive care units or in
areas such as convalescent wards where little nursing is required, would provide
a suitable setting for pre-Certificate course work.

Work for the Certificate in Nursing Practice would begin with a four-week
introductory course which would include:

(a) a survey of the educational programme to be followed and an explanation
    of how the different elements in it are related to each other;
(b) an introduction to the organisation, operations and forward plans of the
    National Health Service;
(c) an introduction to the organisation and objectives of the social services
    and other supporting services in the area;
(d) an introduction to some of the main problems of social change, with
    particular reference to health, disease, medicine and the place of nursing
    in the caring professions;

(e) an introduction to human growth, development and reproduction in their physical and psychological aspects;
(f) an introduction to human relations and communication;
(g) a discussion of the role of the nurse and of professional ethics; and
(h) an introduction to Whitley Council, consultative and grievance procedures and an explanation of the work of trade unions and professional associations.

Following this introductory course nursing students would pursue a programme of study and work related to a core of four twelve-week 'modules'. This term has been widely used in recent years, and we referred to it in Chapter III, paragraphs 222 *et seq*. We adopt it not because it is fashionable but because it is useful. We believe that the 'modular' system enables the individual through the study of units of experience and related teaching gradually to build up knowledge and skills and acquire a deeper and larger understanding of the practice of nursing. Thereby it allows the greatest flexibility in programming. At the same time, in the course of its preparation, systematic analysis of the necessary components in a teaching programme is encouraged.

The four twelve-week modules would comprise experience in each of the four main clinical areas of medical, surgical, psychiatric and community nursing, and in each module theory and practice would be dealt with concurrently; additionally there would be at least twenty weeks' further clinical experience. Although we consider that the basic nursing skills can be learnt substantially in any of the principal settings in which nurses practise, we have chosen our four modules in such a way that the student becomes familiar with a variety of settings. We feel certain that with this experience behind them Certificated nurses will thereafter be able to perform adequately at the basic level in the nursing team in any field.

As far as possible, nursing students should be allowed to choose the type of experience covered in their first module. Thereafter the modules could be taken in any order according to local circumstances.

All students should have the equivalent of two weeks out of the twelve weeks spent on each module safeguarded exclusively for education. Determining the use and distribution of this time would be a matter for the Colleges of Nursing and Midwifery, but in every case the time set aside should provide for:

(a) an introduction to new areas of clinical experience;
(b) an element of continuing teaching during clinical experience;
(c) an opportunity for the student to summarise knowledge acquired and to clarify subjects not completely understood.

Having completed their four core modules, nursing students would need to spend a period of time acquiring clinical experience under educational guidance in order to increase their competence and confidence up to the level required of a Certificated nurse. For able students, twenty weeks would, in our view, be a sufficient period of consolidation. This consolidation period would involve one or two 'units' of clinical experience and these could be taken in any clinical setting which would provide further experience in basic nursing skills. Not more than one-third of this period should be spent on night duty.

In the selection of these further areas of clinical experience the following factors would be taken into account:

(*a*) the student's own preference and aptitudes;

(*b*) an assessment by the College of Nursing and Midwifery of the type of experience needed to ensure that the student would have been given a satisfactory balance of experience between the nursing of acute and of longer-term illness and disability and between the nursing of people in different age groups;

(*c*) the kind of clinical experience actually available locally in hospital and community nursing. The Colleges of Nursing and Midwifery would list the 'training units' available which would then have to be approved by the Nursing and Midwifery Education Boards.

The minimum period leading up to the award of the Certificate in Nursing Practice would be eighteen months, and we consider that a properly designed and efficiently implemented programme of basic education in nursing with the requisite clinical experience can be completed within this period. It will be essential for Colleges of Nursing and Midwifery to design their courses and plan their teaching in a thorough yet imaginative way. In particular, they should bear in mind from the outset that while all students will be following a common programme, they will be following it at different rates of progress and with different degrees of understanding and assimilation. Colleges should be free, therefore, to experiment with 'groupings' of students, when necessary re-grouping them from one module to another in the light of students' progress. They should ensure that individual guidance is given to each student to make the best use of his or her aptitudes. Students should be told at each stage how the Certificate course is related to later work, and with the more able students it would be possible at an early stage to discuss education beyond the first Certificate and to develop a sense of perspective and involvement in the learning process. Less able students might be required to repeat one of the core modules or to lengthen the period spent on acquiring clinical experience. We stress here the importance of providing a good system of academic and personal counselling, a subject developed further in Chapter VI. Throughout the whole process of learning, students should be encouraged to work cooperatively together and be made to feel they are members of the nursing team as they will be later on as qualified nurses.

paras. 270–81

REGISTRATION

We recommend that students who have the ability and the desire to train further after completing their statutory Certificate in Nursing Practice would apply to proceed through the next eighteen months to Registration. We see great value in also providing during this period a more academically demanding course which would lead to the award of a Higher Certificate as well as Registration. This dual course would be particularly suitable for those nursing students who had shown above-average ability in the course for the Certificate in Nursing Practice.

The Colleges of Nursing and Midwifery would guide selected Certificated students either into courses leading to Registration or into a dual course. We emphasise that a good academic counselling system, necessary during the early stages of pre-Certificate training, when the new entrant is making her or his way through often unfamiliar problems, is indispensable also at this stage when important individual choices have to be made.

The course leading to Registration should be a coherent and meaningful educational experience both for nurses wishing to concentrate on community health and those wishing to work in hospitals. There is considerable value, in our opinion, in continuity of experience, with students proceeding immediately to post-Certificate courses in the same Colleges where they had studied and worked for their Certificate. At the same time, the way should be open for mobility between institutions and for a postponement of going further ahead with professional education. Certificated nurses should be able to proceed at a later time in their lives to the Registration course and Registered nurses could take the Higher Certificate course later in their lives. We believe that given the continuation of present social trends the number of people wishing to acquire these qualifications later in life will increase.

The Registration course would include three modules of education in nursing above the level of basic skills where greater depth of study is involved. The nursing student would study two modules in the field of his or her choice and one balancing module; the balancing module for nurses interested primarily in the care of the physically ill should be a psychiatric module and vice versa. We discuss the choice of modules in more detail in paragraph 294 below. The modules would be followed by further selected units of clinical experience, and shortly before Registration all students would take part in a two-week team management course.

All students would have been given one module of psychiatric nursing during the course leading to the Certificate and this might have been obtained in a mental or a mental handicap setting. We think it desirable also that wherever possible those students who do not select psychiatric nursing as their field of choice in the course leading to Registration should have a balancing module of psychiatric experience. We suggest that where the pre-Certificate module was taken in a mental illness setting the balancing pre-Registration module might be in a mental handicap setting, and vice versa. Not only would this shift of settings and presumptions widen students' horizons and be a valuable nursing experience, but it would also shorten the additional length of time they would have to spend on post-Registration courses if and when they moved from one field of nursing to another.

Wherever experience is available an obstetric/neonatal module should be included for post-Certificate students. Paediatric experience would be obtained as a necessary part of training, as would experience of nursing elderly patients, which need not take place in specialised geriatric units. Students wishing to obtain most of their experience in sick children's hospitals or wards should be encouraged to do so when such experience is available, and hospitals for the mentally handicapped could usefully be included in the provision of this experience. The more flexible the system the better. Nevertheless, as the availability of paediatric experience will be limited, it is essential that Colleges should give priority in allocating such practical experience to those students wishing to take a Higher Certificate in paediatric nursing.

paras. 285-90

THE HIGHER CERTIFICATE

We recommend that the courses for the Higher Certificate should last six months. This Certificate would provide an additional qualification for the nurse. An eighteen-month course leading to the dual qualification might take the form of two Registration course modules followed by the six-month course for the Higher Certificate (which would include the third module) followed by one or two units of clinical experience.

The different elements in the Higher Certificate course would be studied in greater depth than subjects either in the curriculum of the Certificate in Nursing Practice or in the modules leading to Registration. They would be related both to hospital and community nursing and to the development of an integrated National Health Service. They would include:

(a) human morphology, physiology, biochemistry and microbiology;
(b) psychology (including child development) and an introduction to the social sciences;
(c) nutrition;
(d) preventive medicine and health education;
(e) the principles of treatment including the action and uses of drugs and their administration;
(f) the history and development of the nursing profession.

Nursing students following the dual course or taking a Higher Certificate after Registration would also take a clinical course in *one* of the following subjects:

(a) the nursing of medical patients;
(b) the nursing of surgical patients;
(c) the nursing of patients with orthopaedic and traumatic conditions;
(d) the nursing of mentally ill patients;
(e) the nursing of mentally handicapped patients;
(f) residential care for the mentally handicapped (arranged in conjunction with social service departments);
(g) the nursing of sick children;
(h) the nursing of geriatric patients;
(i) clinical nursing in the community;
(j) preventive nursing in the community.

At the post-Registration stage further clinical courses could be added to this list, and a second course could be taken without repetition of the common element. All midwifery courses would also include a Higher Certificate, and we expand on this in paragraphs 304 and 305.

paras. 296–8

8 The Paramedical Professions

Introduction

Although doctors and nurses are still numerically by far the largest groups of professional staff employed in the health service, new professions and technical specialisms are emerging almost every year. A year or two ago, Kissick, of the surgeon-general's department in Washington, estimated that there were close on 200 health professions in America, and it may be that the British situation is not very dissimilar. It depends of course partly on one's definition of 'profession', but probably no useful purpose is served by defining it narrowly. Historically, a number of the paramedical groups are splinter groups from either medicine or nursing who have established an independent existence. Others have had humbler origins. Theatre technicians are currently fighting hard for recognition, but not so many years ago most theatre technicians were members of the portering staff who had acquired an interest and skill in the care of anaesthetic apparatus and operating theatre equipment.

Some of the practical and operational problems to which the increasing fragmentation of the paramedical groups gives rise are discussed in the Zuckerman Report, and many of the points made in that report with reference to scientific and technical staff have equal force in relation to the remedial professions—with which of course Zuckerman did not deal. However, the remedial professions are perhaps particularly prone to feeling misunderstood and undervalued by their colleagues in the medical and nursing professions. There is a clear social hierarchy, too, with physiotherapy having the highest proportion of its members drawn from upper middle-class backgrounds, with occupational therapists next, and radiographers at the bottom of the table. Again, training is linked to status, and the professions have persistently pushed for longer periods of training.

The position of the paramedical groups, and particularly the remedial professions, is organizationally an ambiguous one. In hospitals they tend to look to medical consultants for professional leadership and support, but the consultant designated as 'in charge' of a deparment may take little interest in its detailed running. Some control will be exercised by the lay administration, but there is ample opportunity for a skilful departmental head to claim maximum autonomy by playing one off against the other. Equally, she (or he) may find herself in the unhappy position of being passed from one to the other, and getting no real support from either.

The ingenuity of the Zuckerman solution for the scientific and technical grades prompts the thought that a unified structure for all those professions directly concerned with the treatment and care of the patient—medicine, nursing and remedial professions—might offer a solution to some of the problems of training, morale and deployment which are so much in evidence to even the casual observer. So far, however, there has been little enthusiasm for the idea of a 'greater medical profession'. The remedial professions would fear that they would be swallowed up and many of them would be reluctant to be too closely associated with the nursing profession—here the question of status comes to the fore again.

The nurses have a continual crisis of identity and in recent years have redoubled their efforts to prove that their contribution to the treatment and care of patients is that of a profession with its own skills and body of knowledge and not that of a subordinate branch of medicine. So they do not take kindly to the idea. However, the McMillan Report holds out the hope of a more limited integration of the three remedial professions of physiotherapy, occupational therapy and remedial gymnastics.

8.1 Reports of the Committees on Medical Auxiliaries (Cope Reports)

Published: 1951

Chairman of all the committees: *V. Zachary Cope MD, MS, FRCS*

Members common to all the committees: *G. A. Clark VD, MD; A. B. Taylor; J. G. Paterson (secretary to July 1949); T. C. L. Nicole (secretary from August 1949)*

Members of individual committees
Almoners: *Professor F. Grundy MD, DPH; Miss M. M. McInnes; Miss M. J. Roxburgh; Professor C. Wilson MA, MD, MRCP*

Chiropodists: *St J. D. Buxton FRCS; Miss D. Grant Nisbett; Miss C. F. Norrie; J. A. Scott OBE, MD, DPH*

Dietitians: *Mrs M. C. Bowley MBE; Professor S. J. Cowell MA, FRCP, D. P. Cuthbertson MD, DSc, FRSE; G. Graham MA, MD, FRCP; Miss R. Pybus OBE*

Laboratory Technicians: *T. C. Dodds; Professor L. P. Garrod MA, MD, FRCP; J. E. McCartney DSc, MD; A. Norman; G. S. Wilson MD, FRCP, DPH*

Occupational Therapists: *Miss M. D. Barr; Miss E. M. Macdonald; L. W. Plewes MA, MD, FRCS; T. P. Rees OBE, MD, DPM*

Physiotherapists and Remedial Gymnasts: *J. T. Buchan; J. H. C. Colson; J. L. Livingstone MD, FRCP; Miss M. I. V. Mann; Miss M. U. Sharpe; T. T. Stamm FRCS; W. S. Tegner MRCP*

Radiographers: *S. Cochrane Shanks MD, FRCP, FFR; Professor G. Stead MA, DSc; G. Lovell Stiles; R. White; Professor B. W. Windeyer FRCS, FFR, DMRE*

Speech Therapists: *E. J. Boome MRCP, DPH; J. B. Gaylor MA, FRFPS; Miss E. MacLeod; V. E. Negus MS, FRCS; C. C. Worcester-Drought MA, MD, FRCP*

Terms of Reference (1949): *To consider the supply and demand, training and qualifications of certain medical auxiliaries employed in the National Health Service and to make recommendations. The auxiliaries specified were almoners, chiropodists, dietitians, medical laboratory technicians, occupational therapists, physiotherapists (including remedial gymnasts), radiographers and speech therapists.*

The Cope Reports discussed a group of professions which had come into existence for the most part to provide particular forms of treatment or carry out investigations on behalf of medical practitioners who prescribed the treatment, or ordered the investigation, and who took overall responsibility for the patient. The one group that stood out as being rather different from the others were the almoners. It was perhaps rather surprising that they were, even at that time, willing to be regarded as medical auxiliaries. Subsequently they moved away from this position and in the late 1960s allied themselves firmly with their colleagues in other branches of social work as members of a profession on a level with, and by no means auxiliary to, the profession of medicine.

In May 1949 a series of eight committees were set up to consider the supply and demand, training and qualifications of almoners, chiropodists, dietitians, medical laboratory technicians, occupational therapists, physiotherapists (including remedial gymnasts), radiographers and speech therapists employed in the National Health Service. The chairman and two other members were common to all eight committees, which were then made up with people having particular experience of each specialism. As the work progressed it became clear that many of the problems being discussed were common to all eight committees. It was therefore decided to preface the series of eight reports with a general consideration of the matters which seemed to affect each of the professions. This report on 'Matters Common to all Types of Medical Auxiliary Service' was drafted by the members common to all the committees, but at every stage it was submitted to all eight committees for discussion and approval. It was approved unanimously by four of them; in the other four there was general approval on matters of principle, but a minority preferred different administrative solutions. As printed, therefore, the Cope Reports consisted of a general report, eight reports on individual professions, and three minority reports, with a number of appendices giving detailed factual and statistical information.

The main general proposals were that there should be a statutory register of persons qualified for employment as medical auxiliaries in the NHS, and a statutory body should be set up under the aegis of the Privy Council to perform this and other functions. It should be called 'The Council for the Medical Auxiliary Services in the National Health Service'. The Council should be required by statute to set up representative professional committees to furnish it with expert information, advice and assistance. A professional committee should as a rule be concerned with a single medical auxiliary service. The Council and the professional committees should consist of medical, medical auxiliary and other members. Medical auxiliary members should be in a majority on the professional committees. Registration by the Council should be an essential qualification for employment as a medical auxiliary in the NHS.

Each of the eight committees in turn examined existing arrangements for training and qualification in its particular field, making recommendations for improvement where required. The first minority report, signed by two members of the almoners' committee, two members of the occupational therapists' committee, and one member of the committee on speech therapists, dissented from the use of the term 'medical auxiliary'. They felt this carried unprofessional implications and they preferred 'non-medical professional and technical staff'. They felt there were dangers in relating registration to employment in the NHS. If statutory registration were limited to persons qualified for employment in the NHS, two standards of qualification and practice might well emerge. They opposed the suggestion for a central council to co-ordinate and control the work of professional committees and recommended instead the establishment of separate registration boards for each profession and a central council with much more limited functions and more restricted membership. The first minority report also questioned the assumption that doctors, by virtue of their medical training and experience, could satisfactorily plan and control the curricula of training and methods of work of the professions under review, and called for stronger representation from the professions themselves than was proposed in the main report.

The second minority report, signed by four members of the committee on physiotherapists, opposed the establishment of one council for all eight professions. They noted that the five doctors and one lay member on the committee were in favour of one council for all medical auxiliaries, but the three physiotherapists and one remedial gymnast were all against. At the same time as they felt that one council would be unable to deal with the diverse problems of all eight professions, they also felt that the establishment of separate professional committees for physiotherapists, remedial gymnasts and occupational therapists would tend to segregate three professions which ought to move more closely together. They therefore proposed a Council for Physical Therapy in the National Health Service for these three professions alone with (here perhaps they flew in the face of their own reasoning) professional committees to furnish it with expert information and advice. They did not suggest what should be done with the other auxiliary professions which they had discarded from their proposed council.

In the third minority report, two members of the occupational therapists' committee dissociated themselves not only from certain points of the main report but also from the proposals put forward in the second minority report.

The Cope Reports in due course bore fruit in the Professions Supplementary to Medicine Act, 1960. The change of terminology will be noted. The principle of having one council for all the professions, with a separate board, subordinate to the main council, for each, followed closely the main recommendations of the general report, but significantly the almoners were not included in the new arrangements.

8.2 Report of the Committee on Hospital Scientific and Technical Services (Zuckerman Report)

Published: 1968

Chairman: *Sir Solly Zuckerman OM, KCB, MD, DSc, FRCP, FRS*

Members: *Professor A. R. Currie BSc, FRCP (Ed. and Glas.), FCPath, FRS (Ed.); R. Gaddie BSc, PhD, FRIC; Professor J. E. Roberts DSc; A. B. Scott MBE, MA, FHA; Professor J. P. Shillingford MD, FRCP; Professor S. Shone OBE, MD, FRCP; R. P. S. Hughes (secretary)*

Terms of Reference (1967): *To consider the future organization and development of hospital Scientific and Technical services in National Health Service hospitals and the broad pattern of staffing required and to make recommendations.*

At the beginning of the twentieth century medicine was still very largely an art, but by the 1960s one of the major problems of the modern hospital had become how to accommodate, both physically and organizationally, the rapidly growing range of scientific specialities that had grown up in support of medicine; either to provide more precise and searching techniques of investigation than the traditional clinical examination, or to make available specialized science-based treatments. The increasing use and multiplication of such techniques had over the years given rise to a number of professional and sub-professional groups, ranging from the well established radiographers and medical laboratory technicians to the more recently emerging cardiology and physics technicians. New technical developments produced new splinter groups or, even more disturbingly, ran into difficulties because it was not clear which group was best fitted to take responsibility for them. Individual workers in these fields often found hospital life frustrating because there was no proper career structure for them, and workers in the older professions gave them and their work scant recognition.

The Zuckerman Committee did not find it easy to define their field of interest, but listed the activities of hospital scientific and technical services as follows:

(i) The use of apparatus in collaboration with clinicians or on behalf of clinicians for diagnostic, therapeutic or research purposes, and the calibration, care and maintenance of such apparatus;

(ii) the development of new instruments and apparatus for use in patient care or in research;

(iii) the application of fundamental physical, chemical and biological research to medicine;

(iv) examination and analysis of body tissues and fluids;

(v) patient monitoring, measurement and recording, in association with clinical departments;

(vi) the application of statistics, data processing, and computers to medicine and medical research;

(vii) the development, construction and fitting of prosthetic appliances.

The committee identified about thirty groups of staff, numbering about 27,000, as falling within their terms of reference. Their recommendations were designed to substitute for a fragmented, uncoordinated, compartmentalized and inflexible system one in which scientific and technical services would be centralized within hospital groups and coordinated at regional and national level; a career structure would be provided to transcend professional and specialist lines of demarcation; and new technical developments could be absorbed without necessitating the growth of a new profession.

It was proposed that a Hospital Scientific Service should be set up. It should include the four main branches of pathology and the biological sciences, nuclear medicine, medical physics, biomedical engineering and applied physiology. The Department of Health and Social Security and the Scottish Home and Health Department should set up National Hospital Scientific Councils to give them expert advice on the development and organization of the scientific service, on recruitment and training, and should consider the appointment of a chief scientist. Each regional hospital board should appoint a regional scientific advisory committee and a regional scientist who would be the principal scientific officer of the Board. In each district general hospital there should be a 'division of scientific services' and scientific functions should as far as possible be grouped together geographically.

The Service should include medically qualified and non-medically qualified graduate staff, as well as technical staff, who would be re-classified into a few broad functional categories with opportunities for advancement and promotion to the higher classes according to qualifications, experience and ability.

The Zuckerman Committee considered the position of those professions falling under the jurisdiction of the Council and Boards for Professions Supplementary to Medicine which would be affected by their proposals, i.e. medical laboratory technicians, radiographers, dietitians and orthoptists, but not, for example, the rehabilitation professions, physiotherapists, remedial gymnasts, and occupational therapists. They concluded a paragraph with ominous overtones for professional autonomy by saying: 'We can foresee circumstances in which the National Hospital Scientific Council might conclude that the training approved by a Board was unsuitable or too rigid for their purposes and would find it necessary, if the Board were unable to meet their requirements, to recommend to the Ministers other appropriate amendments of the Regulations to remove or modify the requirement that State Registration should be a condition of employment for a particular class.'

The Boards for the Professions Supplementary to Medicine appear to have been set up, the Zuckerman Committee declared, on the assumption that the professions were separate. 'But it is the essence of our proposals that the professions should be brought together into one service.' So while the Zuckerman recommendations were widely welcomed by those most directly affected on the grounds that a Hospital Scientific Service would open up career possibilities that did not exist before (the frustrations of the professions supplementary to medicine have been well documented in Crichton and Crawford's 1963 study for the Welsh Hospital Board, *Disappointed Expectations*), concern was also expressed at the likely loss of professional independence for at least some of the groups involved. At the time of writing no decision on full implementation of the Zuckerman recommendations has been announced, but the DHSS have appointed a chief scientist and regional health authorities have been authorized to appoint regional scientific advisers.

Zuckerman Report, 1968

THE NEED FOR CHANGE
Apart from the pathology element, the present system, with exceptions in some regions, is primitive and unco-ordinated. It is a restrictive and exclusive arrangement in the sense that when a new development is introduced, existing departments and existing grades of staff tend neither to be ready nor able to include it within their framework. New departments may then be formed in isolation, often in improvised accommodation, with new technical classes. Many of the difficulties which hospitals have experienced in staffing their technical departments are attributable to this shortcoming.

para. 3.12

When a new development takes place, staff with the requisite technical experience may not be available either because there is no well developed scientific department in the hospital, or because the technical staff of other departments have been trained only for some particular purpose. Nor is there, as a rule, any administrative arrangement for re-allocating existing staff according to the changing needs of the specialties. As a result new technical occupations, each with its own limited and specialised training and function, come into being as new developments in medicine occur.

It is inevitable that within departments there will be some degree of specialisation, but this need not be incompatible with the development of a more broadly trained and more versatile class of technician. The whole range of hospital technical work could not be undertaken by a single class of technician, but it should be possible for most of it to be covered by two or three classes in place of the present multiplicity of separate occupations. Such a re-organisation would both provide a better technical service, and offer wider experience and more attractive career prospects for the technician.

There are considerable variations in the training arrangements from class to class. The basic training of technicians ranges from three years' full-time training before entering employment, or five years' part-time training whilst in employment, to little or no formal training at all. In some specialties the medical profession has played an active part in the promotion of training, while in others it has been left to the initiative of the technicians themselves, through the formation of staff associations which devise courses of training and award their own qualifications. In the case of medical laboratory technicians, radiographers, dietitians and orthoptists, training is now regulated under the Professions Supplementary to Medicine Act. In recent years the Health Departments, in collaboration with the medical profession, have recommended to hospital authorities schemes of in-service training for certain classes of technician. In very few cases has there been any systematic examination of functions in order to determine the content and form of training required. The general experience is that the establishment of a suitable training scheme follows long after the technical function for which it is required has developed. Further training and advanced qualifications are available in only a few of the classes, and there are no general arrangements by the hospital service for retraining or reorientation to meet changing needs.

paras. 3.16–3.18

The management, operation and servicing of sophisticated equipment, whether in the laboratory, operating theatre or wards, is a scientific and technical function. At present, because of the lack of the necessary scientific and technical service, these tasks often fall to clinicians and nurses, diverting them from the exercise of their proper duties. The deployment of such equipment and, even more, its operation, should not have to be the concern of the clinician. Moreover the present fragmentation of the scientific services is uneconomic not only in the use of manpower (both technical and scientific), but also in the use of accommodation and of equipment which may be duplicated, under-used or not freely available to all departments.

para. 3.20

THE NEW STRUCTURE

We strongly favour, both for operation, organisation and planning and for the classification and training of staff, an 'inclusive' system, i.e. one which permits a new development to be introduced without the generation of a new department or a new *ad hoc* grade of staff. Whilst specialisation is not inhibited by such a system, flexibility is achieved. The functional grouping of small departments and small groups of staff in a large organisation should often lead to greater efficiency and to a better use of resources whether of manpower, equipment or accommodation.

para. 4.5

The professional staff in the Hospital Scientific Service should have two career structures. The medical staff should normally remain, as at present, in the hospital medical staff structure. Science graduates should follow the new parallel scientific staff structure which we recommend on the lines of the scheme in Table 2. This would provide a staffing structure comprising four broad functional levels or classes, distinguished by their levels of responsibility and the training and qualifications normally required. It should be possible for medically qualified staff to join the scientific career structure at the relevant level, subject to appropriate qualifications and experience. We would expect there to be some overlapping of the classes.

Although there will be only one designation of each class, the 'specialty' of the staff, e.g. physicist, biochemist can still be recognised as in the Scientific Civil Service. . . .

There should as far as possible be common initial training for technicians and the maximum flexibility of function. All members of a class should be eligible on merit for supervisory posts, and we envisage posts with managerial responsibility which would be open to personnel of any scientific or technological discipline relevant to hospital work, and for which there would be appropriate education and training.

paras. 5.5–5.7

In our study of the scientific and technical work performed in hospitals we have identified four broad functional levels according to the education and training normally required, the knowledge and experience that have to be acquired, and the responsibilities that are carried. We recommend that for non-medical scientists and technical staff these four classes should be adopted as a framework, and that within each class there should be such grades as might be found necessary. Entrants to any of these classes should be able to make their career within that class, subject to experience and fitness for promotion, but there should also be ample opportunity for advancement to the next higher class either by obtaining the requisite qualifications or by demonstrating the necessary qualities to the satisfaction of an assessment panel drawn from more than one employing authority.

The four classes are:

(a) *Scientific Officer*. Normally recruited from graduates with 1st or 2nd Class Honours degrees or equivalent qualifications. Chartered engineers and sometimes persons with medical qualifications will also belong to this class. There should be opportunity for direct appointment to higher grades for scientists with appropriate experience outside the National Health Service.

(b) *Technical Officer.* Qualifications of the level of the Higher National Certificate. Some members of the class may be graduates.

(c) *Technical Assistant.* Training will normally include practical training, generally provided in-service, and complementary further education through courses for higher qualifications including those leading to promotion to the Technical Officer class.

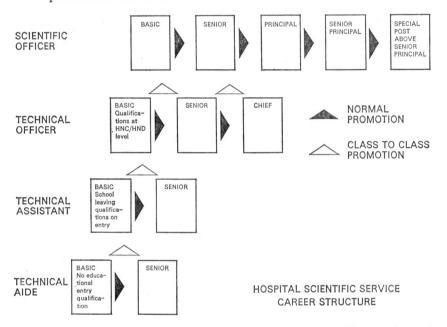

SCIENTIFIC OFFICER

TECHNICAL OFFICER

TECHNICAL ASSISTANT

TECHNICAL AIDE

HOSPITAL SCIENTIFIC SERVICE
CAREER STRUCTURE

(d) *Technical Aide.* No age limits or special qualifications. The members of this class will have the qualities required for simple routine procedures, care of equipment and other work requiring experience of hospital procedures. Training would normally be in-service and promotion by experience and length of service.

In order that Technical Officers and Technical Assistants may be readily deployed to meet new and changing requirements, we have recommended that the aim should be versatility and interchangeability and that deployment at the level of the district hospital should be the responsibility of the Division of Scientific Services. To achieve versatility and interchangeability, there should be a reclassification of present technical functions. Detailed study involving wide consultation with the interested parties will be necessary in order to determine broader vertical divisions of function, such as medical and physics laboratory work, construction and design of equipment and appliances, and the use of monitoring equipment. Those men and women who do not proceed by qualification or selection to a higher class would be eligible for higher grading within their class in respect of supervisory, advanced or specialist work.

... we envisage grades within each class reflecting the different levels of responsibility carried by the technician or the different degrees of knowledge, experience and skill required for the performance of his task. For example we envisage some chief posts entailing managerial responsibility for technical services in which a Technical Officer, as distinct from a Scientific Officer, is responsible for supervising technical services over a wide geographical area or in more than one of the broad functional divisions mentioned in paragraph 7.3. But we have not seen it as being our task to specify in detail the jobs to be done in each class. This job definition will necessarily be a continuous process and it will be a responsibility of the Divisions of Scientific Services to keep under review the work done, and requiring to be done, by technicians, and to provide regular information to those responsible for determining the grading structure of the service, for regulating terms and conditions of service, and for determining the grading of particular posts by appropriate methods including job evaluation. ...

paras. 7.1–7.4

8.3 Report of the Working Party on the Hospital Pharmaceutical Service (Noel Hall Report)

Published: 1970

Chairman: *Sir Noel Hall*

Members: *Miss N. Brierley BEM; W. R. L. Brown BPharm, PhD, FPS; Professor J. Crooks MD, FRCP (Ed.); FRCP (Glas.), FRCP (Lond.); J. S. S. Fairley MD, BChir; E. J. Fitchett FPS; W. Macfarlane; A. Roxburgh FPS; E. A. G. Spanswick; C. C. Stevens LLB; D. M. Thomas FHA, FCIS; A. J. Merifield (secretary)*

Terms of Reference (1968): *To advise on the efficient and economical organization of the hospital pharmaceutical service with particular reference to: (1) the most suitable unit(s) of organization for the whole or parts of the service; (2) the best use of pharmacists, including the need and facilities for their post-graduate training; (3) the best use of supporting staff (including their recruitment and training); (4) a suitable career structure for pharmacists and supporting staff.*

The Noel Hall Report followed a period of rising concern at the shortage of qualified pharmacists in the hospital service. Evidence presented to the working party drew attention to the high wastage and turnover in the basic and senior pharmacist grades, to what was considered the unacceptably high number of part-time pharmaceutical staff, and to shortages in both pharmacist and technician classes. A number of themes which were by then familiar emerged in the report: the need for larger units of organization to make the most effective use of available staff; the delegation of tasks that do not require the skills of a trained pharmacist to less highly qualified staff; the provision of a career structure offering improved promotion possibilities; and the training of pharmacists to meet their increased managerial responsibilities. These themes were familiar because they had already emerged from the Salmon, Hunt and Zuckerman Reports and appeared to embody principles applicable to a wide range of professional activities in the health service. In addition each professional group—which was of course heavily represented on the working party concerned with its particular specialty—was naturally ready to welcome a form of organization which provided more numerous and more lucrative opportunities of promotion for its members.

The reaction of the working party to the suggestion of the Zuckerman Committee that pharmacists and pharmaceutical technicians 'might be appropriate for inclusion' in the proposed hospital scientific service was mixed. It seemed that some members were in favour, and some were not; those who were not pointed out that 'The pharmacist is closely connected with the treatment of the patient, and he has professional responsibilities in this respect which would have to be safeguarded.'

Although evidence was presented to the working party to indicate that there was a serious shortage of pharmacists in the hospital service—figures like 43 per cent of established posts in the basic grade vacant in England and Wales in 1966 were quoted—the report accepted that the difficulties of hospitals were aggravated by failures to put available staff to the best use and to delegate suitable tasks to technicians and other supporting staff. The problems of attracting and retaining younger pharmacists were seen in terms of inadequacies in organization, salary and career structure. Although pay was not included in the working party's terms of reference —this being a matter for the Whitley Council—it was obviously hoped that the improved career structure would provide opportunities for higher earnings.

The report also included recommendations on training at varying levels for both pharmacists and supporting staff.

8.4 Report of a Working Party on the Remedial Professions (McMillan Report)

Published: 1973

Chairman: *E. L. McMillan*

Members: *Dr D. C. Ower; W. D. Paget; Mrs S. E. Reeve (until July 1973); Mrs J. M. Firth (from July 1973); J. H. C. Colson; Miss L. Dyer; Mrs E. M. G. Grove; J. S. Tapsfield; Mrs A. Brown (secretary)*

Terms of Reference (1973): *To make recommendations . . . on the future role of the [remedial] professions in relation to other professions and to the patient, and on the pattern of staffing and training needed to meet this.*

When the McMillan Committee reported, the future of the remedial professions had been a matter of discussion for a number of years. The three professions of occupational therapy, physiotherapy and remedial gymnastics had developed along separate lines for historical reasons, but if it had been possible to start with a clean slate there might not have been any need to create three professions. One—certainly not more than two— might have sufficed. Yet there they were, each with its own professional organization, its qualifying examination, and its own board under the general umbrella of the Council for Professions Supplementary to Medicine. In 1970, a committee set up by the Council under the chairmanship of Dr J. A. Oddie commented in its report that over the years there had been 'expressions of goodwill, and a general wish for a closer relationship, but few if any concrete proposals for action'.

In 1972, a sub-committee on rehabilitation of the Standing Medical Advisory Committee of the Central Health Services Council published a report (the Tunbridge Report on Rehabilitation) recommending that an analysis of the work of the remedial professions in hospitals throughout the country should be undertaken as a matter of urgency and should precede any reorganization of the remedial professions. A few months earlier, the Committee on the Remedial Professions set up by the Health Departments in 1969 had issued a brief statement in lieu of a full report in which they had supported proposals for a degree of integration between the professions, including a common first year of training.

The publication of the Tunbridge Report and the Statement of the Committee on the Remedial Professions was followed by a conference at which representatives of the professions made it clear to the Secretary of State, Sir Keith Joseph, that having waited for some years for constructive proposals for their future they felt they had been let down. They saw no prospects of progress in the development of their professions or proper recognition of the skills and service they had to offer to the community. The Secretary of State's response was to call a meeting of the professional bodies, together with the Council for Professions Supplementary to Medicine, at which he invited them to set up a small informal working party with officers of the Department of Health and Social Security, the task of which would be to produce some firm proposals and to produce them quickly. The working party was convened in March 1973 and reported in October.

In his preface, the chairman (an officer of the DHSS) emphasized the professional representatives' conviction that the three professions were at a point of crisis which could be resolved only by the firm prospect of positive action. The report set out as the most serious problems facing the remedial professions:

(*a*) misuse and waste of professional skills;

(*b*) dissatisfaction with career and salary structure;

(*c*) shortage of trained therapists (caused partly by *a* and *b*) worsened by an increased demand for their services, not matched by an increase in the numbers of those qualifying;

(*d*) inadequate support from clerical, secretarial and portering staff;

(*e*) problems of overlapping of responsibilities, not only between the remedial professions themselves but also between them and other professions, so that it was not always clear, or understood, where responsibilities should lie.

The report noted that the Chartered Society of Physiotherapy and the Society of Remedial Gymnasts were considering amalgamation. It recommended that this should go ahead and should be regarded as the first step towards uniting all three professions to form one comprehensive profession within which there would be scope for specialization. Training should also be integrated, with an integrated basic course, shorter than the existing three-year professional courses, which would equip a therapist to work at the basic level in both physical and psychiatric fields. Those who wished to proceed to more senior posts would then take further, more specialized training; courses would also be provided for those wishing to study for a degree, undertake research, or teach. The report also called for a new career and salary structure reflecting the increased responsibilities which it was envisaged therapists would undertake (*see*, for example, 'Relationship with the Medical Profession'), increased use and recognition of aides and other supporting staff, and more research into the effectiveness of remedial treatment.

McMillan Report, 1973

THE ROLE OF THE PROFESSIONS

The term 'therapist' is used by a number of professions. In this report, unless it is otherwise stated, it refers to a member of the remedial professions of occupational therapy, physiotherapy and remedial gymnastics. The remedial professions treat patients with the object of helping them to achieve maximum functional independence at work, at home, and in society. Treatment includes advice to patients, their relatives, and other members of the rehabilitation team. It can be of value to patients of all ages, it covers a wide range of conditions, and it may be given in the hospital or elsewhere in the community. Remedial therapists can assess and define the objectives of treatment; they also plan and carry out a patient's treatment programme, working in close co-operation with other members of the rehabilitation team. Each profession offers particular skills:

(a) Occupational therapy. The use of appropriate creative and work activities to achieve an improvement in the patient's physical and psychological state; the provision of work or domestic situations in which to assess and prepare the patient for re-settlement. About 50 per cent of occupational therapists work with mental illness or mental handicap, and 50 per cent with physical disability.

(b) Physiotherapy. The use of physical means to prevent injury when possible and to treat the results of injury or disease. Methods include the use of therapeutic movement, electrotherapy, hydrotherapy and manipulation.

(c) Remedial Gymnastics. Group and individual exercise therapy throughout all phases of recovery, including exercise in water. Functional training in preparation for work, recreational therapy in both general and special fields, e.g. mental illness and mental handicap.

Although each has a particular contribution to make, we recognise that there are great similarities between them.

para. 8

RELATIONSHIP WITH THE MEDICAL PROFESSION

In a medical rehabilitation service the doctor who carries primary clinical responsibility for the patient is the key figure. We do not wish in any way to detract from such responsibility but we are concerned that frequently this is interpreted as requiring the doctor to prescribe and supervise in detail the therapy provided by the remedial professions. There are many places where doctor and therapist have a relationship in which both appreciate the complementary contributions of the other, but too often therapists are given insufficient scope to exercise their skills to the best possible advantage of the patient. This attitude is crystallised in paragraph 11(iii) of the note attached to HM(62)18, which states that 'Doctors should prescribe physiotherapy with the same precise therapeutic indications in mind as they have when prescribing drugs, and the dose should be adequate to achieve the desired effect in the shortest time'. It goes on to say 'All too often therapy is prescribed in general terms and the important details such as frequency and progression of treatment, as well as arranging for attendance at medical review clinics, are left to the discretion of the physiotherapists'.

We consider that these views are based on outmoded concepts and recommend that this guidance be reviewed. The Tunbridge Report states 'surprisingly few doctors have sufficient experience of the range of modern occupational therapy, physiotherapy and remedial gymnastics to be able to prescribe in detail the most effective treatment and those who have the necessary experience rarely have time to see the patient sufficiently frequently to vary the treatment as soon as the need arises'. Therapists are not trained to diagnose, nevertheless experienced therapists can undoubtedly make a valuable contribution to diagnosis. Few doctors who refer patients will be skilled in the detailed application by therapists of particular techniques, although there will be exceptions. With this in mind, it should surely be possible for the doctor and the therapist to work together in an atmosphere of mutual respect and appreciation. We attach the greatest importance to this relationship. We think it follows that the therapist can operate more effectively only if given greater responsibility and freedom within a medically orientated team than is general at present; but this freedom must be earned. Junior therapists will not have the experience to work unsupervised, but should assume greater responsibility as their experience increases. Their ability to do so should be assessed by senior therapists.

We recommend that in hospital the arrangements operating between doctor and therapist should be on the following lines:

(a) In referring the patient for therapy the doctor would normally provide a diagnosis, and set out the aims of treatment with its limitations and contra-indications if any. He would probably say when he expected to review the case. Within this framework the nature and duration of treatment should be for the therapist to determine.

(b) Ideally, regular review sessions should be held at which both doctor and therapist should be present. If this is not possible, then the therapist's report should be available when patients are reviewed and the therapist should be kept fully informed of the findings of the review.

(c) It is important that treatment should not be initiated or prolonged unnecessarily. In our view both doctors and therapists often start and continue inappropriate treatment and we consider that both should have equal right to terminate treatment which they consider not to be of value. We recognise that this could lead on occasion to differences of opinion and we hope that the relationship between doctor and therapist will be such as to enable them to discuss the needs of the particular patient and agree on what should be done. Where for one reason or another this is not possible there must be some local means of resolving any differences of professional opinion.

(d) Where there is a properly established rehabilitation team we believe that members other than the doctor, e.g. the nurse or social worker could refer a patient to the therapist who could begin treatment and report to the doctor at the earliest appropriate opportunity.

(e) We consider it essential that the therapist should have direct access to the consultant clinically responsible for the patient.

The principles outlined above are also applicable when health service therapists work in the community, when the medical care might be in the hands of the consultant or of the general practitioner. Where therapists are employed by local authority social service departments it is important that they have access to medical advice and do not become isolated from their health service colleagues. Under the new health services organisation the district community physician might be best placed to check that such liaison is made possible and is operating effectively.

The relationship between the doctor and therapist has sometimes been confused by misunderstandings about legal liability for the consequences of treatment. In this report we are recommending greater responsibilities for therapists, but we do not consider that this affects the present legal position. Doctors have not in the past accepted liability for mistakes made by therapists, there is no reason why this should change.

paras. 20–4

9 Mental Disorder

Introduction

The subject of mental disorder deserves a part to itself not only because of the number of reports and enactments there are to choose from if we wish to compile a selection illustrative of trends in thought and practice over the last 140 years, but also because of the fierce controversies currently raging over the nature of mental disorder and the appropriateness of our traditional ways of describing it and dealing with it. There are vital questions of social policy, too, inherent in the clash between the needs of the individual and the needs of the community which have worried legislators in this field. Relatively recently the right, progressive, solution has seemed to be to adopt an attitude to mental illness that implied it was 'an illness like any other', and to provide hospitals and forms of treatment that approximated as far as possible to those provided for physical illness. Now we hardly know what to think. The 'medical model' is under attack from those who believe the behavioural manifestations of what has been taken to be mental illness to be no more than an almost inevitable response to social pressures and conditioning, rather than evidence of a pathological process in the individual. What is more rational, they argue, than to withdraw totally from an intolerable situation, even if it is into a world of fantasy and torment? Or they point to the manner in which those who are 'labelled' as mentally ill, neurotic or inadequate respond to the expectations of those around them and behave in a way that confirms the diagnosis.

In an effort to remove the stigma attached to mental illness, both outpatient and inpatient facilities have been provided in general hospitals, so that it is possible to say 'That is the eye ward, that is the chest department, and that'—with only a slight additional emphasis—'is the psychiatric unit'. Yet just as we are about to run down and close the great isolated mental hospitals the Victorians built, it is suggested that the busy general hospital might not be the right environment for the mentally ill after all, and that there might be something to be said for the original concept of an 'asylum', a place of rest and shelter.

Public attitudes to the mentally ill, and to the mentally handicapped (for they have a place in this part too), offer considerable scope for discussion. In recent years enlightened people have tried to persuade the community that the mentally ill and handicapped should be housed in the community, rather than in isolated institutions, and that they should take part in the life of the community. When policies based on these beliefs have been put into effect the community has not always been as welcoming as had been hoped. Perhaps people do not want to make the adjustments and bear the burdens that such policies require of them. If this is the case, what answer has the social administrator who has always argued that social service provision should reflect the wishes of the community?

The documents in this section in most cases illustrate trends in thought and national policy, but the Report of the Committee of Inquiry into Whittingham Hospital is one of a number of reports on mental hospital 'scandals' which appeared from 1968 onwards. These reports played an important part both in awakening the public conscience and in persuading the Department of Health to divert additional resources to a sector which had traditionally been under-financed and under-staffed. To what extent this will help solve the basic problems remains to be seen.

9.1 Final Report of the Metropolitan Commissioners in Lunacy

Published: 1844

Chairman: *Lord Ashley*

Members: *Rt Hon. P. Vernon Smith; Robert Gordon; Col William Henry Sykes; James Milnes Gaskell; John Barneby; Frances Barlow; James Robert Gowen; Dr Thomas Turner; Dr John Bright; Dr Henry Herbert Southey; Dr John Robert Hume; Dr Thomas Waterfield; Dr Francis Bisset Hawkins; Dr James Cowles Prichard; James William Mylne; Bryan Waller Procter; John Hancock Hall; R. W. Skeffington Lutwidge; Edward du Bois (clerk and treasurer)*

In 1828 the Madhouse Act, or Gordon's Act as it was sometimes known, set up the Metropolitan Commissioners in Lunacy and charged them with the duty of inspecting private asylums in the London area. Elsewhere in the country these asylums were visited by panels of local magistrates and there was a good deal of evidence that their inspections were somewhat cursory. In 1842 the Metropolitan Commissioners were given power, by the Lunatic Asylums Act of that year, to inspect all asylums and madhouses in the country twice yearly for a period of three years. The chairman of the commissioners by this time was Lord Ashley, later and better known as the seventh earl of Shaftesbury, whose maiden speech in Parliament had been devoted to the cause of the mentally ill and who was fast achieving a reputation as the foremost social reformer of his day.

In order to make feasible the plan of inspection laid down in the Act, authority was given to appoint additional Commissioners, so that there might be not fewer than fifteen and not more than twenty, of whom four were to be lawyers and six or seven medical men. It was hoped that this systematic inspection would reveal the lines which future legislation should follow, and this proved to be the case. The tours of inspection were carried out by the legal and medical commissioners, and the information they provided was used by Ashley to draft, in 1844, a final report which included a number of suggestions for amendment of the law.

The commissioners were critical of the management, as well as the siting and construction, of a number of the county asylums, although there is some evidence that the threat of inspection was itself sufficient to put a stop to a number of abuses. They found that proprietors of private madhouses often disregarded the law, and they confirmed that local magistrates often failed to take seriously their duties of visiting and supervision. Concern was expressed at the number of insane persons confined in workhouses who might have been cured if they had been transferred at a sufficiently early stage to a well-conducted asylum.

The commissioners asked for legislation to make the building of county asylums mandatory instead of permissive, and for a uniform system of inspection by a statutory authority. Reforms were called for in the system of certification so as to prevent collusion between the certifying doctor and relatives of the patient who might have an interest in his being detained. Separate accommodation should be provided for incurable pauper lunatics, so that asylums could concentrate on the treatment of curable cases. The lunacy authority should be responsible for visiting and reporting on the condition of all pauper patients, whether in workhouses or county asylums, and a central authority should be set up to approve sites and plans for all new public asylums.

The Act which followed this report—the Lunatics Act of 1845—set up a Lunacy Commission with eleven members, five lay, three medical and three legal, to constitute a permanent full-time inspectorate for all asylums and houses licensed for the care of the insane in the country (with the single exception of Bethlem Hospital in London). The medical and legal commissioners were to be paid a salary of £1,500 a year (the lay commissioners were unpaid) and a secretary was to be appointed at £800 a year. The chairman was to be elected from among the lay members. (Ashley was in fact elected and remained chairman until his death in 1885.) The commissioners were also empowered to visit gaols, workhouses and other institutions where the mentally afflicted might be found, and in the case of the workhouses they were to report their findings to the Poor Law commissioners. Otherwise their reports were to be submitted to the Lord Chancellor. The Act also revised the forms for certification and laid down records that must be kept in all institutions for the treatment of the insane. The protection of the law was extended to cover single patients being cared for for profit, although not those detained by relatives and friends, and the same certificates were now required for these 'single lunatics' as for patients detained in an institution.

A separate Act, the Lunatic and Pauper Asylums Act, 1845, made it a duty of counties and boroughs to provide asylums for pauper lunatics, or to increase the numbers of beds if there were insufficient. Smaller boroughs were to combine with the counties in which they were situated for the purpose of building an asylum.

Under Ashley's leadership—from 1851 we must call him Shaftesbury —the Lunacy commissioners presided over an era of enlightenment and progress. The commissioners' visits were seen not as mere inspections, to establish whether statutory requirements were being met, but as opportunities to advise and to spread knowledge of good and successful practices which had been introduced elsewhere. Psychiatry was emerging as a respectable medical specialty with its own journals and a specialist association, the Association of Medical Officers of Asylums and Hospitals for the Insane, founded in 1865. This later became the Royal Medico-Psychological Association and pioneered the training and examination of mental nurses on a national basis long before there was any parallel development in general nursing. Progressive doctors like Charlesworth and Gardiner Hill at Lincoln, and John Conolly at Hanwell Asylum, abolished physical methods of restraint in their hospitals, and Conolly and others used occupational therapy and education to rehabilitate their patients. Later this period came to be seen by many as a golden age of British psychiatry, which with the 1890 Lunacy Act suffered a severe setback from which it did not recover until the middle of the twentieth century.

Report of the Metropolitan Commissioners in Lunacy, 1844

THE DIFFERENT CLASSES OF LUNATIC ASYLUMS

The distinctions which exist between the various Lunatic Asylums in England, and the nature and extent of their accommodations, will be better understood, if the Asylums are divided into classes, and a brief enumeration is given of the principal points in which they differ from each other. They may be divided into five classes:—

First.—County Asylums, which have been established under the Acts of 48 Geo. III. c. 96, and 9 Geo. IV. c. 40, and have been erected by Counties, and paid for wholly out of County rates, for the reception of Paupers; but in some of which private Patients have nevertheless been received. In this class, are included the Asylums for the Counties of Bedford, Chester, Dorset, Kent, Lancaster, Middlesex, Norfolk, Suffolk, Surrey, and for the West Riding of the County of York: in this class, also, may be included the Asylum at Haverfordwest, St. Peter's Hospital, Bristol, and the Workhouse at Hull, which have been declared County Asylums under special Acts of Parliament.

Secondly.—County Asylums united with Subscription Asylums, which have been established under the last-mentioned Acts, and have been erected by Counties and subscribers, and paid for partly out of County rates, and partly by private subscription. In this class are included the Asylums for the Counties of Cornwall, Gloucester, Leicester, Nottingham, and Stafford.

Thirdly.—The Lunatic wards of the Royal Military and Naval Hospitals, supported by, and under the control of the Government.

Fourthly.—Public Hospitals, and parts of Hospitals or other Charitable Institutions, supported wholly or partly by voluntary contributions. Of this class are the Lunatic Asylums at Exeter, Lincoln, and Northampton; the Warneford, (formerly called the Radcliffe,) at Oxford, the Retreat at York, the York Asylum, St. Luke's Hospital, the Bethel Hospital at Norwich, the Lunatic ward of Guy's Hospital, the Hospital at Manchester, and the Liverpool Asylum.

Lastly.—Licensed Houses, which receive Private Patients only, Private and Pauper Patients jointly, or Pauper Patients only. This class includes the licensed parts of the following Workhouses, viz., the House of Industry for the Isle of Wight at Carisbrooke, the Workhouse at Devonport, the Houses of Industry at Kingsland near Shrewsbury, and at Morda near Oswestry.

The Royal Hospital of Bethlem is not included in the above enumeration.

Besides the several Asylums already described, there are numerous Workhouses belonging to Parishes and Unions, which are not licensed for the reception of the Insane, but which, nevertheless, contain wards exclusively appropriated to Lunatics, and receive large numbers of Insane persons, dangerous as well as harmless; such as the Workhouses at Birmingham, Manchester, Sheffield, Bath, Leicester, Redruth, in Cornwall, the Infirmary Bethel at Norwich, and others.

pp. 9–10

THE IMPORTANCE OF EARLY TREATMENT

Although it appears that pauper lunatics, in some few districts of England, are sent to Asylums soon after the first attack of mental disease, we have found that the practice of detaining them for long periods subsequently, (either in Workhouses, or as boarders with their friends, or elsewhere,) prevails to a very large extent throughout the kingdom. In order to bring this subject in a more distinct manner, before your lordship, and to show the evils which result from it, we beg to call your lordship's attention to Appendix (C.) at the foot of this report. This appendix contains the answers given to our inquiries, by the Medical Superintendents and Visiting Physicians of the different County Asylums and Public Hospitals for lunatics, and by the proprietors of a large number of licensed houses into which paupers are admitted.

In the Asylums of Lincoln, Leicester, Nottingham, and Northampton, the Superintendents and Visiting Physicians of those institutions have expressed their unanimous opinion, that pauper lunatics are sent there at so late a period of their disease, as to impede or prevent their ultimate recovery. Opinions, to nearly the same effect, have been given by the medical superintendents of every County Lunatic Asylum, with the exception of those of the Asylums for the counties of Bedford and Stafford. It is right to remark that, in some instances, there has been a reluctance to express any opinion as to the bad and hopeless condition in which pauper lunatics have been taken to Asylums, from a fear of offending either parish officers or other persons.

At the Retreat, York, at the Asylums of Lincoln and Northampton, and at the

Asylum for the county of Suffolk, tables are published, exhibiting the large proportion of cures effected in cases where patients are admitted within three
months of their attacks, the less proportion when admitted after three months,
and the almost hopelessness of cure when persons are permitted to remain in
Workhouses or elsewhere, and are not sent into proper Asylums until after the
lapse of a year from the period when they have been first subject to insanity.
The Asylums for the counties of Lancaster and Middlesex and for the West
Riding of the county of York have published statements to the same effect. In
the Dorset County Asylum, out of thirty-seven cases admitted in the year 1842,
only six were received within three months after their first attack. Five of these
six recovered, and were discharged within four months from the time of their
admission, and the sixth, a female, aged seventy-five, was improving at the time
of our visit.

In the year 1842, the cures in St. Luke's Hospital averaged seventy, and in the
year 1843, sixty-five, per cent., a fact which, even taking into account the circumstance of their receiving only recent cases, and such as are supposed to be
curable, is calculated to remove the reluctance commonly felt to send the insane
to Asylums, and to exhibit the great importance of removing Lunatics as soon as
possible after the first appearance of disease, to institutions where proper medical
treatment can be obtained.

The reasons principally assigned for the insane poor being sent so late to
Lunatic Asylums, have been the ignorance of overseers and guardians of the
poor as to the importance of early medical treatment in cases of insanity, and
their reluctance to send paupers to Lunatic Asylums, on account of the great
additional expenses incurred in those establishments beyond the ordinary cost
of maintenance in Workhouses or in lodgings. There can be no doubt that both
these causes have operated to a great extent, in improperly detaining paupers
from Lunatic Asylums. There are, however, other circumstances, which, as we
conceive, have still greater influence in causing this serious evil. Even if there
did exist on the part of guardians and overseers of the poor a full knowledge of
the importance of early treatment, and the most earnest desire to avail themselves
of its advantages, throughout almost the whole of England, and in the whole of
Wales, there is so great a want of accommodation for the reception of the insane
poor, that they could not carry their views into effect.

pp. 80–2

A PLACE OF REFUGE

The disease of Lunacy, it should be observed, is essentially different in its
character from other maladies. In a certain proportion of cases, the Patient
neither recovers nor dies, but remains an incurable lunatic, requiring little
medical skill in respect to his mental disease, and frequently living many years.
A Patient in this state requires a place of refuge; but his disease being beyond
the reach of medical skill, it is quite evident that he should be removed from
Asylums instituted for the cure of insanity, in order to make room for others
whose cases have not yet become hopeless. If some plan of this sort be not
adopted, the Asylums admitting Paupers will necessarily continue full of Incurable Patients; and those whose cases still admit of cure, will be unable to
obtain admission, until they themselves become incurable; and the skill and
labour of the physician will thus be wasted upon improper objects.

Under all these circumstances, it seems absolutely necessary that distinct places of refuge should be provided for Lunatic Patients who have become incurable. The great expenses of a Lunatic Hospital are unnecessary for Incurable Patients: the medical staff, the number of attendants, the minute classification, and the other requisites of a Hospital for the cure of disease, are not required to the same extent. An establishment, therefore, upon a much less expensive scale would be sufficient.

In illustration of these remarks we call to your Lordship's notice the rapidity with which the accumulation of patients has taken place at the Asylum for the County of Lancaster:—From the 25th June, 1842, to the 24th June, 1843, 267 patients were admitted into this Asylum. The discharges during the same period amounted to 103, and the deaths to 71, and thus were added, in that year, 93 persons, whose chance of recovery was diminished by the circumstance of it not having been effected within the first twelve months. A similar accumulation is taking place, although not to the same extent, in nearly all the county Asylums; so that a certain and progressive increase of chronic or incurable cases is produced, in all houses which have no outlet for them, a circumstance which seems never to have been contemplated by those who have the management of these large public Asylums, and for which no relief or remedy has hitherto been provided.

We are glad to remark that the Visiting Justices of the Asylums for the West Riding of the county of York, and for the counties of Nottingham and Stafford, permit the substitution of recent for old cases.

The disposal of incurable patients, however, although a very serious and difficult question, is certainly of less moment than the exclusion of curable cases from Lunatic Hospitals, which have been erected at great public cost, and are fitted up with every convenience for the purpose of cure.

pp. 92–3

OCCUPATIONS, AMUSEMENTS AND EXERCISE

By the Acts 2 & 3 Will. IV. c. 107, s. 37, and 5 & 6 Vict. c. 87, ss. 10, 34, we are directed to inquire what occupations and amusements are provided for Insane Patients; and (by the latter Act) to state the effect thereof, in-door and out-door respectively.

The answers which we have received to our inquiries have been generally, that occupations and amusements, especially such as take place in the open air, are beneficial to the bodies as well as to the minds of the Patients. Indeed, all intelligent persons who are well acquainted with the disease of Lunacy, by having seen it in its different stages and varieties, and can therefore form some opinion as to the chance of its relief or ultimate cure, are strenuous in advising that insane patients should be employed as much as possible. From the observations which we have been enabled to make on the subject, in the course of our visits through the several public and private Asylums of this country, we are disposed to concur fully in this opinion. It appears to us that employment should be afforded to all patients, whether pauper or private; and that they should be induced to occupy themselves as much as is consistent with their bodily health: not, however, with the view of deriving any profit from their labour, but solely for the purpose of relief or cure. There can be little doubt but that by amusing the mind of a patient, and diverting his attention from any idea, either painful or delusive, which occupies it, that much good may be effected. The longer a delusion is dwelt upon, the stronger and more inveterate it becomes. It is important, therefore, that it should be displaced (though only for a time) as soon as possible, by a fresh and healthy train of thought, and by occupations which may improve the patient's bodily condition, with which his state of mind is often connected, especially in the early stages of insanity. Employment, therefore, in cases of long standing, tends to the tranquillity, and in recent cases contributes materially to the recovery, of the patient.

In most instances, it is desirable to place at the disposal of the patient, the same species of occupation that he has been accustomed to follow, previously to his entering the asylum; and if he has not been brought up to any profession or trade, it may be even proper that he should be instructed in some regular pursuit, in order fully to engage his attention. It is at all times important, that as much exercise and employment as possible, in the open air, should be afforded, and that for this purpose, gardening and agricultural labour should be provided.

Without reference, however, to any pecuniary advantage that may result to the rate-payer, or to the proprietor of the Asylum, we deem it most necessary that employment should be provided for the lunatic. In fact, the labour of a Patient neither can, nor ought to, be reckoned upon as a regular source of profit. In the first place, it is uncertain; depending upon his health, temper, and disposition. A Lunatic, moreover, is a person afflicted with a positive malady, which frequently circumscribes his physical powers, and at other times exhibits itself in the shape of dangerous or violent excitement, suspending for a time, the capability of making himself useful. The object of employing a patient is not that he should make a return in value for the money expended upon him, but that his tranquillity and comfort should be promoted, and the disease with which he is afflicted, consequently mitigated or even removed. For this purpose, moderate labour only should be resorted to, and that as much as possible in the open air, in order to strengthen without fatiguing the body; and it should be of such a nature as will afford amusement, without any risk of harassing the mind.

With a view to these objects, spacious and cheerful yards, and also pleasure-grounds, should be provided, for the purposes of exercise, and of yielding the patient opportunities, at all seasonable times, of occupation and amusement in keeping them in order. But as, by these means only, sufficient employment cannot at all times be afforded to any considerable number of persons, it seems necessary that a farm, or extensive gardens, (proportioned to the number of patients), should be attached to every large Asylum, and that a variety of in-door employments should also be provided. In order to promote exercise and occupation, it is also advisable that some trifling indulgencies should be given to such patients as are willing to perform a moderate quantity of labour.

Music, dancing, and various games (as many as possible in the open air) may be resorted to with advantage, in most cases, except where the patient is too exciteable. No Asylum should be without a library. Books, judiciously chosen, especially such as will not encourage any morbid ideas already existing, are an important help in promoting a happy and serene state of mind. In cases of great depression, and particularly of religious melancholy, books of a cheerful character should be placed, to a much greater extent than is generally done, at the disposal of the patients. In most of the Asylums that we have visited, we have found an abundance of religious publications, and in some few of them little else. However useful such works may be, we have frequently urged upon the various proprietors and superintendents, the duty of their also procuring books and publications of an entertaining character, adapted to the capacity of the patients under their care.

In the better-conducted Asylums, these views are apparently acted upon to a considerable extent. Books are procured and placed at the disposal of the patients; the exercise of trades and other in-door employments is encouraged,—in some cases rewarded; and out-of-door occupation is provided by means of large gardens or farms, in which patients regularly labour in the proper seasons.

pp. 128–31

RESTRAINT

In every licensed house and county Lunatic Asylum, and also in every public hospital, and other place containing insane persons, which we have visited, we have made minute inquiries as to the particulars of every person found under restraint, and as to the system adopted in the establishment in this respect.

In some Asylums, both public and private, the superintendents and proprietors state that they manage their patients without having recourse to any kind of restraint whatever. In other Asylums, it is affirmed that the disuse of restraint is their rule and system, and that its use, in cases of necessity or expediency, forms the exception to the rule. Those who profess the entire disuse of restraint, employ manual force and seclusion as parts of their method of management, maintaining that such measures are consistent with a system of non-restraint. It is said by these persons that when any of the limbs (as the legs or hands of a patient) are confined by the strait-jacket, the belt, or by straps or gloves, he is under restraint. But in cases where he is held by the hands of attendants, or when he is for any excitement or violence forced by manual strength into a small chamber or cell, and left there, it is said that restraint is not employed, and the method adopted in these cases, is called 'the non-restraint system.' In those cases where the patient is overpowered by a number of keepers holding his hands or arms during a paroxysm of violence, it is said that there is no mechanical restraint. Here restraint of some sort or other is manifest; and even in those cases where the patient is forced into a cell by manual strength, and prevented from leaving it until his fit of excitement shall have passed, it is difficult to understand how this also can be reconciled with the profession of abstaining from all restraint whatever, so as to be correctly termed 'Non-restraint.' It seems to us that these measures are only particular modes of restraint, the relative advantages of which must depend altogether on the results.— The advocates of these two systems, to which we have called your Lordship's attention, appear to have been actuated by a common desire to improve the condition of the insane. Those who employ, as well as those who do not employ mechanical restraint, adopt an equally mild and conciliatory method of managing their Patients. The usual forms of mechanical restraint are strong dresses, strait-waistcoats, gloves, straps or belts made of linen-cloth or leather.

pp. 137–8

9.2 Idiots Act, 1886

The distinction between the mentally handicapped and the mentally ill is a relatively modern one but in medical circles at least it was well established by the middle of the nineteenth century. Work done in France to explore the possibilities of educating the mentally subnormal to achieve some degree of social competence spread to England and resulted in the founding of a School for Idiots (the term was a recognized and acceptable one at the time) at Bath in 1846, and an 'asylum for idiots' at Highgate in 1847. In 1864 the Starcross Asylum was opened at Exeter and a few years later the Northern Counties Asylum for Idiots and Imbeciles at Lancaster. Nonetheless these institutions cared for only a small proportion of the mentally handicapped, and there were many more in lunatic asylums, undistinguished from the mentally ill, and in workhouses. In 1881 nearly 30,000 mental defectives were said to be in institutional care of one kind or another, but this was widely believed to be a substantial under-estimate.

Through the interest in the problem of Sir Charles Trevelyan, the imperial administrator and civil service reformer, the influential Charity Organization Society were led to press for legislation to make better provision for the 'feeble-minded'. The fundamental philosophy of the COS was to help people to help themselves, and the Society were noted then and later for their firm opposition to the 'pauperising influence' of state aid and indiscriminate charity. Obviously Sir Charles and the medical experts had been able to convince the Society that here was a group of people who were not able to help themselves. The Society's habitual distinction between 'deserving' and 'undeserving' recipients of aid was shown here to be irrelevant.

There was of course nothing to prevent the construction of asylums for the mentally handicapped under existing legislation, which drew no distinction between mental handicap and mental illness. (Nor was such a distinction drawn in the 1890 Lunacy Act, the provisions of which applied to both.) However, it was felt that specific legislation would encourage local authorities to build, and the Local Government Board were persuaded to introduce a Bill. The Bill attracted no controversy in either House and became law in June 1886.

The Idiots Act allowed, but did not compel, local authorities to erect special asylums for the mentally handicapped ('idiots' and 'imbeciles' were the terms used in the Act) and offered the incentive of a grant of four shillings (20p) a head from the Government for every patient placed in a special institution. This was the same arrangement as was already in existence for lunatic asylums. Similar provisions as to certification and supervision by the Lunacy Commissioners were made as applied to the mentally ill. Because the Act was permissive it achieved little and few authorities made use of its provisions.

9.3 Lunacy (Consolidation) Act, 1890

The passage of the 1890 Lunacy Act has been described as 'the triumph of legalism'. It was also the triumph not merely of legalism as an abstract principle, but of the lawyers who had campaigned for many years, against the opposition of Lord Shaftesbury—the principal author of the 1845 Lunatics Act and chairman of the Lunacy Commissioners—for the introduction of more comprehensive safeguards for the liberty of the subject. It may seem strange that Shaftesbury, the great philanthropist and reformer, should oppose such a desire, but in fact Shaftesbury not only knew much of the agitation to be ill-informed, he also saw the measures the lawyers wanted to introduce as a threat to the possibility of treating mental illness in its early stages, while it was still curable. The Alleged Lunatics' Friend Society was founded in 1845 as a pressure group to arouse public opinion to the dangers of 'unjust confinement on the grounds of mental derangement'. At this date it was of course too early to see whether the provisions of the 1845 Act designed to control the abuses which Shaftesbury and others had exposed, particularly with regard to private asylums, would in the event prove effective, but the society and its successor, the Lunacy Laws Amendment Association, harassed Shaftesbury and his commissioners for the next forty years, visiting asylums and demanding the immediate discharge of any patient who appeared at the time of the visit to be capable of rational conversation.

Novelists seized on the theme of 'unjust confinement' and Charles Reade, in his *Hard Cash*, used in thinly disguised form a number of true stories dating from the early part of the century, and showing how a wealthy man might be wrongfully accused of being insane by relatives who wanted his money, but he placed his novel after 1845, as if the conditions he described were contemporary. In the 1880s an eccentric lady named Mrs Weldon, whose behaviour certainly seems to have provided *prima facie* evidence that she was in need of psychiatric treatment, brought a series of court cases against her husband, against doctors he had called in to certify her, and against various papers that had commented on the case. Some of these cases she won, others she lost, but she was a skilful

publicist and public opinion moved against the doctors. At one of the
trials the presiding judge, Baron Huddleston, expressed his concern that
the formalities required before a person could be confined in an asylum
were not more stringent.

The lawyers, headed by successive Lord Chancellors, wanted a requirement that a magistrate must be involved in the certification proceedings.
The Lunacy Commissioners opposed this because their policies, and the
policies of enlightened specialists in mental disorder, required flexibility. To the lawyers, the liberty of the subject was the prime concern,
to the Lunacy Commissioners and the doctors mental disorder was a
medical matter and could often only be detected in its early stages by the
trained judgment of the medical man. If it was necessary to wait until
the signs of disorder were so gross that they were obvious to a lay magistrate, then it would often be too late to institute effective treatment.

The question had been thrashed out before a select committee of the
House of Commons in 1859 and on the recommendation of Gilbert Bolden,
the secretary of the Alleged Lunatics' Friend Society, the committee
had incorporated in its report the proposal that a magistrate's order
should be necessary in private cases of certification, as it already was with
respect to paupers. The opposition of Shaftesbury and the Lunacy Commissioners ensured that for the time being this recommendation was not
acted upon, but in 1877 another select committee was set up with a
specific brief to consider the Lunacy Law 'so far as regards security
afforded for it against violations of personal liberty'. Public opinion continued to be disturbed by allegations that not only was it too easy for
interested relatives and complaisant doctors to secure committal to an
asylum, but also that once there the person was likely to be abused and
ill-treated by ignorant and careless attendants. It did not pause to reflect
that much of the evidence of neglect and ill-treatment related to the
thousands of the mentally ill who were housed in workhouses and workhouse
infirmaries, rather than in asylums which came under the regulation and
inspection of the Lunacy Commissioners.

Nonetheless conditions in the asylums varied enormously. The standards which obtained at Hanwell in the days of Conolly, at Lincoln, at
the Surrey asylum at Wandsworth and at the Retreat at York were by no
means universal, and Shaftesbury himself admitted that the private asylums
were always a problem because of the lack of incentive to the doctor in
charge to release any patient who was a source of profit to him. The Select
Committee were, however, convinced by his evidence that compared with
earlier days the abuses were trifling, and they did not recommend that
a magistrate's signature should be required for certification.

The report of a fact-finding inquiry commissioned by the *Lancet* in
the same year went further and recommended that admission to both
public and private asylums should be completely without formality, as

was the case with general hospitals. Dr Mortimer Grenville, under whose direction the inquiry was carried out, was of the opinion that lack of the personal touch and lack of money were the real evils of the contemporary system of caring for the insane, not insufficient safeguards for personal liberty. Judging by the subsequent course of legislation, his views were about seventy-five years ahead of his time.

Lord Shaftesbury died in 1885. Earlier in that year he had, by threatening to resign as chairman of the Lunacy Commissioners, persuaded the Government to drop a Bill designed to increase the legal formalities required for certification, but the following year two further Bills were introduced, one to consolidate existing law, the other to introduce a magistrate's order in non-pauper cases. In 1888 a new Bill was introduced, combining the chief features of both the previous Bills, and after further vicissitudes was passed in the summer of 1889. Almost immediately a Lunacy (Consolidation) Bill was introduced to consolidate all previous enactments, and this was the Bill which became the Act of 1890.

Under the Act there were four methods of admission to an asylum or house licensed for the care of lunatics: (i) reception order on petition by a relative or friend to a justice of the peace, supported by two medical certificates; (ii) urgency order, requiring a relative's petition and one medical certificate only, but valid for no more than seven days; (iii) summary reception order, the normal method for pauper patients, requiring a justice's order and two medical certificates; (iv) admission by inquisition, a complex procedure for use in cases where substantial property was involved. There were detailed regulations governing the signing of certificates and orders, and stringent requirements for visiting and inspection of all asylums and licensed houses were laid down. Patients had the right to send letters to the Lord Chancellor, a Judge in Chancery, a Secretary of State, a Lunacy Commissioner or a Chancery Visitor, and these were to be forwarded unopened. Notices explaining these rights had to be exhibited as directed by the Lunacy Commissioners. There were provisions for patients to be discharged by the Lunacy Commissioners, even against the opinion of the responsible medical officer, and any patient who escaped from an asylum and succeeded in remaining free for fourteen days had either to be discharged or re-certified.

Not surprisingly, with all this legal apparatus, doctors came to consider admission to an asylum as the last resort in the treatment of mental illness. Both mental nurses and doctors who wished to specialize in psychiatry found that matters of law and procedure figured as prominently in their training as did the causes and treatment of mental illness. Together with the tendency to build very much larger mental hospitals about this time, the Lunacy Act has been held responsible for the era of custodial care which succeeded much that was hopeful and forward-looking in British psychiatry in the mid-nineteenth century.

9.4 Mental Deficiency Act, 1913

The 1913 Mental Deficiency Act implemented, after a five-year delay, the main recommendations of the 1908 Report of the Royal Commission on Mental Deficiency. The reluctance of the Government to rush into legislation was exasperating to those who believed legislation was urgently required both to protect the mentally defective from exploitation and to protect society as a whole from their uncontrolled increase and from the delinquency into which they could be so easily led, but it was understandable. The Government had a great deal else on their hands and the trouble encountered by a private member's Bill on the subject in 1912 gave a foretaste of the bitter opposition which was to be mounted against the Government's own measure by MPs and others who saw in it a threat to the liberty of the subject. There were in fact two private members' Bills introduced in 1912 before the first Governmnet Bill was brought in in May. This Bill lapsed at the end of the session and a new Bill, which eventually became the Mental Deficiency Act, was introduced in March 1913. It was tenaciously opposed through all its stages by a small group of MPs who represented it as putting 'into prison 100,000 people who are at present at liberty', and as setting up 'a horde of salaried officials'. After numerous divisions and some all-night sittings the Bill was eventually passed and received the Royal Assent in August.

The Act set up a Board of Control, who in addition to supervising the new provisions for mental defect were to take over all the powers previously vested in the Lunacy Commissioners as far as the mentally ill were concerned. The Board would consist of fifteen members, twelve of them salaried, and would include the existing four medical and four legal Lunacy Commissioners. The Board were to supervise local authorities in their discharge of duties under the Act, to visit and inspect all institutions for the care of the mentally defective, and to visit every defective under guardianship twice a year. Special institutions were to be provided by the Board for mental defectives considered to be violent and dangerous. The Board were to report annually to the Home Secretary and the Home Secretary was himself empowered to make regulations regarding certification, institutional management, classification and treatment of patients, inspection and visitation, discharge and absence on licence, guardianship and research.

Each county or county borough council were to set up a mental deficiency committee to ascertain persons subject to be dealt with under the Act within the authority's area, provide and maintain institutions, and care for or supervise mental defectives in the community. Subsequently many authorities made use of the powers given them by the Act to finance the work of voluntary mental welfare associations rather than carry out the work themselves, and thus there came about a fruitful partnership between statutory provision and voluntary effort, a partnership which was for many years much more marked in the case of mental deficiency than in mental illness.

Four grades of mental deficiency were defined in the Act: idiots, imbeciles, the feeble-minded, and moral defectives. Moral defectives were those who from an early age showed 'some permanent mental defect coupled with strong vicious or criminal propensities on which punishment had little or no effect', a group similar in most respects to those who later came to be regarded as 'psychopaths', a category notoriously difficult to define (mental defect as such was not necessarily present in later definitions) but apparently necessary as a residual category for those whose behaviour indicates that they do not respond to normal social controls. The other three grades represented degrees of intelligence, with idiots as the lowest grade, and the feeble-minded as those who later came to be referred to as 'high-grade' defectives. For many years these 'high-grades' did much of the day-to-day work of most hospitals and colonies for the mentally handicapped and the economy and staffing of these institutions underwent a drastic change when policies were adopted which resulted in the discharge of such patients into the community.

The circumstances in which a mental defective became 'subject to be dealt with', i.e. sent to an institution or placed under statutory guardianship, were set out in the Act. Normally the initiative lay with the parent or guardian to petition the local authority; two medical certificates were necessary and unless the patient was certified as being an idiot or an imbecile, a magistrate's order was also required. If the patient was neglected, abandoned, cruelly treated or without visible means of support the local authority could seek a magistrate's order, again with two medical certificates. In other circumstances the patient might be detained under a court order, for instance if he had committed a criminal offence and was found to be defective. Orders for detention or guardianship (which conferred on the guardian the powers normally exercised over a child, whatever the chronological age of the patient) were for one year in the first instance, and then for five years at a time.

Following the passage of the Act local authorities were chivvied both by the Board of Control and by the Central Association for the Care of the Mentally Defective (later the Central Association for Mental Welfare) to meet their obligations under the new legislation. The building of new hospitals was slowed down by the outbreak of war but between 1914 and 1927 the number of beds provided rose from 2,163 to 5,301. Institutional care was of course available for only a small proportion of the defectives ascertained by local authorities—over 60,000 at the latter date—and it was thought in many quarters that there were as many again who had not been ascertained but who ought to have been. They were to be found struggling at the bottom of classes in schools where teachers did not recognize the problem as one of innate deficiency, in the wards of mental hospitals, from which they could not be discharged because there was no alternative accommodation for them, and in workhouses. In successive reports the Board of Control urged local authorities to improve their ascertainment, to employ properly trained officers for the work—the Central Association had organized a range of training courses for work with mental defectives— to set up occupation centres and industrial centres for defectives who needed supervision but did not need to be admitted to an institution.

The change of emphasis from institutional to community care reflected both the difficulty of getting local authorities to spend large sums of the ratepayers' money on providing and maintaining residential institutions, and a growing belief that many mental defectives were better cared for in the community. The old belief in the necessity for segregation which had informed much of the evidence to the Royal Commission of 1908 was dying away. The opportunity to stress local authorities' duties of super- vision in the community, and to lay on them a duty to provide occupation and training as well as supervision, was therefore taken in the Mental Deficiency Act of 1927, which was passed primarily to bring within the scope of legislation a class of patient that had not previously been con- sidered. This was the person who suffered from a defect brought about by arrested development, caused by disease or injury. The wording of the 1913 Act, which specified that the defect must be present 'from birth or from an early age' had excluded these cases, but the necessity to include them was brought home to the nation by the 1926 epidemic of *encephalitis lethargica* (sleeping sickness), and so mental defectiveness was redefined as 'a condition of arrested or incomplete development of mind existing before the age of eighteen years, whether arising from inherent causes or induced by disease or injury'. Otherwise the definitions of the various classes of defect in the 1913 Act were left undisturbed.

9.5 Report of the Royal Commission on Lunacy and Mental Disorder (Macmillan Report)

Published: 1926

Chairman: *H. P. Macmillan PC, KC*

Members: *Earl Russell; Lord Eustace Percy MP;* Sir Humphry Rolleston Bt, KCB, DM, PRCP; Sir Thomas Hutchison Bt;† Sir Ernest Hiley KBE; Sir David Drummond KBE, DM; W. A. Jowitt KC; F. D. MacKinnon KC;‡ H. Snell MP; Mrs Anna Mathew; Miss Madeleine Jane Symons; P. Barter (secretary); W. Fairley (assistant secretary).*

*Resigned November 1924 on his appointment as President of the Board of Education
†Died April 1925
‡Succeeded by N. Micklem on his appointment as a High Court Judge

Terms of Reference (1924): *To inquire as regards England and Wales into the existing law and administrative machinery in connexion with the certification, detention and care of persons who are or are alleged to be of unsound mind; to consider as regards England and Wales the extent to which provision is or should be made for the treatment without certification of persons suffering from mental disorder; and to make recommendations.*

The Macmillan Report laid the foundations for the Mental Treatment Act of 1930 and for a new approach to the treatment and care of the mentally ill. This approach was based on what was in its day an enlightened understanding of the nature of mental illness and on a balanced view of the conflict between the patient's need for treatment and the necessity of safeguarding his civil liberties. Two eminent doctors—Sir Humphrey Rolleston and Sir David Drummond—served on the Commission, and the lucid statement of up-to-date views on mental illness and its treatment which appeared in the second chapter of the report made an important contribution to educating public opinion on the subject. The line taken in this statement was that mental disorder was an illness, more or less like any other, which should be regarded, and as far as possible treated, like any other illness. Gradual acceptance of this view of mental illness over the next three decades was responsible both for some improvement in public attitudes to mental illness and the mentally ill, and for a growing desire on the part of progressive mental hospitals to become as much like general hospitals as possible. It was not until the 1960s that this medical model of mental disorder as a determinate disease process with an underlying pathology—physical or mental—amenable to treatment if the cause could be correctly ascertained, was seriously challenged, and by that time the whole concept of disease, even in physical medicine, was undergoing profound modification. By then it could be argued that mental hospitals should stop trying to ape general hospitals, that the very title 'nurse' was a handicap to those who cared for the mentally ill by virtue of the inappropriate expectations that it generated, and that a generation of psychiatrists which had emphasized disease categories and the efficacy of certain forms of physical treatment had seriously misled the public about the true nature of mental illness.

However, this is to leap ahead. At the time the Macmillan Commission were appointed there was a good deal of public uneasiness relating to the administration of the lunacy laws and allegations were being made both that large numbers of sane people were being detained as insane, and that cruelty was widespread in the public mental hospitals. From this, no doubt, sprang the fact that the majority of members of the Royal Commission were lawyers, but it was to their credit that they did not take a narrowly legalistic view of the problem and made recommendations for changes in the law designed to facilitate early treatment of mental illness. They laid down the principle that the law, in dealing with cases of mental illness, should extend no further than was necessary to ensure: (a) that no mental patient's liberty was infringed longer or to a greater extent than his symptoms necessitated in his own or the public interest; (b) that advantage was not taken of his disabilities to neglect or ill-treat him; and (c) that he received proper treatment for his ailment.

The Royal Commission were bombarded with applications from mental hospital patients and former patients wishing to give evidence pointing to abuses in the system, and the National Society for Lunacy Reform also put forward a number of former patients as witnesses. After a somewhat stormy two and a half days' public examination of the first of the Society's witnesses the commissioners announced that as this expenditure of time and effort had resulted 'in the eliciting of only a few material facts which the commissioners could have themselves obtained in at most an hour or two', they would examine further witnesses in private. They subsequently examined twelve former patients and two former nurses, but did not find 'that the evidence received from this source made any constructive contribution of material value to the main purpose of our Inquiry'. The commissioners also received a 'voluminous' correspondence; many of the letters were requests for the discharge of a particular patient, a number were unintelligible. Finally they visited, without notice, twenty-five institutions in various parts of the country, and spoke with many patients, including some who had written letters to them.

The Commission found the existing law complex and recommended that any changes should be in the direction of simplification and of approximating the treatment of mental illness as far as possible to that of physical ailments. Certification should be a last resort, and not a necessary preliminary to treatment. The procedure for certification when it had to be invoked should be simplified, should be made the same for private and rate-aided patients, and should be dissociated from the Poor Law. Under the existing legislation a patient who could not afford to pay the full cost of private treatment found that certification carried with it automatic classification as a pauper, even though he was contributing to his own maintenance. Thus he suffered from the double stigma of certification and the Poor Law.

There should be two classes of case: voluntary and involuntary. Any person should be eligible for treatment as a voluntary boarder on making a written application. Such patients should be allowed admission to any public mental hospital, registered hospital, licensed house, general hospital or nursing home, and should be entitled to discharge themselves on seventy-two hours' notice in writing. An involuntary patient with an early prospect of recovery should be treated under a provisional treatment order, which could be kept in force for up to six months; otherwise certification would be necessary. In addition, there should be emergency procedures to enable a patient to be detained for up to seven days while steps were taken to secure either a provisional treatment order or a reception order.

The report considered the position of the Board of Control but rejected the suggestion that it should be absorbed into the Ministry of Health. To meet the criticism that the Board was inaccessible because its fifteen members were always on visitation it was recommended that a smaller Board, of four members, all of whom would be based in London, should be created, and the visiting should be carried out by fifteen assistant commissioners.

The commissioners declared themselves well satisfied with the general standards of care in the twenty-five hospitals they visited and gave their opinion that 'the wholesale allegations of neglect and ill-treatment which are sometimes made in regard to the present system' were unjustified. However, some improvements were required, including greater contact with the outside world; relief of the medical superintendents from administrative details which then occupied too much of their time; increases in medical staff and more opportunities for them to study for post-graduate qualifications; the more widespread use of women nurses on male wards; better classification of patients within hospitals to allow for the segregation of noisy or objectionable cases and the provision of separate admission wards; improvements in lavatory and toilet accommodation; and greater facilities for employment and recreation. The commissioners also recommended that no more hospitals of more than 1,000 beds should be built and that the design of future mental hospitals should be based on the villa system.

Macmillan Report, 1926

GENERAL CONSIDERATIONS OF POLICY

We think it desirable to place on record at this stage certain general impressions which our study of the problems before us has left upon our minds.

It has become increasingly evident to us that there is no clear line of demarcation between mental illness and physical illness. The distinction as commonly drawn is based on a difference in symptoms. In ordinary parlance a disease is described as mental if its symptoms manifest themselves predominantly in derangement of conduct, and as physical if its symptoms manifest themselves predominantly in derangement of bodily function. This classification is manifestly imperfect. A mental illness may have physical concomitants; probably it always has, though they may be difficult of detection. A physical illness on the other hand may have, and probably always has, mental concomitants. And there are many cases in which it is a question whether the physical or the mental symptoms predominate.

The rough and ready distinction drawn by the public between mental and physical ailments, notwithstanding its merely empirical character, is no doubt practically convenient but, as the sequel will show, it has had an undue influence in the development of our lunacy system.

The derangement of conduct with which the idea of mental illness is popularly associated may take many forms. It may manifest itself in irrationality of speech, abnormality of emotion, extravagance or violence of behaviour. But the common feature is the inability of the patient to maintain his social equilibrium; he has lost his balance, as the phrase goes. It is this special characteristic of his symptoms which has led to the setting apart of the mentally afflicted from all other sufferers. Human society is intolerant of the abnormal and instinctively seeks to protect itself from the aberrations of such of its members as will not or cannot conform to the accepted code of social conduct, by expelling them from its company and confining them in isolation. The first impulse of society has been to safeguard itself against the menace to its comfort and security which such persons constitute by putting them out of harm's way.

A survey of the early history of the treatment of the insane in this country thus discloses, as might be expected, a predominance of the idea of detention.

The primitive and crude methods of dealing with the problem which formerly obtained were fostered by inherited superstitions which regarded the insane as the victims of a mysterious visitation of Providence. With the advance of medical science and the growth of more enlightened views insanity is coming to be regarded from an entirely different standpoint. It is being perceived that insanity is, after all, only a disease like other diseases, though with distinctive symptoms of its own, and that a mind diseased can be ministered to no less effectively than a body diseased. But the old conception of insanity dies hard and its traces are still persistent. The modern conception calls for the eradication of old established prejudices and a complete revision of the attitude of society in the matter of its duty to the mentally afflicted.

paras. 38-40

The keynote of the past has been detention; the keynote of the future should be prevention and treatment. But it is just here that the crucial difficulty of the whole matter resides. Owing to the special nature of the symptoms of mental illness, treatment must in many cases involve compulsion and restraint. This is the element which differentiates the treatment of insanity from the treatment of other illnesses. The patient suffering from an ordinary ailment is generally an intelligent co-operator in his own treatment and cure; he is able to appreciate what is being done for him and no coercive restriction of his liberty is needed. In many cases of insanity this is not so. The illness has affected the patient's intelligence and his ability to appreciate his position. His will has ceased for the time being to be rational. In such cases where there can be no voluntary submission to treatment, the treatment must needs be compulsory.

It is round this problem of compulsion that the main controversies of our subject have centred. The liberty of the individual to manage himself and his property is a cardinal principle of our law. But it must always be remembered that the principle is not an inviolable one. No man can be a member of society without sacrificing some of his liberty. He is entitled to exercise his liberty of action in so far only as he does not thereby infringe the liberty of others. If he insists on exercising his liberty so as to cause danger to others he must suffer restraint. The price of liberty is conformity to the social order of conduct. Thus the citizen who abuses his liberty by infringing the criminal law has his liberty restricted by imprisonment. In the case of certain infectious diseases the sufferer has his liberty restricted by the requirement that he must be isolated from his neighbours lest he infect them with his malady. And so, in the case of the insane who may do injury to themselves or to others some infringement of their liberty is essential both in their own interest and in that of the community. In the case of the criminal, no doubt, his temporary isolation from the life of his fellows is dictated by the motive of deterrent punishment. This element was not altogether absent from the primitive methods of dealing with the insane. But in this connection it is entirely wrong. As regards the mental patient himself, compulsory detention ought to have one object and one object only, the protection, treatment and, if possible, cure of the patient.

The accommodation then of these two conflicting principles, the principle of the liberty of the subject on the one hand and the principle that the treatment of the disease of insanity frequently necessitates the restriction of that liberty on the other hand, constitutes the problem of the legislature in this department of the law. The existing lunacy code represents the present stage of the compromise. It recognises that there must be power to infringe the liberty of the subject in the case of the insane and its concern is to ensure that such necessary infringement shall be safeguarded from abuse. It is manifest from a perusal of the anxious provisions of the code that it is designed to secure that the liberty of the subject shall be restricted only so far as and so long as the condition of the patient necessitates it. We shall hereafter consider its efficacy in this respect. Meantime we may observe that the very pre-occupation of the legislature with this aspect of the matter, important as it is, would seem to have led to some neglect of the other, and not less important, matter of the treatment and cure of the patient.

From the foregoing considerations a practical conclusion emerges, namely that every facility and encouragement should be afforded to mental patients of submitting themselves voluntarily to treatment. The public, and the legislature reflecting public opinion, have been too prone to draw a definite line between the sane and the insane and to prescribe freedom for the sane and detention for the insane. There is no such line. Complete irresponsibility even among the admittedly insane is by no means universal. The degrees of mental instability are infinite. Restriction of liberty is necessary only where the instability has reached the stage of being a danger to the sufferer himself or to his neighbours or is such that the patient is incapable of managing himself. In slight or incipient cases compulsion is unnecessary and harmful. But it is in such cases and at that stage that curative treatment is most valuable and is likely to be productive of the best results.

In this connection an anomaly which has much struck us is that except in the case of registered hospitals and licensed houses the doors of our institutions for the treatment of the mentally afflicted are closed to all but certified cases. In order that a patient may qualify for the benefit of treatment in any of the mental hospitals maintained with public money (with the exception of Maudsley Hospital and the City of London Mental Hospital) he must first be certified. But the pre-requisite of certification is that the patient's disease shall be so definite and well-established that he can be declared by a medical practitioner to be actually of unsound mind and in a condition justifying compulsory detention. In the case of every other type of institution for the treatment of disease the aim is to get in touch with the patient at the earliest possible stage of his attack and by care and treatment to ward it off or at least mitigate its effects. Not so in the case of insanity. Contrary to the accepted canons of preventive medicine, the mental patient is not admissible to most of the institutions provided for his treatment until his disease has progressed so far that he has become a certifiable lunatic. Then and then only is he eligible for treatment. It is perhaps not remarkable in these circumstances that the percentage of recoveries in public mental hospitals is low. In our view the position should be precisely reversed. Certification should be the last resort in treatment, not the pre-requisite of treatment. Hence the necessity in our opinion not only of making all institutions available for the reception of voluntary uncertified patients, subject to proper safeguards against abuse, but also of making provision either in connection with existing institutions or by the provision of new institutions, for the treatment of mental disease from the very earliest moment of the appearance of its symptoms.

The explanation of the anomaly to which we have alluded is no doubt to be found in the anxiety of the public mind with regard to the exercise of compulsion. The idea persists of a mental institution as a place where people are confined against their will. Hence the rule of law that none shall be confined in them but such as require confinement. But if the asylum be regarded, as it ought to be, not as a place of detention but as a hospital for a special type of disease, the symptoms of which in only a proportion of the cases necessitate compulsory detention as an incident of treatment, the whole outlook is changed. Compulsory detention will no doubt always be necessary in a large number of cases, but it should be regarded not as an object in itself but only as incidental to the treatment of the case.

We are in no way disposed to belittle the importance of protecting the public against the possibility of unlawful detention, but we are inclined to think that the emphasis laid upon this aspect of the matter has tended to obscure other equally important aspects. The existing lunacy code bristles with precautions against improper detention. No safeguards that can be devised can be absolute. The proposals we have to make for the treatment and observation of incipient cases and for the postponement of certification will, we venture to think, provide additional safeguards. At present, when a case must in general be either certified or not certified and can only be received in a public mental hospital for treatment if certified, both doctors and judicial authority may in doubtful cases be influenced to take the course attended with least risk to the patient and the public. The truth is that insanity is not a definitely ascertainable state. It is a matter of degree, upon which there must often be room for honest difference of opinion. Yet the task imposed upon the doctor is either to certify or not to certify, in either case at his peril. We shall endeavour to suggest means for remedying this state of matters.

paras. 42–6

Another aspect of the present day treatment of insanity which has been brought home to us is the extent to which it is associated with the poor law. For this there are no doubt historical reasons and reasons of convenience. Without in any way disparaging the great services rendered by boards of guardians and poor law officials in the administration of the lunacy laws we cannot but feel that this association is unfortunate. It is another of the causes which have tended to accentuate the differentiation of the mentally afflicted from other sufferers. Many households make their first acquaintance with the relieving officer in connection with the occurrence in the family of a mental case. It is not a concomitant of other illnesses that the patient in order to obtain treatment must necessarily become in law a pauper. The present legal status of the great bulk of the insane persons in this country is that of paupers. They have become in law paupers because they have been overtaken by this particular form of illness, although they may never before have been in contact with the poor law. Indeed, patients of means may in certain circumstances have to pass through a stage which renders them in law paupers before they regain the status of private patients. There runs, moreover, through the whole existing lunacy code a distinction in procedure between the pauper case and the private case, the justification for which has largely disappeared under modern social conditions. We desire to see the treatment of mental disease freed as far as possible from its present association with the poor law. We recognise, however, that the whole question of the poor law is at the moment under consideration and its abolition, indeed, contemplated. It will be necessary in any scheme designed to this end to take cognisance of the extent to which the machinery of the poor law is utilised by our lunacy system and to provide new machinery in substitution.

para. 49

We are satisfied that under the present system a considerable number of persons are certified who might avoid certification if certification were preceded by a period of observation and treatment, coupled if necessary with temporary or provisional powers of detention. Statistics with which we have been furnished show that a substantial number of cases, often very acute cases, recover completely within a short time. Such patients if provisionally detained under a modified system might avoid certification altogether. The number who would avoid certification would also undoubtedly be increased if greater facilities existed for persons who are willing to submit themselves to treatment and if access to treatment were not preceded by the necessity of taking the irrevocable step of certification.

para. 51

9.6 Mental Treatment Act, 1930

The Mental Treatment Act made the first real breach in the legal fortress erected by the 1890 Lunacy Act, although the latter Act continued in force and was not repealed until 1959. For those professionally engaged in the care of the mentally ill one disadvantage of this was that the new Act meant yet another set of procedures and regulations to memorize without being able to abandon any of those already in force. To the category of certified patients, still governed by the 1890 Act, the Mental Treatment Act added the categories of 'voluntary' and 'temporary' patients. A voluntary patient was one who himself made application for treatment in a mental hospital, and who retained the right to discharge himself at any time on giving seventy-two hours' notice. In the case of a child the parent or guardian could make application. While voluntary patients had to be capable of expressing volition to qualify as such (mere failure to object to admission, as in the case of a confused or delirious patient, was not sufficient), a temporary patient was defined as one who was suffering from mental illness and likely to benefit from treatment, but who was for the time being incapable of expressing himself as willing or unwilling to accept treatment. Temporary patients could be detained for six months in the first instance, and then for two further periods of three months, but at the end of a year had either to be discharged or certified under the provisions of the Lunacy Act. In any case if a patient regained the power of volition he was entitled, unless he expressed a wish to continue to receive treatment as a voluntary patient, to be discharged within twenty-eight days.

The Act thus catered for two important classes of patient in a more satisfactory way than had hitherto been possible. Entry to hospital as a voluntary patient was not entirely without formality, but it was hoped that it would be without stigma. (Unfortunately, for many years and even perhaps up to the present day, stigma attached to mental hospitals as such and not merely to the mode of admission, although of course certification did carry an additional stigma of its own.) Thus it became possible to treat in hospital both patients in the early stages of serious mental disorder which, if untreated, might necessitate certification, and patients suffering from less serious mental and emotional disturbances and behaviour disorders who would never be certifiable but who could be helped by hospital treatment. The temporary classification avoided the stigma of certification for those patients whose mental disorder had an underlying physical cause and who could be expected to recover when that cause was treated. Patients suffering, for example, from puerperal psychosis, who had formerly often had to be certified for their own safety and that of the child, were now normally treated as temporary patients.

The admission of voluntary patients to mental hospitals had, from the point of view of the other patients, both advantages and disadvantages. They benefited from increased freedom in cases where progressive doctors and administrators saw the need to adopt a less restrictive regime than in the past, when it was a serious matter to allow a patient to 'escape'. This development should not be over-stated, however. In most hospitals it was another three decades before a jangling bunch of keys ceased to be the symbol of office of the mental nurse. A less happy consequence of the Act was the emergence of two standards of accommodation, staffing and treatment, with those wards set aside for voluntary patients becoming the showpieces where the psychiatrists spent most of their time, and where the younger and more intelligent mental nurses were put to work.

Other provisions of the Act permitted local health authorities to provide psychiatric out-patient clinics at general or mental hospitals, to make arrangements for the after-care of discharged mental patients, and to foster research into mental illness. The Act also reorganized the Board of Control, reducing it to a chairman and not more than five members, all of them paid and to be known as Senior Commissioners, assisted by a staff of full-time salaried commissioners, and it brought the terminology of mental illness up to date. The word 'asylum' was replaced by 'mental hospital' and the 'lunatic' became the 'patient' or 'a person of unsound mind'.

The Mental Treatment Act did not go as far as the Royal Commission on Lunacy and Mental Disorder had urged but the Government's caution was rewarded with a relatively easy passage through both Houses of Parliament. The lawyers were disarmed by the moderate nature of the changes proposed and by the assurance of the Government spokesman, himself a barrister, that a doctor was 'not the sinister figure which in former times he was represented to be, anxious to confine a man in a dungeon for life'. In fact many doctors were anxious to take advantage of the opportunities the Act gave them to treat mental disorder on an out-patient basis and in its early stages. During the 1920s and 1930s a number of physical treatments were introduced—electro-convulsive therapy, leucotomy, insulin and malarial therapy—which appeared to offer more hope when used before patients had sunk into long-term mental deterioration. (It was not widely realized at the time how much of this deterioration was

due to the regime imposed by the institution rather than to factors inherent in the patient's illness.) The rediscovery of occupational therapy
and the development of therapeutic techniques based on the teachings of
Freud also appeared to have more relevance to the needs of those suffering
from acute short-term illnesses and from neurotic disorders than to those
of patients who had been in the hospital for perhaps ten, twenty or thirty
years.

9.7 Report of the Royal Commission on the Law Relating to Mental Illness and Mental Deficiency (Percy Report)

Published: 1957

Chairman: *Baron Percy of Newcastle*

Members: *Sir Cecil Oakes CBE; Sir Walter Russell Brain MD, PRCP; T. P. Rees MD, MRCS, MRCP; Hester Adrian; Claude Bartlett; Elizabeth Margaret Braddock; Harry Braustyn Hylton Hylton-Foster QC; Richard Meredith Jackson LLD; David Howell Hugh Thomas MRCS, LRCP; John Greenwood Wilson MD, FRCP, MRCS; Jocelyn Edward Salis Simon QC; H. M. Hedley (secretary)*

Terms of Reference (1954): *To inquire, as regards England and Wales, into the existing law and administrative machinery governing the certification, detention, care (other than hospital care or treatment under the National Health Service Acts, 1946–52), absence on trial or licence, discharge and supervision of persons who are or are alleged to be suffering from mental illness or mental defect, other than Broadmoor patients; to consider as regards England and Wales, the extent to which it is now, or should be made, statutorily possible for such persons to be treated, as voluntary patients, without certification; and to make recommendations.*

The Percy Report took up the unfinished business of the Macmillan Commission of 1924–6, recommended sweeping changes in mental health legislation, and led in due time to the passing of the Mental Health Act, 1959. On only a few points did the Act diverge from the recommendations of the Royal Commission and, unlike that of the Macmillan Commission, the work of the Percy Commission really did inaugurate a new era in the care of the mentally ill and the mentally handicapped. While the 1930 Mental Treatment Act represented an important advance, the 1890 Lunacy Act continued in force as the basic legislation, perpetuating what Kathleen Jones has described as 'the triumph of legalism'.

The appointment of the Royal Commission was announced in October 1953, and early in 1954 a debate took place in the House of Commons on a motion by Kenneth Robinson—then in Opposition but later to become a Labour Minister of Health—which called for the modernization of the mental health service. Robinson focused on four main shortages—of beds, suitable buildings, staff and money. Later speakers challenged the idea of a shortage of beds, pointing out that modern trends were towards increasing community care rather than keeping patients in hospitals. The debate showed the House of Commons at its best, discussing a non-party question in an informed and thoughtful way, and it played an important part in capturing public attention for the kind of problems which the Royal Commission were to consider.

The Royal Commission's terms of reference, however, limited them to legal and administrative issues, of which there were plenty, for as the report pointed out the existing tangle of legislation was so complex that expert witnesses at times went wrong over details, and it was difficult for magistrates, doctors, social workers and other officials to acquire a sound general knowledge of the law relating to mental illness and mental defect. (Mental deficiency was of course the term embodied in statute law until the Mental Health Act, 1959, substituted the term 'mental subnormality'. At the time of writing the term 'mental subnormality' has been displaced among workers in the field—though not of course in legal usage—by the term 'mental handicap', which is somehow felt to be less stigmatizing. In just the same way the ugly word 'psychiatric' is often preferred to the perfectly good term 'mental', and so we get 'psychiatric nurses' and 'psychiatric hospitals'. It is difficult at times to keep up with the fashionable euphemisms.)

The existing law was in fact so complex that when the Ministry of Health and the Board of Control submitted evidence to the Royal Commission it required a chart some fifteen inches square, printed in very small type, to summarize existing procedures for the admission of patients; the law also imposed on the Board the duty of scrutinizing over 4,000 documents connected with the admission, care or discharge of patients every week. Another aspect of this legal jungle on which the Royal Commission laid emphasis in their report was the stigma attached to certification and the extent to which this was aggravated by the involvement of a magistrate.

The recommendations of the Royal Commission represented a massive move away from legalism. It was necessary, the report said, to have compulsory powers to override the normal personal rights of individuals in certain circumstances, when mental disorder made them incapable of protecting themselves or their interests, or when it was in their own interests or those of other people or society in general that they should be removed for treatment even against their will. Special legislation was therefore needed (a) to define the circumstances in which such powers might be used and to provide safeguards against their abuse; (b) to protect patients' property when they were incapable of managing their own affairs; and (c) in connection with criminal cases. These were the only purposes, the Royal Commission held, in which special mental health legislation was still needed. The existing Lunacy, Mental Treatment and Mental Deficiency Acts should be repealed and a single new Act should lay down the circumstances in which compulsion might be used and the procedures to be followed, in as simple a way as possible. There was no need for separate legislation for mental illness and mental deficiency, because however different these two conditions might be medically and socially the safeguards required when compulsion was used were basically the same.

Apart from the question of compulsion, the mentally disordered should be treated in the same way as other sick people and admitted to hospitals which had the facilities for treating them, regardless of any rigid designation of hospitals for particular categories of patient. They should be protected as far as standards of care were concerned in exactly the same way as other patients, that is by the responsibility of the Minister of Health and other health service authorities to provide proper services, and not by special legislation and a special body such as the Board of Control. The mental health services should as far as possible be integrated with the general health and welfare services. Local authorities should further develop their preventive work and community care facilities.

The Percy Report introduced a new terminology. The term 'mental disorder' was used as a generic term to cover all forms of mental ill-health, mental illness, mental deficiency, and the psychopathic states. Three types of mental disorder were recognized for legal and administrative purposes: (1) mental illness, which included the mental infirmity that may be associated with old age; (2) psychopathic personality, a term used to include all types of aggressive or inadequate behaviour which did not render the patient severely subnormal and which was 'recognized medically as a pathological condition'; (3) severe subnormality, when the general personality is so severely subnormal that the patient is incapable of leading an independent life, a category which included those formerly known as idiots and imbeciles, and some, but not all, feeble-minded persons.

It was recommended that where compulsion was not necessary patients should be admitted to mental hospitals and mental deficiency institutions without formalities of any kind. It should no longer be necessary, as under the 1930 Act, for a patient to sign a form requesting admission, nor should it be necessary for him to give seventy-two hours' notice of an intention to discharge himself. This meant that it would no longer be needful to use compulsory powers for the fairly large class of patients who were not capable of expressing volition, but who equally had no specific objection to treatment. 'Compulsory powers should then be used only when they are positively necessary to override the wishes of the patient or his relatives for the patient's own welfare or for the protection of others.' Procedures for compulsory admission and for the discharge of detained patients should be streamlined, and should not involve the intervention of a magistrate, and Mental Health Review Tribunals should be set up in each area to review individual cases.

Percy Report, 1957

THE NEED FOR NEW LEGISLATION

In our view, as in the view of almost all our witnesses, individual people who need care because of mental disorder should be able to receive it as far as possible with no more restriction of liberty or legal formality than is applied to people who need care because of other types of illness, disability or social or economic difficulty. But mental disorder has special features which sometimes require special measures. Mental disorder makes many patients incapable of protecting themselves or their interests, so that if they are neglected or exploited it may be necessary to have authority to insist on providing them with proper care. In many cases it affects the patient's judgment so that he does not realise that he is ill, and the illness can only be treated against his wishes at the time. In many cases too it affects the patient's behaviour in such a way that it is necessary in the interests of other people or of society in general to insist on removing him for treatment even if he is unwilling. **This makes it necessary to have compulsory powers to override the normal personal rights of individuals in certain circumstances. Special legislation is necessary (a) to define the circumstances in which such powers may be used and to provide safeguards against their abuse; (b) to protect patients' property when they are incapable of managing their own affairs; and (c) in connection with criminal cases. In our view these are the only purposes for which special mental health legislation is still needed.**

Procedures to regulate the application of compulsory powers to individual patients are still necessary, and must be laid down in special legislation. The present procedures (which we discuss in detail in Parts IV and VI of our report) contain many unsatisfactory features. It would not be possible to remove these simply by amending the present Lunacy and Mental Treatments Acts and Mental Deficiency Acts. Completely new legislation is needed. **The present Acts incorporate some general assumptions and attitudes current in the late nineteenth and early twentieth centuries, many of which are no longer generally accepted.** These underlie not only particular procedures but the arrangement, spirit and language of the Acts as a whole and of the Rules, Regulations and statutory forms. It would not be possible to remove these without repealing the present Acts completely.

The attitudes and assumptions which are now out of date include, for example, the assumption that 'persons of unsound mind' and 'defectives' admitted to 'institutions' must be subject to detention, except those patients in mental hospitals who are 'suitable' to be voluntary patients. This assumption also lies behind the use of such expressions as 'escape', 'recapture' and other similar phrases. There is also a lack of discrimination between the needs of individual patients for particular forms of care. The Acts emphasise the need for doctors to provide grounds for an opinion that a person is 'of unsound mind' or 'defective', but do not require them to specify the reasons why the patient requires institutional rather than community care. Under the Mental Deficiency Acts no distinction is made between the circumstances in which a defective may be sent to an institution or placed under guardianship. The procedures applied to mentally ill patients emphasise the importance of the patient's 'status', that is to say, whether he is 'certified', 'temporary' or 'voluntary'. When a patient's 'status' is changed—as when a temporary patient regains volition—he is said to be 'discharged' and 're-admitted' even though he does not leave the hospital. There are also still many vestiges in the Lunacy and Mental Treatment Acts and Rules of the distinctions originally drawn between pauper and non-pauper patients. Although the main procedures for admission and discharge now apply equally to paying and non-paying patients, the transfer of a patient from the 'health service' to the 'private' class must be notified to the Board of Control and other authorities. There are different procedures for moving 'private' and 'health service' patients from one hospital to another, and the statutory notices of admission and discharge state whether a patient is of the 'private', 'health service' or 'Broadmoor' class.

Another reason for repeal and partial re-enactment is the great complexity of the present Acts. The Royal Commission on Lunacy and Mental Disorder, reporting in 1926 on the Lunacy Acts alone, expressed the view that 'the existing code . . . is in certain respects too complicated for the comprehension of those who have daily to administer it.' Since then it has become much more complicated by amendments and new legislation, and in addition there is the separate mental deficiency code which deals with some of the same principles in a different way. We noticed that some of our witnesses had little knowledge of aspects of the law and of the administration of the mental health services other than those with which they themselves are particularly concerned. Others, in describing the present law to us, sometimes went wrong over details. We do not blame them; we only hope we have avoided errors ourselves. In this report we deal mainly with general principles and have tried not to become involved more than we must in detail, but if anyone doubts that the present Acts are unnecessarily complicated, especially on comparatively minor matters, let him look at the provisions of the Acts and Rules governing the absence of mentally ill patients from hospital on short leave, on trial, for reasons of health or boarded out. . . .

paras. 136–9

CLASSIFICATION

We recommend that three main groups of patients should be recognised in future for legal and administrative purposes:

(a) Mentally ill patients. The term 'mental illness' would be used in the same sense as at present, including the mental infirmity of old age. The term 'person of unsound mind' would no longer be used.

(b) Psychopathic patients, or patients with psychopathic personality. We use the term 'psychopathic personality' in a wider sense than that in which it is often used at present and intend it to include any type of aggressive or inadequate personality which does not render the patient severely subnormal in the sense of group (c) below but which is recognised medically as a pathological condition. Our psychopathic group includes all patients at present classified as feebleminded or moral defectives who need care but do not fall into group (c), and also some other psychopaths who are pathologically mentally abnormal but are not covered by the present legal definition of mentally defective persons. We use the term 'feebleminded psychopath' when referring to psychopaths whose disorder includes a marked limitation of intelligence but still does not bring them into group (c).

(c) Patients of severely subnormal personality. This term would be used when the general personality is so severely sub-normal that the patient is incapable of leading an independent life. This group includes all patients at present classified as idiots and imbeciles and some of those now classified as feeble-minded. The terms 'idiot' and 'imbecile' and the terms 'mental defectiveness' and 'defective' would no longer need to be used.

There should be no rigid legal designation of hospitals for any one of these groups of patients only. The extent to which particular hospitals specialise in treating particular types of disorder should be a matter for medical and administrative arrangement, in the psychiatric field as in other branches of medicine. The arrangements should be capable of adaptation as medical developments may require, and there should be no legal barrier preventing the admission of any patient to any hospital which provides the sort of treatment he is thought to need.

The law should define the circumstances in which patients in each of these three groups should be liable to compulsory admission to and detention in hospital or to legal control while living in the general community; these would not be the same for all three groups of patients (see paragraphs 24–33). We recommend various procedures appropriate to the varying circumstances in which compulsory powers may need to be used; these form a single set of procedures which do not introduce further distinctions between the three main groups of patients when other circumstances are similar. . . . These new procedures should be laid down in a single new Act.

paras. 17–19

COMMUNITY CARE

There is increasing medical emphasis on forms of treatment and training and social services which can be given without bringing patients into hospital as in-patients or which make it possible to discharge them from hospital sooner than was usual in the past. It is not now generally considered in the best interests of patients who are fit to live in the general community that they should be in large or remote institutions such as the present mental and mental deficiency hospitals. Nor is it a proper function of the hospital authorities to provide residential accommodation for patients who do not require hospital or specialist services, nor to provide other care for patients who have left hospital apart from necessary medical follow-up or out-patient services. The division of functions between the hospitals, local authorities and other official bodies should be broadly the same in relation to mentally disordered patients as in relation to others.

The general division of functions between hospitals and local authorities should be:

(i) The hospitals should provide in-patient and out-patient services for patients who need specialist medical treatment or continual nursing attention. This includes the care of helpless patients in the severely sub-normal group who need continual nursing, if proper care cannot be provided at home. It also includes in-patient training designed to promote the mental or physical development of severely sub-normal and psychopathic patients if such training requires individual psychiatric supervision, by which we mean that the patient's individual progress needs to be watched and if possible controlled by a psychiatrist. The aim of treatment or training is to make the patient fit to live in the general community. No patient should be retained as a hospital in-patient when he has reached the stage at which he could return home if he had a reasonably good home to go to. At that stage the provision of residential care becomes the responsibility of the local authority.

(ii) The local authorities should be responsible for preventive services and for all types of community care for patients who do not require in-patient hospital services or who have had a period of treatment or training in hospital and are ready to return to the community. This may involve the provision of day or residential training centres for some severely sub-normal children; training or occupation centres and social centres for adult severely sub-normal patients, psychopathic patients or patients with residual disability after a mental illness; residential accommodation in private homes or in homes or hostels provided by voluntary societies or by the local authorities themselves for many types of patients including old people with mild mental infirmity; and general social help and advice to patients of all types and ages and to their relatives.

(iii) Social work for patients who are not receiving hospital treatment, including patients who have left hospital, is essentially the responsibility of the local authorities, who can also do a great deal in co-operation with the hospital staff for hospital out-patients and even for in-patients. There must be very close co-operation between the medical staff and social workers of the hospitals and local authorities to ensure the best use of the resources of each and maximum continuity in the care of individual patients. Arrangements to ensure such co-operation should be made in each local area. After-care should be provided by the local authorities as long as it is needed, and should not be dependent on the continuation of compulsory powers such as licence or guardianship.

This would involve a considerable expansion of residential and non-residential community health and welfare services. In developing these services the local authorities have a major part to play in the prevention and relief of all forms of mental disorder. It is essential that medical officers of health should take a personal interest in this work and have suitably experienced medical officers and social workers on their staff.

paras. 46–8

9.8 Mental Health Act, 1959

Only eighteen months after the Royal Commission on the Law Relating to Mental Illness and Mental Deficiency had published their report (the Percy Report), the Mental Health Bill was introduced in the House of Commons. In its broad lines it followed the main recommendations of the Royal Commission. It made a clean sweep of existing mental health legislation, repealing fifteen Acts completely and thirty-seven Acts in part. It dealt, as the Royal Commission had recommended, with both mental illness and mental deficiency, providing a single code for all types of mental disorder. There were only two points of substance where the Act differed from the recommendations of the Royal Commission. The first was the addition of a fourth category of patient, the subnormal, to the three—mentally ill, psychopathic and severely subnormal—which appeared in the Percy Report. This was to embrace those feeble-minded persons who required care, but who would not have been included in the Royal Commission's fairly stringent definition of 'severely subnormal'.

The second difference was over financial provision for the services which were the responsibility of local authorities. The Royal Commission had recommended that there should be a specific grant from the Government to local authorities for capital development—the provision of hostels, training centres and the like—but government thinking had moved away from the idea of specific grants earmarked for particular purposes. The Government's subsidy to local authority mental health services was now part of a general grant, and the Government did not propose to reopen the question of general versus specific grants at this stage. This caused a good deal of concern during the debate on the Bill because many members felt that local authorities would not spend sufficient on their mental health services to make possible the shift in emphasis from hospital to community care that the Royal Commission and the sponsors of the Bill envisaged, if they were not induced to do so by earmarked grants or other forms of central government pressure. Local authority powers in this field derived from legislation which permitted them to do much but compelled them to do little, and many of them had done very little indeed. On the other hand, the Minister pointed out that local authorities as a whole were spending much more on their mental health services; in 1954–5 the figure had been a little over £2¼ million, but in 1957–8 it was over £3½ million, and it was estimated that in 1958–9 it would be over £4 million. No major amendments were made to the Bill in either House, although there were a number of small but useful refinements and improvements.

Following the passage of the Act the Minister of Health, using powers given to him by the Act and by the National Health Service Act, 1946, laid on local health authorities a duty to provide a full range of community services for the mentally handicapped, including residential services, thus restoring a function which local authorities had lost in 1948 when all their residential establishments for the mentally handicapped had been transferred to the hospital authorities (there was no apportionment between health and welfare services as there was in the case of residential accommodation for the elderly). Nor were any institutions run by hospital authorities transferred back to local authorities in 1959. The local authorities were faced with the task of building up their stock of residential accommodation from scratch, and progress in many areas was very slow indeed. The local authority record was, however, rather better where training facilities were concerned. The number of places in junior training centres rose from 12,200 in 1960 to 23,500 in 1970. In 1971 these centres were transferred from health authorities to education authorities as education authorities were made responsible for the education and training of all mentally handicapped children—the more severely handicapped had previously been excluded from the educational system as such. The number of training places for mentally handicapped adults rose from 10,100 in 1960 to 26,400 in 1970, although even at the later date there was still a considerable shortage.

9.9 White Paper on Better Services for the Mentally Handicapped

Published: 1971

The White Paper, *Better Services for the Mentally Handicapped*, set out the principles by which the Conservative government which came into office in June 1970 proposed to be guided in its development of services for those who were still known statutorily—even though many of those working in the field chose to reject the term as one that conveyed unnecessary stigma—as the mentally subnormal. The White Paper owed much to the work in the early 1960s of Professor Jack Tizard of the Medical Research Council Social Psychiatry Unit at the Maudsley Hospital. Tizard had shown that mentally handicapped children could improve enormously in behaviour and social adjustment if given the opportunity to form one-to-one relationships with adults and that many of the problems experienced in institutions for the mentally handicapped were the result of institutional conditioning and emotional deprivation rather than an inherent feature of mental handicap. Tizard argued that the extent to which the mentally handicapped were segregated from the rest of the community should be minimized. Wherever possible they should be cared for at home or in small family-type units, and the distinction between institutional care and home care should be minimized by allowing residents in institutions to make use of the same diagnostic and treatment services, the same schools, day centres, sheltered workshops and training centres as those who lived at home.

Tizard's criticisms of institutional care were given additional point by the reports of the Ely and Farleigh inquiries in the later 1960s and by Dr Pauline Morris's book *Put Away*, published in 1969. Dr Morris reported a survey of thirty-five hospitals commissioned by the National Society for Mentally Handicapped Children, a survey which showed that not only were conditions often squalid and standards of care low, but those responsible for the administration of these hospitals often failed to see anything wrong. Dr Morris rejected the idea that the mentally handicapped should be cared for in institutions that were medically oriented and doctor dominated and suggested that the purpose of institutions for the mentally handicapped—where institutional care was unavoidable—should be seen as socio-therapeutic rather than clinical, with an emphasis on training and education at least as great as that placed upon medical treatment and nursing care. Like Tizard, she called for increased provision of community care and small-group homes.

The White Paper went part of the way with those who thought like Pauline Morris, but it did not go the whole way, and for this it was bitterly attacked by Professor Peter Townsend, who had written an introduction to her study. It proposed a major shift from hospital to community, involving a substantial run-down in the number of hospital beds—it was estimated that only 27,000 beds ought to be required for adult mentally handicapped patients compared with 52,100 currently provided—and a massive increase in the provision of residential places in the community. The White Paper acknowledged that there were 'different opinions, even among the experts, on the extent to which local authority services can meet the needs of people with substantial but not profound mental handicap, with or without associated physical handicap, and on the extent to which such people require medical, nursing or other skills which it is the function of hospitals to provide', and it took a relatively cautious view of the extent to which it would be possible to provide for these people in the community.

Chapter 6 of the White Paper set out a programme of action embracing services provided by the Government, by local authorities, by hospital authorities and by voluntary bodies. As far as local authorities were concerned no new policies were called for, only faster progress in the implementation of those already agreed, and the White Paper set targets which were in most cases 'far beyond what the authorities have yet planned to provide'. In an earlier chapter it was made clear that failure on the part of local authorities to provide sufficient residential places and community services was responsible on the one hand for 'almost unbearable stress' suffered by families with mentally handicapped members living at home, and on the other for gross overcrowding in hospitals which were under unrelenting pressure to admit more patients to already overcrowded wards. The paragraph referring to the financing of further development in the local authority sector and of the improvements and reorganization called for in the hospital service were a trifle confused, but in November 1970 the Government announced the allocation of £110 million additional resources for the health and social services in the years 1971-2 to 1974-5, and the White Paper stated that about £40 million of this was to be spent on services for the mentally handicapped.

The hospital service faced the dual task of relieving overcrowding and improving sub-standard conditions in existing hospitals while at the same time working towards the long-term reorganization of services. Even though fewer beds would be required in the future they would frequently be required in different places. No new large hospitals were to be built, and no hospital of more than 500 beds was to be enlarged. New buildings to relieve overcrowding at hospitals of more than 500 beds were to be located in areas of population elsewhere in the hospital's catchment area. New accommodation for in-patients would be provided either in units for the mentally handicapped within a hospital also containing other departments, or in separate hospitals of not more than 100–200 beds closely associated with a general hospital, but not usually on the same site. The general hospital might contain the assessment and treatment unit, but space for occupational activities and leisure activities and a homely type of building could more easily be achieved on a separate site. New facilities for children would normally be separate from those for adults, have close links with the children's department of a general hospital and be provided in small domestic units. They might be either on or off the site of the general hospital. In planning all these facilities regional hospital boards were to work closely with the relevant local authorities and to relate their hospital units to defined populations. Teaching hospitals were also called upon to play their part in providing in-patient, day patient and out-patient facilities for the mentally handicapped, both as part of their service to their districts and in order to make future doctors familiar with problems of mental handicap.

White Paper on Better Services for the Mentally Handicapped

GENERAL PRINCIPLES

Chapter 4 describes the state of our present services for mental handicap. Chapters 5 and 6 discuss in detail present views on the services required and how they should be organised. Chapter 7 discusses the important role of voluntary services. The main principles on which current thinking about mental handicap is based need first to be stated.

These can be summarised as follows:

(i) A family with a handicapped member has the same needs for general social services as all other families. The family and the handicapped child or adult also need special additional help, which varies according to the severity of the handicap, whether there are associated physical handicaps or behaviour problems, the age of the handicapped person and his family situation.

(ii) Mentally handicapped children and adults should not be segregated unnecessarily from other people of similar age, nor from the general life of the local community.

(iii) Full use should be made of available knowledge which can help to prevent mental handicap or to reduce the severity of its effects.

(iv) There should be a comprehensive initial assessment and periodic re-assessment of the needs of each handicapped person and his family.

(v) Each handicapped person needs stimulation, social training and education and purposeful occupation or employment in order to develop to his maximum capacity and to exercise all the skills he acquires, however limited they may be.

(vi) Each handicapped person should live with his own family as long as this does not impose an undue burden on them or him, and he and his family should receive full advice and support. If he has to leave home for a foster home, residential home or hospital, temporarily or permanently, links with his own family should normally be maintained.

(vii) The range of services in every area should be such that the family can be sure that their handicapped member will be properly cared for when it becomes necessary for him to leave the family home.

(viii) When a handicapped person has to leave his family home, temporarily or permanently, the substitute home should be as homelike as possible, even if it is also a hospital. It should provide sympathetic and constant human relationships.

(ix) There should be proper co-ordination in the application of relevant professional skills for the benefit of individual handicapped people and their families, and in the planning and administration of relevant services, whether or not these cross administrative frontiers.

(x) Local authority personal social services for the mentally handicapped should develop as an integral part of the services recently brought together under the Local Authority Social Services Act, 1970.

(xi) There should be close collaboration between these services and those provided by other local authority departments (*e.g.* child health services and education), and with general practitioners, hospitals and other services for the disabled.

(xii) Hospital services for the mentally handicapped should be easily accessible to the population they serve. They should be associated with other hospital services, so that a full range of specialist skills is easily available when needed for assessment or treatment.

(xiii) Hospital and local authority services should be planned and operated in partnership; the Government's proposals for the reorganisation of the National Health Service will encourage the closest co-operation.

(xiv) Voluntary service can make a contribution to the welfare of mentally handicapped people and their families at all stages of their lives and wherever they are living.

(xv) Understanding and help from friends and neighbours and from the community at large are needed to help the family to maintain a normal social life and to give the handicapped member as nearly normal a life as the handicap or handicaps permit.

paras. 39–40

ROLE OF THE HOSPITAL

When a mentally handicapped person requires hospital treatment for a physical illness, or surgery, or treatment for mental illness, he should normally receive this in the appropriate department of a general or mental illness hospital. There may however be cases where psychiatric treatment for a mental illness associated with severe mental handicap, or occasionally treatment for physical illness, is better provided in a hospital or unit accustomed to dealing with the severely mentally handicapped.

Paragraphs 130 to 141 mention the need for hospital staff to participate in the prevention, early detection and comprehensive assessment and reassessment of mental and other handicaps. Children's departments of general hospitals have an important part to play in diagnosis and assessment and early remedial measures. Psychiatric out-patient clinics in local hospitals are also useful for this purpose. The contacts thus established between hospital psychiatrists and handicapped children or adults and their parents also help to support the family while the handicapped member lives at home, and to ease the transition to hospital if he needs to be admitted later.

Day hospital services are needed for handicapped children or adults who can live at home but need assessment in a hospital setting. They are also required for some of those with severe physical handicaps or behaviour problems whose families can keep them at home if relieved of their care for a few hours each day. For such patients day services may replace or postpone in-patient admissions, or allow discharge after a period as an in-patient.

Day patients may attend hospitals which also treat in-patients, or separate day hospitals. Any hospital taking day patients must of course be easily accessible to the population it serves. For some patients relatively simple accommodation will suffice, and may be in a small local unit. Others will need treatment facilities which can be provided only in a larger hospital. In addition to whatever medical, nursing and other specialist services are needed, there must be facilities in the hospital or nearby for education for children and suitable occupation and training for adults, and also meals and recreation. Paragraph 63 refers to the possibility of associating day hospital services in some areas with a training centre or special school provided by the local authority.

In-patient services are needed for those who can no longer remain in the family home or in other residential care and require treatment or training under specialist medical supervision or constant nursing care. A high proportion will need this because their mental handicap is associated with severe physical disability or behaviour disorder.

The aim is to help all patients, including the most severely handicapped, to develop to their full potential and to achieve as positive and independent a life as their handicaps allow. After a period of treatment or training some will be able to be discharged back to life in the community with support from the local authorities or hospital out-patient or day-patient services.

The hospitals should be staffed to provide all necessary medical, dental and para-medical services. In addition to doctors, dentists and nurses, this may require, according to individual patients' needs, the services of whole-time or part-time psychologists, physiotherapists, speech therapists and other specialists. A range of educational services for patients of all ages should be provided by or in consultation with the local education authority, together with industrial and occupational therapy and a range of leisure activities for which appropriate staff need to be employed.

paras. 176–82

Admission to hospital should have no air of a final break with the patient's family, as it often has at present. The hospital staff should be at pains to ensure that their own professional services do not make the relatives feel superfluous, nor guilty at shedding their immediate responsibility for the handicapped person. A family's inability to carry on caring for a severely handicapped child or adult should not be seen by them as a failure, or as an occasion for them to withdraw their interest. . . .

If the hospital employs its own social workers, they should maintain close links with the local authority social services departments to ensure a continuing service to families while their relative is in hospital, and to secure proper arrangements if and when he is discharged. Another possible arrangement is for the local authority to provide a social work service, used jointly with the hospital, for patients from the authority's area and their families; the same social workers would then be responsible whether or not the handicapped member of the family becomes a hospital in-patient. If a hospital in-patient has no family links, the local authority social worker can provide a contact with the community; this may be particularly necessary if the patient is a child.

If contacts with the family are to be maintained, the hospitals must be accessible to the populations they serve. This will affect both the location and the size of hospitals or hospital units for the mentally handicapped, which are discussed in paragraphs 189 to 192 and in Chapter 6.

Contact should be maintained with life outside hospital through contacts with the local community around the hospital, as well as with patients' families. Voluntary help and visitors from the local community should be encouraged to come into the hospital. Patients should go out to shop, to use local parks and playgrounds and join in social events; even severely handicapped patients can benefit from the interest and stimulus this provides. Some may also go out of the hospital regularly to work or to attend adult training centres or special schools.

paras. 185–8

VOLUNTARY SERVICE IN THE HOSPITAL

Voluntary services are indispensable for maintaining links between the general community and hospital patients and staff. This is particularly important for patients who stay in hospital for years—as many mentally handicapped patients do—and for staff of isolated hospitals, many of whom live in the hospital grounds and can become isolated and inward-looking.

Volunteers can come into the hospitals and contribute to their internal life. They can take patients out locally or for longer excursions or holidays. They can help relatives to visit and can visit patients who have no interested relatives of their own.

No hospital unit is too large or too small to need such help. When hospital services are reorganised into smaller units, as foreshadowed in Chapter 6, voluntary help in maintaining contacts with the surrounding community will still be essential. A small hospital unit or residential home can be as isolated as a large one if it has no visitors.

Voluntary service can be directed to groups of patients or to individuals, or to raising funds for amenities for patients generally or for staff. All these are needed. Voluntary work should be planned in consultation with the hospital's staff. The appointment of a voluntary help organiser ... can improve the scope for co-operation.

Group activities and services. Activities for small groups of patients which can be organised and led by volunteers include games of all sorts, drama, music, painting, modelling, and other hobbies, play groups, horse-riding—to name but a few. Voluntary organisations run library services and hospital shops and canteens. A most valuable service is the organisation of transport to help relatives visit patients in hospitals which are not easy to get to.

Groups of patients can also be given opportunities to join in activities outside hospital. Holiday camps can be organised, or day-trips, shopping expeditions, visits to cinemas, fun-fairs, football matches and other sports. And perhaps best of all, invitations to people's own houses, singly or in small groups.

Friendship for individual patients. At least a third of the 60,000 patients who now live in hospital are never visited. Others have only occasional visits from relatives. To befriend an individual patient is one of the most worthwhile forms of voluntary service. It is also one of the most difficult. Many patients, particularly the more severely handicapped, have difficulty in communication. Lack of an early response can be discouraging; it takes time and patience to form a useful relationship.

Funds for amenities. Fund-raising was one of the earliest forms of voluntary service, and is still indispensible. Funds have been raised for amenities for patients such as swimming pools, social centres, hairdressing salons, toys, aquariums, budgerigars and other pets, record players, and colour television. Contributions to Christmas festivities are welcome, and Christmas and birthday presents for patients. Amenities for staff (such as a building for a staff club) have also been provided, and are much needed, especially in the older hospitals.

Help for isolated hospitals. The hospitals most in need of help may be geographically isolated and difficult to reach by public transport. The surrounding community may be small, so that the local volunteers are necessarily few, often belong to several organisations and are heavily committed. The large isolated hospitals serve very large populations; with interest and ingenuity it should be possible to stimulate voluntary services of one sort or another from many different parts of a large 'catchment area'. Leaders of local communities served by such hospitals could encourage this, and it will become more meaningful when the large hospitals are organised in units each serving a particular area, as mentioned in paragraph 267.

Voluntary help is especially important for these hospitals, where many patients are far from their homes and relatives, and staff are short. They need more volunteers to organise outings and excursions, to help in educational and recreational activities, to visit patients. Help at weekends and evenings is particularly important, when teachers, instructors and therapists are off duty.

New sources of voluntary help. The work of the established associations is being augmented by an increasing variety of other groups. School children raised money to buy roller skates for patients at one hospital, and went to the hospital every weekend to help the children to use them. The 'regulars' at a public house have adopted a ward. Local people without young children of their own befriend young patients, visit them regularly and take them out. Groups of students have spent some weeks of their vacations at various hospitals, helping in whatever ways the staff suggest and in new activities which they initiate. There is almost unlimited scope for more help for more people.

Voluntary help organisers. The employment by hospitals of paid voluntary help organisers, usually full-time, is an important new development. Working alongside the voluntary organisations, their aim is to ensure that the contributions of the organisations and of individual volunteers are used to the best advantage. Such appointments have generally been very successful in helping to increase the numbers of volunteers and extend the range of their activities. As with most new developments there have been occasional difficulties; and not unnaturally there have been some doubts among those voluntary organisations already active in the field. This has shown how important it is that the right sort of person should be chosen. Advice is being issued to hospital authorities about the selection of people for this work and the qualities to be looked for.

paras. 285–96

9.10 Report of the Committee of Inquiry into Whittingham Hospital (Payne Report)

Published: 1972

Chairman: *Sir Robert Payne*

Members: *W. A. L. Bowen FRC Psych; J. R. Elliott MBE, FHA; R. Kempster SRN, RMN, RMPA; Miss M. B. H. Whyte MA, MBASW; L. C. Wilcher CBE; Michael Foster (secretary); Miss Joyce Martin (assistant secretary)*

Terms of Reference (1971): *To inquire into the administration of and conditions at Whittingham Hospital and to make recommendations.*

Following the publication in 1967 of the book *Sans Everything*, a savage indictment of conditions in a number of long-stay hospitals, a letter was sent from the Permanent Secretary to the Ministry of Health to all regional hospital boards asking them to 'satisfy themselves that there are not grounds for complaint in their hospitals'. The chairman of the Manchester RHB thereupon wrote in similar vein to chairmen of hospital management committees in the region, adding, 'I know that, with me, you will be only too anxious to establish that patients in the hospitals in our region are not treated in this way and that you will wish to be personally satisfied that there is no evidence of inhuman treatment in any of the hospitals for which your Management Committee are responsible'. Among the HMCs to which this letter was sent was Whittingham HMC, responsible for the 2,000-bed Whittingham Hospital, near Preston, Lancs. From this committee, as from others, suitable assurances were in due course sent to the chairman of the regional board; yet, only a few days before, the hospital's branch of the Student Nurses' Association had held a meeting at which a number of allegations of ill-treatment and fraud were made. It was more than two years before news of this meeting reached the HMC chairman, although senior members of the nursing administration were present.

By this time the hospital was already the subject of inquiries set in train by the Department of Health following the receipt of letters from an assistant psychiatrist and a psychologist employed there which made allegations of ill-treatment, fraud and maladministration, including the suppression of complaints from student nurses. A team of auditors quickly uncovered a number of financial irregularities, and allegations of ill-treatment were referred to the police. In the summer of 1970 two male nurses were convicted of theft and shortly afterwards a male nurse who attacked two patients, one of whom died, was convicted of manslaughter and imprisoned. As soon as the trial was over the Secretary of State announced his intention of setting up an official inquiry into conditions at Whittingham Hospital. The committee of inquiry was constituted in February 1971, its report submitted to the Secretary of State in November, and published in February of the following year.

The committee took evidence in public and, unlike the earlier committee of inquiry into Ely Hospital, it had a solicitor to assemble and present the evidence. Many of the most serious allegations were upheld. The committee were convinced that allegations that patients received the 'wet towel treatment'—a wet towel was twisted round the patient's neck until he lost consciousness—when they were troublesome, and that methylated spirit was poured over patients' clothing and then set alight, were substantially true. They found that large-scale pilfering of patients' money had taken place and that this was made possible by the absence of any adequate system of financial control.

However, the committee of inquiry ranged far beyond these detailed allegations and the most telling passages in the report spoke of the 'administration by labyrinth' and lack of medical leadership that made it possible for such situations to develop. The resignation of the hospital management committee was called for—and did in fact follow publication of the report. It was recommended that day-to-day management of the hospital should be undertaken by a 'professional executive' consisting of the chairman of the medical staff, the chief nursing officer, group secretary and senior members of other professions working in the hospital. This was a similar system to that which had been introduced in the mental handicap division of the East Birmingham hospital group when James Elliott—a member of the committee of inquiry—was group secretary. Other recommendations were designed to ensure that the reconstituted management committee delegated authority for day-to-day management to the officers, thus remaining free for their proper task of deciding policy objectives and monitoring performance.

The regional hospital board did not escape criticism, for Manchester RHB had pioneered the policy of transferring short-stay psychiatric treatment to psychiatric departments in general hospitals, with the consequence that hospitals like Whittingham—which it was assumed would run down and eventually close—became almost exclusively long-stay and were starved of resources, particularly of medical staff. The committee hit hard at the 'two-tier' system of psychiatry and held that the task of re-habilitating long-stay patients required at least as much specialized psychiatric skill as the treatment of short-stay patients. The HMC and staff at Whittingham were in fact doubtful whether the policy of running down and closing the hospital would ever be carried out and the HMC chairman expressed to the committee of inquiry his belief that there would always be a need to accommodate long-stay patients, to provide, as he put it, 'asylum in the true sense of the word'. This conflict between the regional board's policies and the beliefs of the Whittingham HMC and officers was never brought into the open, still less resolved, and appeared to the committee of inquiry to be a fundamental cause of the hospital's malaise.

The committee of inquiry acknowledged that much good work was done at Whittingham, and there were many devoted staff. It was 'a hospital of wide contrasts'. But if the patients were institutionalized, so were the staff—one ward sister had remained in charge of the same ward for forty-seven years. There were few opportunities for new ideas to be introduced; the nursing administration was in-bred and authoritarian in tone. One member of the management committee had served for twenty-five years. Individuals who complained or criticized were regarded as troublemakers. This led to the Gilbertian situation where a woman psychologist who had championed the student nurses who had first drawn attention to cruelty and malpractice on the wards was asked by the HMC to resign; eighteen months later she had not done so and the request for her resignation still stood. The entire Whittingham Report is in fact a classic text in the sociology of closed institutions.

Payne Report, 1972

ADMINISTRATION BY LABYRINTH
Whittingham Hospital Management Committee consists of 15 members. . . . They were said by the Chairman of the Regional Hospital Board to be the best psychiatric Hospital Management Committee in the Manchester region. Certainly they do not lack experience. Six have been members for ten years or more; and of these three, including the Chairman, have been members for fifteen years or more. One, the Chairman of the Nurse Education Committee, has served since 1948. Six are over 65 and three over 70. The long periods in office of key members, and their ages, may not be unconnected with the comments that follow.

The sub-committee structure is complex and, surprisingly, shows no change in the light of advice from the Farquharson-Lang Report* on the rationalisation

* See p. 195.

of hospital management structures, circulated under H.M.(66)28. . . . There are no less than six sub-committees. Apart from Establishment, Finance, Planning and Estates and Statutory, there are special recently set up sub-committees on 'Catering and Visiting' and 'Patients' Rehabilitation and Visiting'. There is a Joint Consultative Committee, consisting of management and staff sides (including student nurses), and a Nurse Education Committee, whose Chairman since 1963 has been Mrs. Goodwright, which itself has a Nurse Procedures Sub-Committee. Medical policy is dealt with by a Medical Advisory Committee consisting of the hospital consultants; its Chairman until March 1971 was Dr. Silverman of Blackburn Hospital, who had no clinical commitments at Whittingham and only one session per week for administrative purposes only. Mr. Phipps told us that the Medical Advisory Committee made requests and recommendations to the Hospital Management Committee, who took the ultimate decisions. In addition there is a 'Principal Officers' Meeting', comprising the Group Secretary, all consultants and (until they were replaced by a Chief Nursing Officer) the twin nursing heads—the Chief Male Nurse and the Matron. This appears to have taken over some of the policy functions normally exercised by the Medical Advisory Committee.

The complexity of the committee structure in our view has greatly handicapped the conduct of business. First, it is by no means clear where the responsibility for decision on major issues lies. Secondly, many matters need reference to more than one sub-committee and this inevitably entails delay and difficulty in reaching decisions. Thirdly, it imposes an unnecessary burden of work on both members and administrative staff. Farquharson-Lang recommended two, and certainly not more than three, sub-committees; but although the Hospital Management Committee discussed the Department's advice at the time no recommendation for any fundamental change was made. In giving evidence, the Chairman of the Hospital Management Committee, Mr. Phipps, did not recall this advice and said that in his view 'the more committees you have the more involved you are'.

This apparently explicit acknowledgment of 'administration by labyrinth' is confirmed by examination of the minutes of the Hospital Management Committee and its sub-committees in recent years. The picture is of vague policy formation, splintered decision-making, inadequate delegation to officers and no systematic monitoring of performance. In fact the management structure represents very much the kind of administration criticised by Farquharson-Lang. Instead of discussing major policy objectives such as unlocking doors, opening up airing courts and progress in extending rehabilitation to all patients, the minutes are packed with day-to-day decisions on trivia such as tenders for loads of gravel and purchases of lavatory basins or flower and vegetable seed. The programme for up-grading wards has been pushed forward with vigour, and this is greatly to the Hospital Management Committee's credit, but it is difficult to discern its link with any planned therapeutic programme. Certainly there seems to have been no recognition how far Whittingham had drifted behind the tide of progress in psychiatry.

Minutes of Hospital Management Committee meetings often seem so brief and elliptical as to convey no meaningful consideration or decision. Indeed it is possible to read some of them without discovering what subjects were under discussion and what decisions were reached. Reference between the various sub-committees seems too often to have been a substitute for grasping nettles. An example is the students' complaints about training conditions of October 1968. These were referred from the Nurse Education to the Nurse Procedures Committee; rejected as unfounded; re-opened by the Hospital Management Committee itself as a result of written protests via the Training School; considered by a 'Sub-Committee of Enquiry' which met once and promised investigation; and then 'lost'. There are other instances of lack of effective action. The students' complaints of July 1967, when the auditors eventually brought them to light at the end of 1969, were placed before the Hospital Management Committee; the Committee reprimanded the Chief Male Nurse and the Matron; but the opportunity to deal with the problems raised was missed. The functions of some sub-committees seem to have been oddly exercised. The Nurse Procedures Committee has been less involved in standardising 'procedures' than in dealing with training and other matters more appropriate to an Education Committee. Hospital Management Committee members of the Catering Sub-Committee rarely visited wards during mealtimes. The Rehabilitation Sub-Committee included no occupational therapists; nor did it co-ordinate rehabilitation activities or even meet the therapists regularly. The Joint Consultative Committee seems to have met only rarely.

More striking still was the lack of co-ordination—in some cases even communication—between different parts of the management structure. The assurances we were given that the Hospital Management Committee Chairman and the Group Secretary were not informed, and learned nothing, of meetings called by the student nurses and the nursing administration about serious allegations of ill-treatment are almost incredible when those concerned were in daily contact. More serious was the lack of effective advice from the Medical Advisory Committee to the Hospital Management Committee. The Chairman of the Hospital Management Committee said in evidence that he consulted the Group Secretary about everything; he also frequently consulted the Chief Male Nurse and the Matron, who attended Hospital Management Committee meetings. But he never consulted Dr. Silverman 'except on one or two occasions when I had definite problems' during the eight years while the latter was Chairman of the Medical Advisory Committee. The fact that Dr. Silverman had only one session per week at the hospital no doubt made it difficult for them to meet. This failure of communication substantially contributed to the therapeutic inertia on long-stay wards which gave rise to the students' complaints of July 1967. We deal with the question of medical leadership, or the lack of it, in Chapter 5.

In this complex structure, with a serious weakness at this critical point, the Group Secretary's role was crucial. Our assessment is that Mr. Makinson (who succeeded Mr. Higgs in May 1967, shortly before the students' complaints) did a loyal and conscientious job in matters of routine but, perhaps because he was burdened with so many problems arising from lack of effective medical leadership, contented himself with keeping the administrative machine running with the minimum of trouble rather than seeking to identify policy objectives, solve essential problems or correct the basic weaknesses of the management structure.

paras. 46–52

TWO-TIER PSYCHIATRY

But perhaps the most lamentable feature of Whittingham's medical organisation has been the low level and uneven distribution of staffing. Although five consultants work at the hospital, because of outside commitments there are in reality fewer than three to care for its 2,000 patients. Even more disturbing is the fact that little more than the equivalent of one whole-time consultant's services is devoted to the care of the 86 per cent. who are 'long-stay'.

Dr. Oakley and Dr. Glynn run the admission unit of 240 beds at Whittingham and the equivalent female unit at Sharoe Green (100 beds) in the Preston Group; they deal with no long-stay wards. Dr. Parker also has responsibility at Preston (6 sessions per week) in addition to his charge of 292 long-stay beds and the medical electronics unit at Whittingham (3 sessions). Dr. Robinson is the only consultant to work almost full-time on long-stay patients (10 sessions) and he is required to look after no less than 780 beds at Whittingham and 100 'rehabilitation' beds at Ribchester. Most remarkable of all, is the case of Dr. Denmark, who has eight sessions per week at Whittingham, of which seven have been allocated to his deaf unit of 26 beds and only one to 625 long-stay beds. In support, at 30 September 1970, there were only one part-time medical assistant and three registrars, also part-time, but no less than eleven general practitioner clinical assistants. . . . On the other hand it has to be recognised that the Manchester Region as a whole has only 0·94 consultants in mental illness per 100,000 population in comparison with a national average of 1·45 and the Department's target of 1·66.

From the evidence given at our hearing it was clear that neither the Hospital Management Committee nor the Regional Hospital Board officers fully appreciated the gross inadequacy of this level of medical staffing; or, if they did so, had done enough to press their concern. Dr. Silverman agreed with Dr. Denmark and Dr. Masters that consultants did not visit long-stay wards because of their heavy commitments elsewhere and acknowledged that Whittingham 'could probably utilise another two consultants quite happily'; but he was not prepared to admit that Whittingham was grossly understaffed in comparison with, say, hospitals in the south of England. He said that there had been a delay at the Board of more than two years about the job specification for a new consultant post, the difficulty being that without 'acute' work as an inducement, it would be very difficult to attract anyone to the post. Dr. Marshall, the former S.A.M.O., would go no further than saying, 'Of course one would like more but quality, I think, is as important as quantity'. He felt that for many long-stay patients the services of general practitioner assistants was all that was needed. He did not feel that the Board had unduly delayed drawing up the job specification; nor did he appear to think that medical staffing was seriously inadequate on the basis of under three consultants for 2,000 patients.

Our own view, contrary to that of the Regional Hospital Board and the Hospital Management Committee, is that rehabilitating long-stay chronic or psychotic patients is no less complex and demanding a task, and requires at least as much specialised psychiatric skill, as the treatment of short-stay patients; and that the Board should not have acquiesced in a policy of medical laissez faire which left the care of patients, their physical health apart, to nurses, subject to an annual medical checkup and occasional visits. It was perhaps only to be expected that, without the consultant strength to organise active rehabilitation for more than a fraction of the long-stay population, minimal care has been the lot of most long-stay patients during their years at Whittingham. But it astounded us, on our visits, to see such abundant signs of locked doors between wards or even, within the old three-decker wards, locked doors between different areas, with nurses brandishing large bunches of keys; the still persisting use of airing courts and, in some parts of the hospital, of the antiquated parole system; and the pitifully inadequate use of the hospital's beautiful and spacious grounds.

We also feel that the Board's planning has been at fault. From the evidence of Dr. Marshall, the former S.A.M.O., we are sure that the Board are aware of the complex problems that arise from running down specialist mental illness hospitals and replacing them by departments in general hospitals. But it is by no means clear that they have so far thought out the solutions and incorporated them in their planning. It is not enough to say that, with the opening of district general hospital units 'Whittingham can close in 15–20 years'. Deprived of its remaining short-stay patients by the establishment of psychiatric units at Sharoe Green and Preston, as planned, Whittingham can certainly run down so far as this category of patient is concerned. But the admission to Whittingham of long-stay patients continues; that of elderly patients rises as longevity in Lancashire, as elsewhere, continues to increase; and without alternative provision for these patients the closure of the old hospital will remain a pipe-dream. Instead, a 'two-tier' system of psychiatry will be perpetuated, with therapeutic activity concentrated on the short-stay patients in the new psychiatric units while the accumulation of long-stay patients at Whittingham receives no more than residual care. This system is as demoralising for staff as it is bad for patients and we were glad to hear from the new Senior Administrative Medical Officer that he was fully appreciative of the need to make provision for all categories of patient in the current reorganisation of services in this part of Lancashire.

paras. 58–62

In our view the first step in sorting out the medical organisation and policies is for the senior medical staff, together with representatives of other medical staff, to constitute a Medical Executive Committee, electing a Chairman whose appointment should be subject to yearly renewal. The Chief Nursing Officer and other professional heads, including local Directors of Social Services, would no doubt be invited to attend as appropriate and it would ease communications if the Group Secretary were to be appointed its Secretary. This Medical Executive Committee should be closely linked with the rest of the management structure through the Professional Executive described in Chapter 4.

The second requirement is a substantial increase in numbers of consultants and their supporting medical staff. At least four additional consultants are needed, together with support from a geriatrician in the Preston Group.

The third is the reorganisation of the whole medical staff. Each consultant should have a share of long- and short-stay patients; and this should be achieved by forming 'multi-disciplinary therapeutic teams' consisting of consultants and their medical staff, nurses, social workers, psychologists and occupational therapists, each responsible for a defined geographical district. Some may be based at Whittingham, some in general hospital units in Preston and later, perhaps at Chorley.

Lastly there should be a clear plan for the hospital's future, co-ordinated by the Hospital Management Committee and agreed with the Regional Hospital Board, based on evaluation by statistical analysis of existing patients and their future needs. This should include, for the short term, a co-ordinated rehabilitation programme for all long-stay patients—which we see as an important creative task, not an unattractive residual exercise; for the medium term, diversification of patients to make maximum use of the hospital as its numbers of psychiatric patients run down; and, for the long term, replacement of the hospital as and when required. The work of the deaf unit should be dovetailed into this plan, whose aim should be to integrate all psychiatric services for the Preston area. It should provide for the gradual cessation of admissions to Whittingham, district by district, as new units open in general hospitals, and should allow for alternative provision for elderly mentally ill patients so as to avoid the accumulation of long-stay psychotic, elderly confused and geriatric cases at Whittingham. In so far as psycho-geriatric assessment facilities will be needed these should be, not at Whittingham, but in the Preston Group. Ribchester is, in its size and situation, a useful hospital that deserves continuation, perhaps for geriatric patients in the long term. When the plan is completed it should be published in the hospital and explained to the staff. In this way the Board, the Hospital Management Committee and all their officers and professional people, with the other hospitals concerned, will be working together towards a common objective.

paras. 64–7

10 Social Work and Family Welfare

Introduction

It is usual and convenient to date the emergence of social work as a profession and of social casework as a skill from the founding of the Charity Organization Society in 1869. The term social casework has a modern sound, but from the beginning the COS described itself as 'a general family casework agency', and while much of the work actually done must have consisted in the distribution of material help, the early workers stressed—to a perhaps disproportionate extent—the importance they attached to establishing a relationship and to offering personal service, before going on to mobilize material help in cash and kind.

From the 1880s the COS was concerning itself explicitly with social work training, and in 1903 it established a School of Sociology and Social Economics to train social workers. The School, later absorbed into the London School of Economics, offered courses in sociology, social theory, and Poor Law administration, but stressed that the training provided was a general basic training for social work, not to be confused with specialized vocational training for a specific job. The training was therefore, in the present-day sense, generic. The proliferation of specialized courses, and the fragmentation of social work which in more recent years posed so many problems came later, though not so very much later.

Writing in 1953, Miss (later Dame) Eileen Younghusband summed up the position in these words:

> How promising and full of vigour was social work in England fifty years ago! The essential initial discoveries about its nature and processes and the methods by which social workers should be trained had been made. All seemed set for a steady advance into territory which had been soundly surveyed. Then for reasons which it is difficult to determine a blight set in, and, with one exception, social work in this country remained almost static, compared with the preceding half century, until after the second world war.

The one exception Miss Younghusband made to that picture of stagna-
tion between the wars was highly significant. It was the establishment in
1929 of the London Mental Health Course, offering the first recognized
training for psychiatric social workers. It was through this course and other
developments allied to it that British social workers became acquainted
with the influence that new teachings in psychiatry and psychology were
having on social work in the USA. Not only psychiatric social work, but
most other forms of casework, and indeed social work as a whole, were in
due course revolutionized by the teachings of Freud, Jung, Adler and their
disciples. In most branches of social work the revolution did not come
about until the late 1940s, but by 1955 it was possible for Barbara Wootton
to attack the prevailing wisdom in social work in these forthright terms:

> Rather than search for 'something deeper underneath' when her help is
> sought in external practical emergencies, the social worker would do
> better to look for something more superficial on top when she is con-
> fronted with problems of behaviour. If she uses a request for practical
> help as an opportunity to intrude into other aspects of her client's life,
> she does so, or should do so, at her peril.'

Elsewhere, Lady Wootton, as she later became, quoted an extended
definition of the social work process by Dame Eileen Younghusband of
which, to avoid being wearisome, I will quote only the last two sentences:

> [The social worker] must enter into [her client's] problems as he sees
> them, his relationships as he experiences them, with their frustrations,
> their deprivations, their satisfactions, and see him, or his different
> selves, as they appear to him himself. Yet at the same time she must also
> be clearly aware of the realities of the situation and through her pro-
> fessional skill in relationships enable him to come to a better under-
> standing of himself and others.

Lady Wootton commented: 'It might well be thought that the social
worker's best, indeed perhaps her only, chance of achieving aims at once so
intimate and so ambitious would be to marry her client.'

Since the 1950s the emphasis of social work has shifted, or at any rate
diversified. There is now much greater willingness to recognize that the
social worker can have a role as a middleman in an increasingly complex
welfare state without compromising her professional status. In addition,
the claustrophobic concentration on the individual casework relationship has for many social workers given way to working with families, with
groups, and with communities to help them adapt to social change, or
even to promote social change. Within the framework provided by the
local authority social service departments set up under the Local Authority
Social Services Act, 1970, there is scope for variety and opportunity for
innovation. Many of the previous legislative constraints on innovation to

meet emerging social needs have been swept away. Only the problems of settling down to do a job of work following yet another reorganization, as a result of the 1974 recasting of the structure of local government, stand in the way of an era of consolidation and achievement.

10.1 Children Act, 1908

The tally of nineteenth century legislation designed to protect children from exploitation and cruelty and to make provision for those who had lost their parents would include the Health and Morals of Apprentices Act, 1803—designed to limit the working hours of pauper apprentices, to ensure proper sanitary arrangements, and to provide them with a minimal education—the Industrial Schools Act, the Prevention of Cruelty to Children Act, 1889, the Infant Life Protection Acts of 1872 and 1896, as well as several pieces of factory legislation and various local by-laws governing the employment of children. As far as the Factory Acts were concerned, measures to protect children were on several occasions used as the thin edge of the wedge leading ultimately to improvement in the working conditions of adults. Many of the noted philanthropists of the age, Shaftesbury pre-eminent among them, were particularly active for the benefit of orphaned and other deprived children. Philanthropic organizations were set up to provide homes for orphans and to train the children of the poor in useful trades. The National Society for the Prevention of Cruelty to Children was founded in 1884.

The public conscience was perhaps more easily stirred on behalf of children than on behalf of any other group. At a time when it was widely felt that adults should be left to fend for themselves it was acknowledged to be a legitimate concern of the State to regulate the working conditions of children. The disclosure of the scandals of baby-farming—the fostering of children for reward—to the Parliamentary Committee on the Protection of Infant Life in 1871 led immediately to the Infant Life Protection Act of 1872 and when this measure proved inadequate to prevent the wilful neglect of these children, further legislation was passed in 1896.

The hardships endured by children in workhouses were brought to popular attention by Charles Dickens, but from the very beginning it had been the intention of the New Poor Law that children, as well as the sick and infirm, should be housed separately from the able-bodied paupers. The persistence of the general mixed workhouse in which all were subject to the same regime was flatly against the principles which had been spelled out in the report of the 1834 Commission. Even so, the more progressive boards of guardians took the lead in providing education for pauper children, even before the Education Act of 1870, and as the century wore on some of them moved the workhouse children into cottage homes where they could live in small groups with a more family-like atmosphere than was possible in the large institution. These cottage homes had been pioneered by voluntary organizations for the care of children, numbers of which were founded in the latter half of the nineteenth century. Dr Barnado opened his first home in 1866 and in 1869 the National Children's Homes were founded. The organization which later became known as the Church of England Children's Society was founded in 1881.

There was therefore a considerable background of concern and of attempts to ameliorate the lot of deprived and neglected children by the time the 1906 Liberal Government embarked on their programme of social legislation. Previous legislation had been piecemeal. Attempts to be more thoroughgoing had been hindered by reluctance to interfere with parental rights and by considerations of economy as far as those children who were the responsibility of boards of guardians were concerned. There was also the very size of the problem. One of the marked differences between the Victorian era and our own is the tremendous decline in mortality between fifteen and forty-five, the years when parents are bringing up children. Most of the children in the care of public authorities today have living parents. In Victorian times 'Orphan Annie' was all too familiar a figure.

The Children Act of 1908, the 'Children's Charter', consolidated previous legislation and took a number of important steps forward. It was the basic statute governing the welfare of children until it was repealed by— and a number of its provisions incorporated in—the Children and Young Persons Act, 1933. The Act implemented the main recommendations of the Committee on the Treatment of Young Offenders, which reported in 1907. The Bill was steered through the House of Commons by Herbert Samuel, later Lord Samuel, then Parliamentary Under-Secretary at the Home Office, where he had also shared responsibility for the introduction of borstals and the launching of the probation service. Earlier legislation on infant life protection and the prevention of cruelty to children was incorporated in the Act and the law was strengthened to cover neglect as well as actual cruelty. It was provided that children being neglected by their parents could be removed to a place of safety. The overlaying of a child by a drunken mother was made a criminal offence, as was the giving of alcoholic liquor to a child under five. Children under fourteen were not to be allowed on licensed premises during opening hours. Children were also forbidden to smoke. The Act provided penalties for allowing children or young persons to be in brothels, for causing them to beg, and for taking goods into pawn from children. A person looking after a child for reward was forbidden to insure the child's life, and strict procedures were laid down for notifying the death of a child both to the local authority and to the coroner.

All these and other measures for the protection of children were accompanied by provisions to temper the previous rigour of the law in dealing with child offenders. No child or young person could be sentenced to death or to penal servitude, and no child could be sent to prison. A young person was not to be sent to prison unless no other form of punishment was suitable. Local authorities were given a duty to provide remand homes to keep children and young persons out of prison while awaiting trial, and it was laid down that juveniles were to be tried in specially constituted juvenile courts.

Children Act, 1908

INFANT LIFE PROTECTION

1.—(1) Where a person undertakes for reward the nursing and maintenance of one or more infants under the age of seven years apart from their parents or having no parents, he shall, within forty-eight hours from the reception of any such infant, give notice in writing thereof to the local authority:

Provided that this section shall not apply, as respects any infant, where the period for which it is received is forty-eight hours or less.

(2) Where a person undertakes for reward the nursing and maintenance of an infant already in his care without reward, the entering into the undertaking shall, for the purposes of this Part of this Act, be treated as a reception of the infant.

(3) The notice shall state the name, sex, and date and place of birth of the infant, the name of the person receiving the infant, and the dwelling within which the infant is being kept, and the name and address of the person from whom the infant has been received.

(4) If a person who has undertaken the nursing and maintenance of any such infant changes his residence, he shall within forty-eight hours thereof give to the local authority notice in writing of the change, and, where the residence to which he moves is situate in the district of another local authority, he shall give to that local authority the like notice as respects each infant in his care as he is by this section required to give on the first reception of the infant.

(5) If any such infant dies or is removed from the care of the person who has undertaken its nursing and maintenance, that person shall, within forty-eight hours thereof, give to the local authority notice in writing of the death or removal, and in the latter case also the name and address of the person to whose care the infant has been transferred. . . .

2.—(1) It shall be the duty of every local authority to provide for the execution of this Part of this Act within their district, and for that purpose they shall from time to time make inquiry whether there are any persons residing therein who undertake the nursing and maintenance of infants in respect of whom notice is required to be given under the foregoing section.

(2) If in the district of any local authority any persons are found to undertake the nursing and maintenance of such infants as aforesaid, the local authority shall appoint one or more persons of either sex to be infant protection visitors, whose duty it shall be from time to time to visit any infants referred to in any notice given under this Part of this Act, and the premises in which they are kept, in order to satisfy themselves as to the proper nursing and maintenance of the infants or to give any necessary advice or directions as to their nursing and maintenance:

Provided that the local authority may, either in addition to or in lieu of appointing infant protection visitors, authorise in writing one or more suitable persons of either sex to exercise the powers of infant protection visitors under this Part of this Act, subject to such terms and conditions as may be stated in the authorisation, and, where any infants have been placed out to nurse in the district of the authority by any philanthropic society, may, if satisfied that the interests of the infants are properly safeguarded, so authorise the society to exercise those powers as respects those infants, subject, however, to the obligation to furnish periodical reports to the local authority.

(3) A local authority may combine with any other local authority for the purpose of executing the provisions of this Part of this Act, and for defraying the expenses thereof.

(4) A local authority may exempt from being visited, either unconditionally or subject to such conditions as they think fit, any particular premises within their district which appear to them to be so conducted that it is unnecessary that they should be visited.

(5) If any person undertaking the nursing and maintenance of any such infants refuses to allow any such visitor or other person to visit or examine the infants or the premises in which they are kept, he shall be guilty of an offence under this Part of this Act.

(6) If any such visitor or other person is refused admittance to any premises in contravention of this Part of this Act, or has reason to believe that any infants under the age of seven years are being kept in any house or premises in contravention of this Part of this Act, he may apply to a justice, who, on being satisfied, on information in writing on oath, that there is reasonable ground for believing that an offence under this Part of this Act has been committed, may grant a warrant authorising the visitor or other person to enter the premises for the purpose of ascertaining whether any offence under this Part of this Act has been committed, and, if the occupier of the premises or any other person obstructs or causes or procures to be obstructed any visitor or other person acting in pursuance of such a warrant, he shall be guilty of an offence under this Part of this Act.

3. An infant, in respect of which notice is required to be given under this Part of this Act, shall not, without the written sanction of the local authority, be kept—

(a) by any person from whose care any infant has been removed under this Part of this Act or the Infant Life Protection Act, 1897; or

(b) in any premises from which any infant has been removed under this Part of this Act by reason of the premises being dangerous or insanitary, or has been removed under the Infant Life Protection Act, 1897, by reason of the premises being so unfit as to endanger its health; or

(c) by any person who has been convicted of any offence under Part II. of this Act or under the Prevention of Cruelty to Children Act, 1904;

and any person keeping or causing to be kept an infant contrary to this section shall be guilty of an offence under this Part of this Act.

4. The local authority may fix the number of infants under the age of seven years which may be kept in any dwelling in respect of which a notice has been received under this Part of this Act, and any person keeping any infant in excess of the number so fixed shall be guilty of an offence under this Part of this Act.

5.—(1) If any infant, in respect of which notice is required to be given under this Part of this Act is kept,—

(a) in any premises which are overcrowded, dangerous or insanitary; or

(b) by any person who, by reason of negligence, ignorance, inebriety, immorality, criminal conduct, or other similar cause, is unfit to have care of it; or

(c) by any person or in any premises in contravention of any of the provisions of this Part of this Act,

any visitor or other person appointed or authorised to execute the provisions of this Part of this Act may apply either to a justice or to the local authority for an order directing him to remove the infant to a place of safety until it can be restored to its relatives or be otherwise lawfully disposed of.

(2) Any person refusing to comply with such an order upon its being produced and read over to him, or obstructing or causing or procuring to be obstructed the visitor or such other person in the execution thereof, shall be guilty of an offence under this Part of this Act, and

(a) if the order was made by a justice, the order may be enforced by the visitor or by any constable; and

(b) if the order was made by the local authority the visitor or other person may apply to any justice for an order directing the removal of the infant, which order may be enforced by the visitor or by any constable.

6.—(1) In the case of the death of any infant respecting which notice is required to be given under this Part of this Act, the person who had the care of the infant shall, within twenty-four hours of the death, give notice in writing thereof to the coroner of the district within which the body of the infant lies, and the coroner shall hold an inquest thereon, unless a certificate under the hand of a duly qualified medical practitioner is produced to him, certifying that he has personally attended the infant during its last illness, and specifying the cause of death, and the coroner is satisfied that there is no ground for holding an inquest.

(2) If any person required to give a notice under this section fails to give the notice within the time specified for giving the notice, he shall be guilty of an offence under this Part of this Act.

7. A person by whom an infant in respect of which notice is required to be

given under this Part of this Act is kept shall be deemed to have no interest in the life of the child for the purposes of the Life Assurance Act, 1774, and, if any such person directly or indirectly insures or attempts to insure the life of such an infant, he shall be guilty of an offence under this Part of this Act, and, if a company, within the meaning of the Life Assurance Companies Acts, 1870 to 1872, or any other company, society, or person, knowingly issues, or procures or attempts to procure to be issued, to or for the benefit of such a person as aforesaid or to any person on his behalf, a policy on the life of such an infant, the company, society, or person shall be guilty of an offence under this Part of this Act.

S. 1–7

A PLACE OF SAFETY

20.—(1) A constable, or any person authorised by a justice, may take to a place of safety any child or young person in respect of whom an offence under this Part of this Act, or any of the offences mentioned in the First Schedule to this Act, has been, or there is reason to believe has been, committed.

(2) A child or young person so taken to a place of safety, and also any child or young person who seeks refuge in a place of safety, may there be detained until he can be brought before a court of summary jurisdiction, and that court may make such order as is mentioned in the next following subsection, or may cause the child or young person to be dealt with as circumstances may admit and require, until the charge made against any person in respect of any offence as aforesaid with regard to the child or young person has been determined by the conviction or discharge of such person.

(3) Where it appears to a court of summary jurisdiction or any justice that an offence under this Part of this Act, or any of the offences mentioned in the First Schedule to this Act, has been committed in respect of any child or young person who is brought before the court or justice, and that it is expedient in the interests of the child or young person that an order should be made under this subsection, the court of justice may, without prejudice to any other power under this Act, make such order as circumstances require for the care and detention of the child or young person until a reasonable time has elapsed for a charge to be made against some person for having committed the offence, and, if a charge is made against any person within that time, until the charge has been determined by the conviction or discharge of that person, and in case of conviction for such further time not exceeding twenty-one days as the court which convicted may direct, and any such order may be carried out notwithstanding that any person claims the custody of the child or young person.

S. 20

10.2 Report of the Care of Children Committee (Curtis Report)

Published: 1946

Chairman: *Miss Myra Curtis*

Members: *S. Clement Brown; R. J. Evans; Lucy G. Fildes; M. L. Harford; Somerville Hastings; Mary L. Kingsmill Jones; John H. Litten; John Moss; Helen Murtagh; Muriel E. Nicol; Henry Salt; J. C. Spence; Francis Temple; S. O. Walmsley; H. Graham White; Miss D. M. Rosling and G. T. Milne (joint secretaries)*

Terms of Reference (1945): *To inquire into existing methods of providing for children who from loss of parents or from any cause whatever are deprived of a normal home life with their own parents or relatives; and to consider what further measures should be taken to ensure that these children are brought up under conditions best calculated to compensate them for the lack of parental care.*

The Curtis Report ranks as one of the great reforming documents of the twentieth century. The work of the Curtis Committee represented, as they themselves pointed out, the first major inquiry directed specifically to the care of children deprived of a normal home life, and covering all groups of such children. The major recommendations were almost immediately implemented in the Children Act of 1948. The committee owed their existence and terms of reference to widespread public and parliamentary concern about the quality of care given to deprived children, concern which was eloquently expressed by Lady Allen of Hurtwood in a letter to *The Times* in 1944, and which was intensified by the O'Neill case the following year. Dennis O'Neill, a child boarded out by a local authority on a lonely Shropshire farm, died from ill-treatment and neglect, and the subsequent inquiry by Sir Walter Monckton KC told a sad tale of administrative muddle and failure to provide effective supervision. The tragic case guaranteed a sympathetic reception for any proposals designed to safeguard the welfare of children in the care of public authorities and other agencies.

It is important to remember that the terms of reference given to the committee limited discussion to children who were already in need of care by someone other than their own parents or relatives. The committee were not charged to consider how children came to be in need of such care, or how situations necessitating such care might be prevented. This limitation ensured that legislation based on the committee's recommendations did not pay much attention to these aspects either, and so the early years of most local authority children's departments were spent receiving children into care rather freely—with in fact no legal powers to spend money on preventing family breakdown—and in ensuring that the care they received was of a high standard. In ensuring this high standard of care they were guided by the belief of the Curtis Committee that 'The need of the deprived child is for a home or a good substitute for a home'. The committee went on to elaborate the concept of the 'substitute home':

If the substitute home is to give the child what he gets from a good normal home it must supply—

(i) affection and personal interest; understanding of his defects; care for his future; respect for his personality and regard for his self esteem.

(ii) stability; the feeling that he can expect to remain with those who will continue to care for him till he goes out into the world on his own feet.

(iii) opportunity of making the best of his ability and aptitudes, whatever they may be, as such opportunity is made available to the child in the normal home.

(iv) a share in the common life of a small group of people in a homely environment.

The most completely satisfactory method of providing a child with a substitute home was, the Curtis Committee felt, adoption, The best method short of adoption was boarding out in a foster home, provided that the foster home was of a satisfactory standard and that sufficient supervision was available to ensure that it continued to be so. However, where not enough good foster parents were available, institutional care was preferable to subjecting the child to the risks of a bad or indifferent foster home. Where institutional care was necessary, the committee favoured the small group home, with the exception that it was thought maladjusted children might do better in a larger group of say about thirty. Children's homes should, however, always be separated from the public assistance institutions—the former workhouses—with which a number of them were still linked, both physically and administratively, in 1946. A further recommendation was the setting up in all areas of reception homes to enable the child to be observed and his needs assessed before he was boarded out or transferred to a small group home.

The greater part of the Curtis Report was devoted to the description of existing statutory provisions and administrative arrangements and of existing standards of care. Members of the committee visited 451 institutions of various kinds, including workhouses, other local authority institutions, voluntary homes, approved schools and remand homes, in all parts of the country, and interviewed officials and members of fifty-eight local authorities. They also visited a number of children in foster homes. Section II of the report drew heavily on reports of these visits and set out the best and the worst for all to see. The worst was very bad indeed. No cases of actual cruelty were observed, although as the committee remarked it was unlikely that actual cruelty would be seen by visitors, even those arriving unannounced, as members of the committee tried to do. There were, however, instances of neglect sufficiently serious to make it necessary to draw the immediate attention of the authorities to the conditions observed. The most widespread failing was a lack of interest and affection for the child as an individual, with his own rights and possessions, his own life to live and his own contribution to offer. Conditions in the large institution often made it difficult to provide this individual care, but the committee were able to quote instances of a very high standard of care which showed what could be done.

Much good work was being done, the committee concluded, but the standard was so variable and at the lower level so poor, that a determined effort had to be made to lift the whole treatment of the child without a home on to a new, more even, and higher level. Failures were generally due to faults of administration and imperfect selection and training of staff. The suggested remedies, therefore, lay mainly in the sphere of administration and personnel. So urgent did the committee feel the question of staff training to be that they issued an interim report on the training of staff of residential homes. The main report followed this with an appendix setting out recommendations for the training of boarding-out visitors, or as they later came to be known, child care officers.

The report criticized the division and confusion of responsibility for deprived children which resulted from the patchwork pattern of existing legislation. A child might be subjected to completely different treatment, depending on which legal category he was placed in, yet this itself was often a matter almost of chance. He could be shuttled between different local authority departments, each of which might be supervised by a different government department, or by none at all. The Curtis Committee therefore recommended that there should be unified responsibility for all deprived children, both at national and local level. They rejected the suggestion of a national authority to take full responsibility, because they felt that constant local interest in the children of a locality was a very important element in their welfare, and local authorities should not be divested of responsibility for their own children who were without normal homes. But in place of the existing division of responsibility between the Ministries of Health and Education and the Home Office, the committee recommended that responsibilities and powers under the Poor Law Act, Children and Young Persons Acts, Public Health Act and Adoption of Children Acts should be concentrated in one central department, which would define and maintain standards at local level by inspection, advice and direction. The committee made no recommendation as to which central department this should be, but in the event it was decided it should be the Home Office. It was also recommended that all services by local authorities to deprived children should be subject to Exchequer grant and that the inspecting staff of the central department should be brought up to the number necessary to ensure the inspection of all children's homes, including those in the hands of voluntary organizations, at least once a year.

At local level the Curtis Committee recommended that county and county borough councils should normally be the responsible authorities, although where the number of children to be cared for was very small, joint boards might be formed. Each authority should have a children's committee which would be responsible for the provision and administration of children's homes, for boarding out, for child life protection, for the local authority's functions with regard to adoption, and for the keeping of records of all deprived children in the area, including particulars of those in voluntary homes. Each children's committee would appoint as its chief officer a children's officer who would be a specialist in child care, and whose appointment would be subject to approval by the central authority.

There was one reservation to the report, signed by six members of the committee. This referred to a paragraph in which the majority of the committee had suggested that existing regulations prohibiting the boarding out of a child with foster parents of a different religious persuasion were unjustifiable if they resulted in a child's being left in an unsatisfactory environment, or being moved to a less satisfactory home, merely on account of this one factor. The minority—Messrs Harford, Litten and Walmsley, together with Miss Kingsmill Jones, Miss Murtagh and Miss Temple, felt, however, that it was a matter of 'the first importance' that all children who were boarded out in foster homes should receive adequate religious care, and not only wanted this regulation retained, but a new one introduced stipulating that where the religious denomination of a child could not be ascertained, he should be boarded out in a foster home where 'adequate religious care is provided'.

Curtis Report, 1946

GENERAL IMPRESSIONS OF EXISTING CARE

We now offer a summary of the general impressions made upon us by witnesses, and by our own survey, with regard to the existing provision made for children deprived of a normal home life. In the first place we are far from satisfied with the immediate provision made for children coming as destitute or in need of care or protection into the care of local authorities. Some authorities indeed receive the children into establishments for temporary care where they can be studied, cleansed and cared for in an adequate and kindly way until they are placed in whatever their permanent substitute home may be but in far too many areas the child is put into a workhouse ward where there is nothing but the barest provision for his physical needs and where the staff have neither the capacity nor the time to relieve his fears, make him feel at ease or give him occupation or interest. What is more, he may remain in such unsatisfactory conditions, temporary though they are supposed to be, not only for weeks, but for months, before something better is found for him.

Turning to the long-term provision, it is evident that more kindly imagination, as well as more scientific thought, has gone into the arrangement and equipment of nurseries than into any other form of care for the healthy child, though a great deal remains to be done in the way of precautions which medical opinion thinks necessary for infants congregated together. Nursery schools, though as yet by no means fully developed, on the whole carry on in the same spirit, and it is evident that their extension will bring brightness and constructive occupation into the lives of the small children in public care. The provision for the older children, in Homes or boarded out, is generally speaking on a lower level both of aim and of achievement. Both these types of provision have recently caused public anxiety—the first because of assertions as to their out of date, harsh or repressive methods, the second because of actual disasters to children so provided for. We think the anxiety was justified, even though the general position is by no means so bad as particular incidents and statements might suggest. We have seen much that is good, and highly creditable to those responsible; but we have also seen much that calls for reform.

It is right to say in the first place, as regards Homes for children, that very little evidence, written or oral, has been tendered to us that there are seriously bad conditions in existing Homes in the sense of conditions involving neglect or harsh usage. Some witnesses have come forward to describe to us their own upbringing as inmates of Homes, and in a few instances the picture drawn was a very dark one. Even allowing for some bias and exaggeration, the treatment of these particular children had clearly not been happy or successful. It must be remarked however that the evidence related to a period of ten or more years ago and that there has been much improvement since then in methods of discipline and other conditions. The whole attitude of society to the treatment of children has been moving towards a gentler and more sympathetic approach, and we had it in evidence from a very experienced inspector that children's Homes and persons responsible for the care of the unfortunate child have shared in this development. We heard moreover other witnesses brought up in institutions who gave evidence of a different purport, even as regards the same period or earlier, and evidently regarded themselves as having been by no means unfortunate in their childhood's experiences. We ourselves have seen excellently conducted Homes run by organisations which have been attacked. We do not therefore feel justified, so far as evidence of this character is concerned, in forming conclusions adverse to the general administration of child care in any organisation or group of institutions. The witnesses in question did however bring home to us the danger, even in an organisation or under an authority with an enlightened policy, that individuals in charge of groups of children may develop harsh or repressive tendencies or false ideas of discipline, and that the children in their care may suffer without the knowledge of the central authority. A code of rules which sets a proper standard is one necessity but it is plain that no code will suffice without regular inspection and constant watchfulness that the right atmosphere of kindness and sympathy is maintained.

Our own survey has given us a firmer basis for conclusions about actual present day conditions. It will be apparent from this Section of our Report that we have seen examples of almost all levels of child care, some very good, some indubitably bad. By far the greater number of Homes were, within the limits of their staffing, accommodation and administrative arrangements, reasonably well run from the standpoint of physical care, and in other ways the child has more material advantages than could have been given to him in the average poor family. Where establishments fell below a satisfactory standard, the defects were not of harshness, but rather of dirt and dreariness, drabness and over-regimentation. We found no child being cruelly used in the ordinary sense, but that was perhaps not a probable discovery on a casual visit. We did find many establishments under both local authority and voluntary management in which children were being brought up by unimaginative methods, without opportunity for developing their full capabilities and with very little brightness or interest in their surroundings. We found in fact many places where the standard of child care was no better, except in respect of disciplinary methods, than that of say 30 years ago; and we found a widespread and deplorable shortage of the right kind of staff, personally qualified and trained to provide the child with a substitute for a home background. The result in many Homes was a lack of personal interest in and affection for the children which we found shocking. The child in these Homes was not recognised as an individual with his own rights and possessions, his own life to live and his own contribution to offer. He was merely one of a large crowd, eating, playing and sleeping with the rest, without any place or possession of his own or any quiet room to which he could retreat. Still more important, he was without the feeling that there was anyone to whom he could turn who was vitally interested in his welfare or who cared for him as a person. The effect of this on the smaller children was reflected in their behaviour towards visitors, which took the form of an almost pathological clamouring for attention and petting. In the older children the effect appeared more in slowness, backwardness and lack of response, and in habits of destructiveness and want of concentration. Where individual love and care had been given, the behaviour of the children was quite different. They showed no undue interest in visitors and were easily and happily engaged in their own occupations and games.

Apart from the absence in many Homes of this essential element in a child's wellbeing, we have found much to criticise in accommodation, equipment and staffing. Even when full allowance is made for wartime shortages and difficulties, it is evident that in many places a higher standard needs to be set. The difference between the results achieved in what would appear to be precisely parallel conditions is often startling. Where a community is successful its success may be accounted for in one of several ways. Enlightened central direction can do much, as is apparent in the approved schools and the best of the voluntary Homes. Good local administration and the interest and support of a competent local committee can do perhaps even more. Full collaboration between the central authority and the local administration is of great importance. We noticed all these factors at one time or another as affecting the quality of a Home. But outstanding among the comments on our visits are references to the good or poor Superintendent, Matron, House mother or other member of the staff in immediate charge of the children. On the personality and skill of these workers depends primarily the happiness of the children in their care. We have seen much admirable and devoted work by people putting their whole heart and energy into this task, sometimes in very unhelpful conditions. But such workers are too few to handle the work to be done, and some of them have had too little preparation for a very difficult task. On the whole, as we indicated in our Interim Report, this task has not been regarded as one calling for any special skill, and many of the children have suffered in consequence.

When we turn to boarding out, we meet a different set of inadequacies and dangers. We found in the children in the foster homes we visited almost complete freedom from the sense of deprivation which we have described among the children in Homes. Indeed the foster homes as a whole made a remarkably favourable impression. While there were some which on one ground or another we did not consider suitable places for the care of a child, there were few in which the child was not a member of the household, or did not appear to be finding affection and happiness. In some cases indeed the fostermother had become too possessive for the relation to be altogether satisfactory. The faults of foster homes are different from those of large communities and very difficult to diagnose at a casual visit. They depend on the attitude of the fosterparents to the child and the accidents of fortune in the home, and a crisis may occur which could not be anticipated from a single inspection.

What impressed us with regard to boarding out was the need for a greater sense of personal interest and responsibility at local authority headquarters, and for more specialist staff there; and for more trained supervisors to visit the children. There is no doubt that the O'Neill case had put authorities on their guard against slackness in administration; and we thought that the individuals in charge of boarding out in the authorities' offices were doing their best, though sometimes in a rather remote and impersonal way, to serve the interests of the children. But the present administrative system seems to us full of pitfalls. Divided responsibility, office delays, misunderstandings and misjudgments of people, irregular visiting and failure to visit promptly in emergency, may easily under present conditions facilitate a tragedy, as they have done in the past. It was moreover clear to us that it was very rare for an authority to feel that it had a choice among a number of thoroughly satisfactory foster homes, though whether more homes would have been available if a greater effort had been made to find them is not so certain. One of the counties in which we saw the most satisfactory foster homes had been able to board out only about a third of the children in the care of the council.

On the whole our judgment is that there is probably a greater risk of acute unhappiness in a foster home, but that a happy foster home is happier than life as generally lived in a large community. Our proposals for improving the quality of both types of substitute home will be found in the next Section of our Report.

paras. 415–22

THE CHILDREN'S OFFICER

Our preference for the single *ad hoc* committee with power to make recommendations and submit estimates direct to the council is based in part on the need we feel for emphasising the function of home-finding as something separate and distinct from the education and health services given to all children; but in part also on our desire that it should have its own executive officer with the standing of an important administrative official of the council, in direct touch with the responsible committee, not a member of the staff of the Education Officer or other head of department, however closely linked with existing departments for purposes of office administration. Needless to say we should regard such close links as indispensable. All the services of the health and education departments should be available to the Children's Officer at need, for example the organiser of school meals as dietetic adviser for the children's Homes, the handicrafts and youth club specialists for the organisation of recreational activities there, and the Health Visitors for advice about children's health. We desire, however, to see the responsibility for the welfare of the deprived children definitely laid on a Children's Officer. This may indeed be said to be our solution of the problem referred to us. Throughout our investigation we have been increasingly impressed by the need for the personal element in the care of children, which Sir Walter Monckton emphasised in his report on the O'Neill case. No office staff dealing with them as case papers can do the work we want done—work which is in part administrative, but also in large part field work, involving many personal contacts and the solution of problems by direct methods, in particular the method of interview rather than official correspondence. All the persons who deal with the child—the Superintendent of the Home, the foster parent and the school teacher—should be known as human beings to the officer of the authority to whom the care of that particular child has been assigned.

So important do we think it that a Children's Officer should be appointed and should be an officer of high standing and qualifications, that where the children in an area are not numerous enough to provide a full load of work we think authorities should combine and set up a joint Children's Board with a joint executive officer. Some of the counties might well combine for this purpose with the county boroughs within their limits. There is something absurd about two officials in different streets of the same town boarding out children, one on behalf of the borough, the other on behalf of the county. Even combined, some of these areas would not, on the present basis, provide a case load for a very responsible officer; the load would, however, be increased if our recommendations with regard to widening the scope of public care were adopted. We have no desire to fix a hard and fast limit, but we think that an area with less than 500 children in the classes requiring periodical visiting should prima facie be combined with another area. The Joint Board should exercise all the functions in relation to deprived children which in the case of a county or county borough council would be exercised through the Children's Committee, including the administration of the children's Homes in the area.

As we envisage the revised organisation which we recommend, the Children's Officer would be its pivot. She (we use the feminine pronoun not with any aim of excluding men from these posts but because we think it may be found that the majority of persons suitable for the work are women) will of course work under the orders of her committee or board, but she will be a specialist in child care as the Medical Officer of Health is a specialist in his own province and the Director of Education is in his; and she will have no other duties to distract her interests. She would represent the council in its parental functions. The committal of the child to the care of a council which takes over parental rights and duties is not without incongruity. To be properly exercised the responsibility must be delegated to an individual, and that individual one whose training has fitted her for child care and whose whole attention is given to it. Though committal by the Court to a 'fit person' should, in order to secure continuity and relieve the officer of an undue burden of liability, be still made to the authority, the Children's Officer would be the *person* to whom the child would look as guardian.

Orphan children not living with legal guardians or near relatives would be her care as war orphans are now the care of the Ministry of Pensions officer. Children would be brought to her notice by the police, relieving officers (or the equivalent under any new arrangement for public assistance), parents, voluntary organisations, and the National Society for the Prevention of Cruelty to Children. She would keep full and careful records of all deprived children for whom her authority is responsible, she would place them in suitable homes where necessary and would care for their welfare until they were independent. All placings of children in foster homes not through her office, whether for reward or not, and whether or not with a view to adoption, would be notified to her, and she would be responsible for the supervision of the children. She would also watch over the welfare of the illegitimate children in the area. She would be notified of all children placed in the voluntary Homes in her area and would arrange for them to be visited. She would maintain close contact with voluntary organisations operating in her area. She would be directly responsible, under her committee, for admissions of children to all Homes in the area owned or managed by the local authority and for the maintenance of these Homes at a proper standard. She would apply in suitable cases to the local education authority for the admission of deprived children to boarding-schools. She would keep a list of suitable foster homes for boarding out and inspect those homes or arrange for their inspection. Other local authorities would not board out in the area except through her and on the understanding that the local Children's Committee would undertake the supervision of these children. She would maintain a record of children for whom her committee was responsible who had been placed in another area, and arrange for them to be visited by the Children's Officer of that area. She would be responsible for the supervision of the staff of the local authority's children's Homes and would have a staff of women and probably at least one man performing the present functions of boarding out visitors and child protection visitors, as well as suitable clerical staff. Though the Children's Officer would be responsible to the committee of her local authority we think it important that her qualifications should be approved by the central department before her appointment and also that she should make an annual report to her committee which should be presented to the council and forwarded to the central department. We should hope that when the organisation we recommend is well established, the Children's Officer would be so well known in her area as the authority on children's welfare questions that individual difficulties and problems would be brought to her as a matter of course.

We attach great importance to establishing and maintaining a continuing personal relation between the child deprived of a home and the official of the local authority responsible for looking after him. This relation with officials of a central department has been achieved by the Ministry of Pensions for its war orphans. It will not be practicable for the Children's Officer of a large county council or county borough council to know and keep in personal touch with all the children under her care, and she should therefore aim at allocating a group of children definitely to each of her subordinates. The subordinate officer would, subject to accidents, illness, change of employment, and the incidence of retirement, be the friend of those particular children through their childhood and adolescence up to the age of sixteen or eighteen as the case might be.

The Children's Officer should in our view be highly qualified academically, if possible a graduate who has also a social science diploma. She should not be under thirty at the time of appointment and should have had some experience of work with children. She should have marked administrative capacity and be able readily to grasp local government procedure and to work easily with local authority committees. Her essential qualifications, however, would be on the personal side. She should be genial and friendly in manner and able to set both children and adults at their ease. She should have a strong interest in the welfare of children and enough faith and enthusiasm to be ready to try methods new and old of compensating by care and affection those who have had a bad start in life. She should have very high standards of physical and moral welfare, but should be flexible enough in temperament to avoid a sterile institutional correctness.

paras. 441–6

10.3 Children Act, 1948

The Children Act, 1948, arose directly from the Report of the Care of Children Committee (the Curtis Report) and embodied a number of its main recommendations. It introduced a system of unified administrative responsibility for the care of deprived children, laying down that 'local authorities shall exercise their functions . . . under the general guidance' of the Home Office, and that each local authority (for this purpose county and county borough councils) should set up a children's committee and appoint a children's officer, the appointment being subject to the approval of the Secretary of State. Two Advisory Councils in Child Care, one for England and Wales and one for Scotland, were appointed to advise the Secretary of State.

The Act made it the duty of the local authority to receive a child into care if the child had no parent or guardian, was abandoned or lost, or if the child's parents or guardians were prevented, either temporarily or permanently, by reason of incapacity or any other circumstances, from looking after the child properly. It was also made a duty of the local authority to restore the child to his parents or guardians as soon as they were able to take him back and it was in the child's interests for them to do so. If the parents or guardians were dead, or permanently unable or unfit to care for the child, then the local authority could, by resolution— subject to appeal to the courts—assume all parental rights over the child who had been taken into care.

The Act paid scrupulous attention to the rights of parents, but the interests of the child were placed paramount, and in accordance with the philosophy of the time there was a good deal of emphasis on fostering and boarding out. Care in a children's home was thought of as a last resort. After the passage of the Act and the appointment of children's officers as the chief officers of the newly formed children's committees, child care officers were appointed to staff the new departments; many of them were at that time known as boarding-out officers. One of the first tasks in many children's departments was to review the children already in local authority children's homes to see how many could be boarded out. At the same time, more children came into care after 1948, largely because the stigma associated with the old Poor Law and its successor, public assistance, had been dissipated. (At least, this appeared to be the case in child care; in other fields, particularly the care of the aged, the stigma of the old Poor Law survived several successive waves of legislation and new nomenclature.) Parents who wished, or were willing, for their children to be received into care found that it could be done with the minimum of formality. Many children's officers were full of zeal to rescue children from unsatisfactory homes, and the whole emphasis of the legislation was on the provision of a high standard of care for the child who had been removed from or abandoned by his parents. Local authorities were given no powers to work or spend money to help a family resolve its difficulties and thus avoid the necessity for a child to be received into care in the first place.

Rescue from an unsatisfactory home, and the provision of the best possible substitute home, with appropriate safeguards for parents' rights, were seen as the objects. Religious susceptibilities were allayed by charging local authorities to see that where possible the person with whom a child was boarded out was either of the same religious persuasion as the child, or prepared to give an undertaking to bring the child up in that persuasion. If the child were placed by the local authority in a children's home run by a voluntary organization, then it had to be a home which provided facilities for him to be brought up in the religious persuasion to which he belonged. These provisions created quite a few problems for child care officers trying to board out children who were members of religious minority groups.

The 1948 Act required a local authority to act as a 'fit person' when a child was committed by a court to the care of a 'fit person' (Fit Person Order) under the Children and Young Persons Act 1933. Thus a child in care might be in care either at the request of his parents, or by order of a court. The Act also laid down that the children's homes provided by a local authority should include reception homes for the temporary accommodation of children, and for observation of their physical and mental condition, before they were boarded out or assigned to some other home. It did not, however, lay down that every child received into care must go to a reception home.

While children were only to remain in the care of the local authority until the age of eighteen, local authorities were empowered by the Act to provide hostels for young people up to the age of twenty-one who were formerly in care, and to help towards the cost of their accommodation and maintenance or of any education or training that they might require between the ages of eighteen and twenty-one. If a young person was still undergoing a course of training when he reached the age of twenty-one, then the local authority might continue to help him until the end of his course.

Finally the Act included provisions for parents to make financial contributions to the maintenance of their children, to allow local authorities to help parents with expenses incurred visiting their children, for the registration and regulation of voluntary homes, for grants to meet the costs of training in child care, and for the extension of earlier child life protection legislation relating to children under the age of nine to those between nine and eighteen.

10.4 Report of the Working Party on Social Workers in the Local Authority Health and Welfare Services (Younghusband Report)

Published: 1959

Chairman: *Miss Eileen Younghusband CBE, LLD, JP*

Members: *Miss Robina S. Addis; Christian Berridge; R. Huws Jones MA, BSc (Econ.); C. M. Scott MRCS, LRCP;* Professor Andrew B. Semple VRD, MD, DPH; Mrs P. E. Steed; Miss Elizabeth Swallow AMIA; P. S. Taylor MA; Thomas Tinto ASAA, DPA; G. I. Crawford and E. L. Hope Murray (joint secretaries)*

Steering Committee: *A. F. Alford CBE, MB, ChB; D. Emery; Miss B. M. Grainger;† James Hutcheon OBE; A. MacLehose;‡ Councillor John Mains OBE, JP; Alderman Eric E. Mole JP; Alderman Miss M. O'Connor OBE; H. L. Oliver;§ G. Ramage MA, MD, DPH; G. Robinson CBE, MC; Alderman Professor F. E. Tylecote MD, FRCP (London), JP; R. J. Whittick‖*

*Appointed in place of Dr P. C. McKinlay, who resigned in September, 1956
†Appointed in place of Miss M. Hayward, who had succeeded Mr E. Harrison
‡Appointed in place of Mr R. Howat
§Appointed in place of Mr D. J. Moxley, who had succeeded Mr R. E. Griffiths
‖Appointed in place of Miss S. Clement Brown

Terms of Reference (1955): *To inquire into the proper field of work and the recruitment and training of social workers at all levels in the local authorities' health and welfare services under the National Health Service and National Assistance Acts, and in particular whether there is a place for a general purpose social worker with an in-service training as a basic grade.*

The Younghusband Report was restricted by its terms of reference to social workers in the local authority health and welfare services and to social workers doing similar jobs with voluntary organizations, but its recommendations were immediately seen to be relevant to almost all branches of social work. The report opened with a historical and general review of existing services, and passed directly to an analysis of the varieties of need for social work. There were three categories:

(1) people with straightforward or obvious needs who require help, some simple service, or a periodic visit;
(2) people with more complex problems who require systematic help from trained social workers;
(3) people with problems of special difficulty requiring skilled help by professionally trained and experienced social workers.

These three categories of need should be matched by three types of worker:

(1) a worker with a short but systematically planned in-service training who would relieve trained and experienced staff of a proportion of the simpler work and straightforward visiting; who would work under the direct supervision of trained social workers and would be trained to recognize indications that more skilled help or a different service was required; they would be known as welfare assistants;
(2) social workers with a general training in social work equivalent to two years' full-time training, who would provide help with the more complex problems which formed the greater part of the social work required in health and welfare departments;
(3) professionally trained and experienced social workers to undertake casework in problems of special difficulty; they would have a professional training in social work following a social science or related qualification.

The working party considered in detail the implications of their proposals for the existing pattern of social work training. The welfare assistant was a new grade, who would have an in-service training. University social science courses followed by professional training of the kind already available for psychiatric social workers, hospital almoners, and generic caseworkers would continue to provide a body of fully professional social workers able to meet the most complex varieties of need. There was, however, no existing course of training to provide the middle-grade workers who would deal with all but the most complex problems on the one hand, and purely routine visiting on the other. It was therefore proposed that a two-year general training should be provided in colleges of further education and should lead to a National Certificate in Social Work. The training would closely relate theory and practice and would be conducted under the supervision of a National Council for Social Work Training.

The National Council would not conduct training courses, but the working party suggested that a national training centre or staff college should be established to pioneer new courses and to provide stimulus and support for other colleges undertaking social work training.

The recommendations of the Younghusband Report were accepted by the Government and the chief of them implemented in the Health Visitors and Social Work (Training) Act, 1962, which provided for the establishment of a Council for the Training of Health Visitors (implementing a recommendation of the Jameson Report: *see* p. 53) and a Council for Training in Social Work. The two Councils were set up with the same chairman and overlapping membership to ensure co-ordination of their activities. The Council for Training in Social Work was initially reponsible only for training in connection with work in local authority health and welfare services, but provision was made in the Act for this scope to be widened by Order in Council at some future date. In 1970 the Council was superseded, along with the Central Training Council in Child Care, by the new Central Council for Education and Training in Social Work set up as a result of the Seebohm Report.

The recommendation that a staff college should be created was in large measure implemented by the setting up in 1961, with the help of the Nuffield Foundation and the Joseph Rowntree Memorial Trust, of the National Institute for Social Work Training.

The two-year general social work courses recommended by the working party were developed during the 1960s under the auspices of the Council, following pilot courses run by the Institute. At the same time, similar courses were sponsored by the Home Office for child care officers, who of course fell outside the Younghusband terms of reference. In order to give some of the many unqualified workers in health, welfare and children's departments the opportunity to become qualified, intensive one-year courses were mounted for those with experience in the field.

Younghusband Report, 1959

THE FUNCTIONS OF SOCIAL WORKERS

In the light of these considerations, we regard the essential functions of social workers in the health and welfare services as being to assess the disturbance of equilibrium in a given handicapped person and in his family and social relationships so as to give appropriate help. The aim will be to offer a supporting relationship in which his and their practical needs, as well as their fears, frustrations and anxieties, are understood and means used to meet or lessen them, and also to further a better personal and social adjustment, and a renewed ability to exercise responsibility, by whatever means are indicated for a given person at a given time. This may often include supplying information and relevant services or concrete help as and when these are needed. We would stress here that the activities we are describing may be simple and straightforward in some instances but complex in others. Our concern is that in all health and welfare departments there should be social workers sufficiently well qualified for thorough initial and subsequent assessments to be made of the needs of each individual and the extent to which these can be met by a social work service.

In short, the purpose of social work as we see it is to help the individual to achieve the best possible personal, family and social adjustment. This will include trying to bring about any necessary improvements in the environment. We have distinguished between personal, family and social adjustments. These are all closely interwoven but it is possible nonetheless to isolate different elements and to intervene at the most appropriate point in the individual case (a 'case' is a situation, not a person). Thus severe physical handicap may occur in someone with a well integrated personality and normal family set-up. In such circumstances the main help needed may be in dealing with the initial shock and with the necessary practical adaptations in living. To break down the total problem of adjustment into its component parts and help the person and his family to see how they could cope with it may be all that is required. In other instances, where, for example, the person is immature and demanding and where there is less strength in the family relationships, much more support, given with greater skill and for a longer period, may be called for. In other cases still, the handicap may occur in someone who already had personality difficulties or who was able to lead a satisfactory life previously but who lacks the inner resources to master the effects of the handicap. These same inabilities to meet misfortune may also occur in someone else in the family as a result of the disturbances caused by the handicap to the family's way of life. For example the shock, coupled with the attention lavished on the handicapped person himself, may cause another member of the family to become more demanding. Many handicapped people will also need help to accept a greater degree of dependence on others, to come to terms with the added burden they must sometimes impose and not to become more dependent than they need.

Social work is directed towards helping individuals and families to cope with their problems and so to achieve at any given time a better personal and social equilibrium, a better chance to face challenges and accept responsibility, than they are able to reach without help. It is in essence a supporting relationship, an extra prop to those who have lost a balance, to help them to regain it. The art of the social worker lies in his use of this relationship and his ability to hold and merit the client's confidence. This means doing things with people rather than for them, not making them dependent but accepting the dependence necessary at a given stage in their disturbed life balance in order that they may be enabled as a result to stand on their own feet again, psychologically speaking, to the extent that lies within their capacities. Some people, particularly those who are or have been mentally ill, may need this support for a very long time, possibly at intervals all through their lives. But to walk with support is better than not to walk at all. The metaphor is perhaps ambiguous at this point, because it is necessary to distinguish between those cases which are 'hopeless', in that no cure is possible in the present state of our knowledge, but where some alleviation or adaptation can be achieved with help, and those where almost no improvement in the person or family is possible, but yet some improvement can be brought about in the situation as a whole by lessening external pressures or by increasing community tolerance. This increase of tolerance applies particularly to 'problem' families, though it is unfortunately true that almost all forms of physical or mental disability lead to varying degrees of avoidance, or to discomfort in the presence of the handicapped person, however much compassion some forms of handicap arouse.

It may well be objected against much we have said that very many people suffer from disturbances in their life adaptation and have to make, and would want to make, adjustments themselves without the help of social workers. This is both true and, when the adjustment can be satisfactorily made, desirable. The factor of time and timing is, however, of primary importance in all social work. The old saying about 'time the great healer' indicates that the living being does come to terms with the shock of loss or deprivation. The real case for social work intervention in this natural process of adaptation is, however, that time is not always on the side of the angels, with the result that if family and personal disturbance is more prolonged than it need be it may have secondary damaging effects which might have been prevented. For example, it is well known that unless a newly blinded or otherwise disabled person is quickly helped to gain confidence through doing things in new ways it may be difficult or even impossible to foster this confidence later. Whether or not to do so requires a high degree of skill in the worker will depend on the particular case.

The essential task of the social worker in helping the individual to establish a fresh equilibrium is thus to know where he and his family are feeling the pressures most and what can be done to relieve these. This means not only supplying necessary services but also knowing enough to be able to do and say those things which help to lessen fear, anxiety, hostility and frustration so that confidence and hope may have a chance to grow. Sometimes this may be achieved in quite simple ways; at other times it may be a skilled process because it may involve sufficient knowledge of human behaviour and of conscious and unconscious motivation, as well as of socially determined attitudes, to make a reasonably accurate assessment of the personal and family strengths and disabilities in a particular case. It always calls for the ability to make a helpful relationship with the person concerned, and to stimulate him to take action to meet his needs, to the extent that this is possible with any necessary help. This means the formulation of a plan, based on an assessment of the situation and aimed at achieving the best possible social and personal improvement in a particular case. In long-term cases there may of course be substantial periods when no action beyond steady support is possible. In many, too, the best that can be done may be to prevent further deterioration in a situation, or to help people and their families to accept inevitable physical or mental deterioration and strain.

This whole social work activity requires skill in helping people to talk about their fears and anxieties which they are often reluctant to express to others, or even to formulate to themselves. This is particularly important with handicapped people, who are often putting on a brave front to others but who badly need to be able to talk about the hopelessness and despair with which they may be struggling alone. We have already referred to the strong verb 'to comfort', meaning to strengthen, having degenerated into bright attempts to reassure, to minimise, or to divert by inadequate means. This is the natural reaction by which many people ward off the full impact of suffering in others. It is, however, no real comfort to the one who suffers. It is often objected that it is much better to try to cheer people up than to let them dwell on their misfortune. This runs counter to old wisdom about 'not bottling things up inside', 'having a good cry', 'feeling better after getting it off one's chest'. Modern psychological knowledge reinforces this view that fear, anxiety and frustration are in fact lessened by being expressed to someone who understands, whose confidence is a source of strength and who is not personally involved as family and friends would be. This calls for skill in helping people to talk about painful things, or small things which may loom large to them, as well as ability to listen sympathetically and to nourish hope and confidence. This sounds easy but in fact may require very considerable skill. These aims are accomplished partly by respect for the person, understanding of him and belief in his capacity to make a better life adjustment. This is likely to communicate itself to him, and make him more able to talk about what troubles him, as well as more confident, and thus more free to make choices about his life. It may often be necessary for a social worker to be concerned with some other member of the family, as well as with the handicapped person himself, in order to bring about this better adjustment. For example, if those on whom the main burden falls can have a good 'blow off' to the worker every now and then about the difficulties of the situation, knowing that their side of the problem is understood, it is less likely that irritation will flare up to the handicapped person himself, particularly if it is also possible to take practical steps to lessen the burden. Work with other members of the families of mentally disturbed people, or where the parent of a handicapped or defective child is either rejecting or over-protective, is particularly important.

Social workers have to learn not only to ask for and give necessary information fully and patiently but also to listen and simultaneously to assess the significance of what is said or not said, and to relate this to previous knowledge of the person and his situation. Sometimes, too, with certain disturbed people, the skill may lie in helping them not to talk, that is, to strengthen their defences against the flood-tides within. In any event, the most difficult stage lies in making it possible to go on, with help, to find constructive ways of dealing with the problems and fears which they have begun to express to the worker. At this and other points, social workers must also be aware of all available statutory and voluntary services which could give the most appropriate help at any given time.

The real purpose of such services, as we see it, is that they should be appropriately used in individual cases at the right point in time in order to strengthen the person through the exercise of his abilities, through increased physical mobility leading to a change of scene, and through group activities which meet a natural human need for companionship outside the family. Individuals may need other services, such as those supplied by the health, welfare, education, children's and housing departments, by the Ministry of Labour and National Service, the National Assistance Board, and by voluntary organisations. It is therefore important for social workers to be well versed in what is available, to use this knowledge appropriately, and to be able to give accurate information about other services. It is also essential that they should understand the functions of other workers and should work in partnership with them.

What we have already said about the social worker's function in accurately assessing a personal, family and social situation from the point of view of the help that might be given to bring about improvements (often in circumstances of stress), indicates that social workers will in the course of their relationship sometimes have to help people to talk about those things which are troubling them, if they wish to do so. For this and other reasons they may know intimate details of peoples' lives. This material may be germane to social remedial action on the case; it may therefore properly be discussed with or passed on to colleagues, usually with the knowledge of the person concerned. It will also be necessary to embody some of it in the case record in order to watch the progress of the case. But beyond this, the strictest preservation of confidence is called for. We believe this principle is already accepted in regard to psychiatric social workers and almoners. We think . . . that it should apply to all social workers, so far as divulging information and safeguarding records are concerned. We refer to this again in Chapter 12 in regard to procedure at co-ordinating committees and case conferences. In any event, no information should be sought which is not relevant to the help which might be given. There is no right to indiscriminate history-taking or discussion of a case, which may sometimes be a polite name for vulgar curiosity.

paras. 615–20

10.5 Report of the Committee on Children and Young Persons (Ingleby Report)

Published: 1960

Chairman: *Viscount Ingleby*

Members: *Lady Adrian JP; The Hon. Mrs P. L. Aitken MBE, JP; R. H. Blundell; Dr D. Carroll; Donald Ford JP; E. H. Gwynn; Dr R. M. Jackson JP; Mrs M. M. C. Kemball JP; G. H. McConnell;* Professor Alan Moncrieff CBE, JP; A. Pickard CBE;† Viscountess Ridley OBE, JP; Dr P. D. Scott;‡ G. A. Wheatley CBE; Alderman Sir Thomas Williams OBE, JP; J. P. Wilson; W. F. Delamare (secretary)*

*replaced E. H. Gwynn, June 1957
†resigned June 1960
‡replaced Dr D. Carroll on the latter's death, December 1956

Terms of Reference (1956): *To be a Committee to inquire into, and make recommendations on: (a) the working of the law, in England and Wales, relating to (i) proceedings, and the powers of the courts, in respect of juveniles brought before the courts as delinquent or as being in need of care or protection or beyond control; (ii) the constitution, jurisdiction and procedure of juvenile courts; (iii) the remand home, approved school and approved probation home systems; (iv) the prevention of cruelty to, and exposure to moral and physical danger of, juveniles; and (b) whether local authorities responsible for child care under the Children Act, 1948, in England and Wales should, taking into account action by voluntary organisations and the responsibilities of existing statutory services, be given new powers and duties to prevent or forestall the suffering of children through neglect in their own homes.*

As experience was gained in working under the 1948 Children Act, it became clear that this could not be the last word in legislation on the subject. The Ingleby Committee was set up to look at the position of juveniles brought before the courts and to consider whether local authorities might be given powers to offer help to families in danger of breaking up before it actually became necessary to receive a child into care. Should they perhaps be enabled to spend money on prevention—even to the extent of offering material help to the family—rather than be forced, as they were by existing law, to sit on the sidelines until the situation became so desperate that it could be shown that a child was neglected or cruelly treated?

The Ingleby Committee recommended the commonsense solution that local authorities should be given power to undertake preventive casework and to give aid to families in danger of breakdown, and this power was promptly bestowed on them in the 1963 Children and Young Persons Act. They also suggested that aid to families might be all the more effective if a unified family service were established in place of the existing fragmented provision, and they pointed out that 'much of the difficulty which at present exists, apart from that attributable to the shortage of skilled casework staff, is due to inter-service rivalries'. They recognized that there were 'obvious and formidable difficulties' in establishing such a unified service, not the least of these being the vested interests of existing departments, but they recommended that the possibility should be explored as a long-term aim. Changes of this kind in organization at local level would also necessitate some reallocation of functions in central government. Meanwhile the committee urged that experimental schemes should be set up to increase the effectiveness of work with families by early detection of families at risk and by giving more publicity to the services available. Such schemes might include the setting up of 'family advice centres' or 'family bureaux'.

The discussion of a unified family service foreshadowed the recommendations of the Seebohm Committee eight years later, but at the time it was no doubt felt that a wider investigation was necessary before such a far-reaching change could be brought about. The terms of reference of the Ingleby Committee were of course limited to services for children, while the later Seebohm Committee had the task of reporting on local authority personal social services as a whole.

As far as child offenders were concerned the committee felt that up to the age of twelve they should not be dealt with as offenders at all, but as children in need of care, protection and control. This meant raising the age of criminal responsibility from eight to twelve. The Government was at first unwilling to take action on this recommendation, but eventually agreed under pressure—notably from Baroness Wootton—to raise the age of criminal responsibility to ten. Provision to this effect was made in Section 2 of the Children and Young Persons Act, 1963, which laid down that children under ten could only be dealt with as 'in need of care or control'.

Ingleby Report, 1960

PREVENTION OF NEGLECT IN THE HOME

In dealing with the prevention of neglect in the home, it is in our opinion essential to distinguish the following three stages:

(a) the detection of families at risk;

(b) the investigation and diagnosis of the particular problem;

(c) treatment: the provision of facilities and services to meet the families' needs and to reduce the stresses and dangers that they face.

It is most important too that arrangements should be made for making the services known to the public and for giving advice so that individuals know where they can apply for help.

From the evidence we received there seemed to be some confusion about these different stages and their relative importance. We in no way wish to suggest that the different stages are always clear cut, or, indeed, that every case needs skilled detailed investigation and treatment. There has been a certain reaction recently against the indiscriminate application of intensive or deep case-work for family or personal difficulties. From the point of view of the family, or of the individual or of economy, attention should first be given to the simple forms of social aid. By analogy, a person who feels ill should first attend his general practitioner rather than a consultant physician; one does not study the blood chemistry of a hungry man, one gives him a meal. Nevertheless there is a proportion of individuals incapable of benefiting from simple aid, and some families have specific characteristics which prevent them from following advice or from applying to the appropriate agency even when this has been clearly indicated to them. Ignorance, shame or discouragement on the part of parents may be overcome by a relatively unskilled friendly approach, but deep antagonism, distrustfulness, perverse satisfaction in degradation, self-damaging tendencies and a desire to evade legal responsibilities, are likely to require a higher order of skill in the worker. In the present state of our knowledge and services, most of these difficult problems will be recognised by the failure of simple remedies. This failure should be accepted as the signal for more careful diagnostic procedures which will require a nucleus of suitably trained staff to be available.

Arrangements for the detection of families at risk should extend over the widest possible front. Many different sorts of agency and worker will function in this rôle. Neighbours, teachers, medical practitioners, ministers of religion, health visitors, district nurses, education welfare officers, probation officers, child care officers, housing officers, officers of the National Assistance Board and other social workers may all spot incipient signs of trouble. It may be that a particular family will come to the attention of a voluntary agency, a local authority department or some other statutory body. It is from this fact that we think much confusion arises. It seems often to be thought that field workers who first make contact with a family at risk should also continue with the next stages. Detection is obviously a vital stage, but it does not follow that the person who makes the discovery is necessarily the one who is best fitted to follow up the case.

The health visitor whose duty it is to visit homes to give advice on the care of young children, of persons suffering from illness, and of expectant or nursing mothers, and on the measures necessary to prevent the spread of infection, is probably the visitor most frequently in touch with families with children and has most opportunity to detect early signs of distress. But as the Working Party on Health Visiting (appointed by the Ministers of Health and Education and the Secretary of State for Scotland) said in their report (1956), it is important that the health visitor should recognise where the help of other workers is needed or is more appropriate than her own, and we understand that the present day training of health visitors encourages this approach.

It was suggested to us that often cases were not referred to trained case-workers because of a shortage of that class of worker. That is no doubt true, but we think it is equally true that there is a reluctance on the part of some workers to seek advice, or a failure to recognise the need. 'Recognition of the point at which another worker should be consulted or a different service is required is essential in social work but this seems to be too rarely accepted.'

The second stage—investigation and diagnosis—is the one which many of our witnesses seemed to overlook; they tended to confuse it with detection, and with treatment. We think it is most important that there should be early reference of cases to a unit within the local authority that can give skilled and objective diagnosis—a unit untrammelled by departmental loyalties, and with authority to decide the best means of providing for each family at risk. The need, of course, is for reference to be made early so that co-ordination can be effected early and at the right point in the attempt to help the family. Co-ordination must begin before treatment, not after treatment has begun. Different skills may need to be brought to bear at this stage, and the process must be such as to ensure that this can be done, and that the best means of providing for the family are devised.

In the larger local authority areas, one way of meeting this important stage might be through the creation of a special unit (a 'family advice centre' or 'family bureau'), which would be a central point of reference both for the various local authority services and for members of the public. Within the setting of the local authority, such a 'centre' should be independent, and we envisage that it would be headed by a senior officer of the authority with as wide an experience as possible. He should be responsible to the clerk to the authority—not to a committee—and would be supported when necessary by officers from other departments with other experience and complementary skills. The procedure must, however, vary from authority to authority, depending upon the size of the authority and the size of the problem it has to face. We therefore make no attempt to stipulate the precise form of the procedure to be followed, but we do urge recognition of the need for early reference of cases for investigation, and the need for impartiality in, and a measure of independence for, those responsible for diagnosis.

The third stage—treatment—should be in the hands of existing agencies both statutory and voluntary, and should be decided upon in consultation with the various departments likely to be concerned. In this connection we should like to emphasise the very valuable work performed by many of the voluntary organisations, and we hope that local authorities will make full use of their powers to make contributions to voluntary bodies engaged in this field.

paras. 38–45

ADDITIONAL POWERS AND DUTIES OF LOCAL AUTHORITIES

A number of organisations concerned with social work expressed the view in their evidence that, for the effective prevention of suffering of children through neglect in their own homes, a skilled intensive case-work service was required (provided either directly by local authorities or through a voluntary agency), and that local authorities should have power to give material assistance where necessary. Some advocated that responsibility for the provision of a preventive casework service should be placed on the local children's authority, on the grounds that the prevention of neglect, the provision of alternative forms of care, and the restoration of a child to his family were all parts of what was fundamentally one task. It was pointed out that children's departments had direct experience of the damage that could be caused to a child by removing him from home, that they were responsible for providing care for the child when preventive measures failed, and that the staffs of children's departments had acquired considerable experience of case-work techniques and were well equipped to undertake preventive work, which many of them were already doing although it was only on the fringe of their statutory functions. Other witnesses considered that the prime responsibility for prevention and rehabilitation should rest with local health departments, and pointed to the importance of the rôle of the health visitor. Still others thought that a new local authority department should be created to take over the work of the existing children's departments and the preventive functions (extended as necessary) of other local authority departments.

It may be that the long-term solution will be in a reorganisation of the various services concerned with the family and their combination into a unified family service, although there would be obvious and formidable difficulties either in bringing all their diverse and often specialised functions into one organisation, or in taking away from the existing services those of their functions relating to family troubles in order to secure unified administration of those functions. Any such reorganisation at local authority level might well involve a corresponding reorganisation of the functions of the different government departments concerned. These are matters well outside our terms of reference, but we urge the importance of their further study by the Government and by the local interests concerned.

Meanwhile, the aim should be to improve co-ordination on the basis of the three-fold division of functions discussed in paragraphs 38 to 45. Departmental boundaries should not be a major consideration in the arrangements, which must be flexible enough to meet the wide variety of situations. To ensure maximum flexibility and an adequacy of power, we recommend that there should be a general duty laid upon local authorities (county and county borough councils) to prevent or forestall the suffering of children through neglect in their own homes. In carrying out this duty local authorities should have powers, apart from those already existing, to do preventive case-work (either themselves or through the agency of a voluntary society) and to provide material needs that cannot be met from other sources. These powers should not be conferred on any particular committee of the local authority, but should be vested generally in the local authority without specifying the committee through which the local authority must act.

We think it is a matter of first importance that there should be adequate arrangements to make known to the public the various services, including voluntary organisations, available to help them in time of need, and where to apply for advice. This question was discussed in a wider context by the Working Party on Social Workers in the Local Health and Welfare Services who thought that there should be a well planned information service as an integral part of the social services provided by local authorities. It is a matter which must be left largely to local initiative, but local authorities should have it constantly in mind and consider in what way their existing publicity arrangements can be improved and kept up to date. In the more densely populated areas particularly, the importance of a central point to which members of the public can turn for advice (the 'family advice centre') seems obvious; citizens' advice bureaux may also perform a most valuable service in this respect.

Because of the varying conditions and requirements in different areas, we do not advocate any uniform machinery for co-ordination of local authority services, but we recommend that there should be a statutory obligation on local authorities (county and county borough councils) to submit for ministerial approval schemes for the prevention of suffering of children through neglect in their homes. The schemes should provide for:—

(a) the detection of families where help is needed;
(b) the co-ordination of information (investigation) and diagnosis of the problem;
(c) the provision of appropriate assistance; and
(d) arrangements for making the services known to the public and for advice as to where individuals can apply for help.

We consider that all local authorities should be required to submit schemes for approval.

In the implementation of this recommendation we are of opinion that it should be made clear to which government department a local authority should look for advice or approval on matters of co-ordination.

paras. 46–51

10.6 Children and Young Persons Act, 1963

The Children and Young Persons Act, 1963, embodied recommendations of the Committee on Children and Young Persons (the Ingleby Committee) and for the first time legalized work that many children's officers had in fact been quietly doing for some years to try to prevent the break-up of families and the necessity to receive children into care. Strictly speaking local authorities had no powers under previous legislation to undertake preventive work of this kind and they would certainly have been *ultra vires* in making cash grants to assist families in danger of break-up. The new Act gave local authorities power to employ staff for preventive work and it gave them power to give assistance to families in kind or cash. This of course was not only more humane than for the children's department to be obliged to stand by helplessly until the family actually broke up and the children had to be received into care, but it was also in almost every case cheaper.

Once the Act had cleared the ground legally, children's departments almost everywhere embraced the opportunity to do preventive casework, and to substitute a family-centred approach for the purely child-centred approach which had earlier characterized much of the service. These shifts in emphasis reflected not only changing legislation, but also the growth of knowledge about the emotional development of children and the consequences of maternal deprivation, and about the importance not only of the family but also of the class and cultural environment to the development of the child. Social workers were now much more hesitant about 'rescuing' a child from an environment which affronted their own values but which might have a value of its own for the child.

Preventive work under the provisions of the 1963 Act could take many forms. A family in danger of eviction might be helped with rent arrears. Some authorities employed day housemothers who could care for children in their own homes during the day until the father came home in the evening if their mother had to go into hospital or was otherwise temporarily unable to care for them. Child care officers could advise families with problems or provide furniture and equipment to help them get on their feet. Some local authorities set up hostels to teach inadequate parents elementary household management. Others used their powers to support preventive work by voluntary organizations.

While Section 1 of the Act was thus concerned with ensuring that reception of a child into the care of the local authority would in future be a last resort rather than the first point at which the children's department could legally step in (local authority welfare departments and to some extent housing departments already had powers which enabled them to do family casework), the remainder of the Act was mainly concerned with sorting out various anomalies and problems which had arisen in the implementation of earlier legislation.

One significant change that was in keeping with the new emphasis on prevention was that the Act made it impossible for a parent to bring his child before a court as in need of 'care, protection or control'. The child could now only be brought before the court by the local authority, and the parent was thus obliged to request the local authority to bring his child before the court if he felt the child was beyond his control. The object of this provision was to give the local authority the opportunity to investigate and try to help the family before the powers of the court were invoked.

The Act also raised the age of criminal responsibility from eight to ten years.

10.7 Report of the Committee on Local Authority and Allied Personal Social Services (Seebohm Report)

Published: 1968

Chairman: *Frederic Seebohm*

Members: *Sir Charles Barratt; Lady James of Rusholme; R. Huws Jones; W. E. Lane; P. Leonard; Professor J. N. Morris; Dr R. A. Parker; Mrs B. Serota;* M. R. F. Simson*

*created Life Peer, 1 January 1967; resigned from the Committee on appointment as Baroness-in-Waiting, 23 April 1968

Terms of Reference (1965): *To review the organisation and responsibilities of the local authority personal social services in England and Wales, and to consider what changes are desirable to secure an effective family service.*

In the 1960s a good many jokes and cautionary tales were being told about families who were being visited by half a dozen or more social workers, each representing a particular service or agency and each concerned with only one aspect of the family's difficulties. This situation had come to pass because of the separate growth of various forms of social provision, some organized centrally, such as the National Assistance Board (later Supplementary Benefits Commission), but many at local authority level. A family might have dealings with representatives of the children's department, the health department, the welfare department, and with social workers attached to the housing and education departments, all under the same local authority. The resulting duplication represented neither the efficient use of resources nor effective service to the family; indeed the family which found itself so unable to cope with the complexity and stresses of modern life that it required all these services was the very family upon which the additional burden of co-ordinating them and of sorting out possibly conflicting advice should not have been thrust. Another aspect of the same problem was the difficulty often experienced by individuals or families in need of help in identifying the service appropriate to their need. One of the most important functions of citizens advice bureaux was to solve this problem for the individual and direct him to the quarter where he could expect to receive help. The voluntary workers in the bureaux required considerable training before they were equipped with the necessary knowledge of the social services to do this.

It was in this context that a feeling grew up that a unified social work department, or family service, might be the answer to the problems of duplication and overlap—and possible gaps in service—which had stemmed from specialization in social work and in social work provision. Specialization in social work had grown up chiefly between the wars, but had been further fostered by some of the post-war social legislation setting up, for example, separate children's departments and thus creating a new and important branch of social work. While early social work training had been generic—a general basic training in social work, not to be confused with specialized vocational training for a specific job—by 1914 a number of specialized vocational courses had been set up, and specialization in training as well as practice was the dominant pattern of the next fifty years or so. By the time the Seebohm Committee reported the pendulum had started to swing back and while virtually all non-university courses in social work prepared workers to enter specific services, mainly child care, probation and local authority health and welfare services, most of the university courses were generic in intent, even if a degree of bias was at times introduced by the fact that students were financially sponsored by authorities which had recruited them for a particular branch of social work.

Again, there were three national councils for training in social work, the Central Training Council in Child Care, the Council for Training in Social Work, and the Advisory Council for Probation and After-Care, and numerous specialized professional bodies. Yet well before 1968 negotiations were going on to create a unified professional organization for social workers, and by the time the Seebohm Report was published only the formalities remained to be completed. In June 1970 the British Association of Social Workers came into being.

The recommendations for the establishment of a unified social service department in each major local authority, for the establishment of one central body to be responsible for promoting the training of the staff of the personal social services and for the provision of a common basic training for all social workers had therefore an air of inevitability. The report recommended that as far as possible a family or individual in need of social care should be served by a single social worker, and the decision on whether to involve other social workers with a family or individual should be taken by the social worker primarily responsible, in consultation with his supervisor and with the client, and not simply because the administrative structure required more than one social worker to be involved. It was acknowledged that specialization would be necessary above the basic field level and during the transitional period would be based on existing expertise. As the service developed, however, new types of specialization would emerge, and these specialists would develop as consultants to the basic field workers.

The Seebohm Committee saw the new unified social service departments as 'community based and family oriented', including in their scope 'the present services provided by children's departments, the welfare services provided under the National Assistance Act 1948, educational welfare and child guidance services, the home help service, mental health social work service, social work services provided by health departments, day nurseries, and certain social welfare work currently undertaken by some housing departments'. But they saw the task of workers within the department as including not merely aid to families and individuals, but also work with groups and communities, a more controversial area which could, as the committee realized, create a difficult situation for the worker who, through his identification with the needs of a community, became involved in situations which led to criticisms of the services provided by his employing authority, or to pressure being brought to bear on the authority to recognize new needs.

The Seebohm Committee placed a high value on the maximum participation of individuals and groups in the community in the planning, organization and provision of the social services, hoping that this would help blur the distinction between consumers and providers. In order that services should be responsive to local needs it was proposed that social service departments should be administered through area offices, serving populations of between 50,000 and 100,000, with teams of at least ten to twelve social workers controlled by a senior professionally trained social worker with a grasp of administrative issues and wide delegated powers of decision.

The report was divided into six parts: I—Introduction and the Present Situation; II—The Need for Change and the Form it Should Take; III—Meeting Needs in a Comprehensive Service; IV—Foundations of an Effective Service; V—Specialisation and Training; VI—Structure and Implementation. The extracts printed below are from Parts II, IV, V and VI; Part III reviewed social needs in chapters devoted to services for children, old people, the physically handicapped, the mentally subnormal and mentally ill, with a final chapter devoted to other services then provided by local health departments, including the home help and health visiting services (it was decided to leave the health visitor on the health side of the divide between health and social services). There were also a number of valuable appendices to the report, including a 57-page review of 'The Personal Social Services as They Are Now', and detailed evidence of the unevenness of existing social service provision over the country as a whole.

The report was given a warm welcome by the social work profession —many were content to describe it as a charter for social workers—and hostile criticism came chiefly from medical officers of health and other workers in the health service, who criticized the perpetuation of the administrative division between health services for the elderly, the mentally ill, and the mentally handicapped, and the welfare services and residential provision for these groups. The main recommendations of the report were, however, accepted almost immediately by the Government and embodied in the Local Authority Social Services Act, 1970.

Seebohm Report, 1968

A SOCIAL SERVICE DEPARTMENT

The need for a more unified provision of personal social services has been made plain by growing knowledge and experience. There is a realisation that it is essential to look beyond the immediate symptoms of social distress to the underlying problems. These frequently prove to be complicated and the outcome of a variety of influences. In many cases people who need help cannot be treated effectively unless this is recognised. Their difficulties do not arise in a social vacuum; they are, have been, or need to be involved in a network of relationships, in social situations. The family and the community are seen as the contexts in which problems arise and in which most of them have to be resolved or contained. Similarly, residential establishments are no longer asylums, separated and insulated from the outside world. They are increasingly expected to maintain contacts with the families of those for whom they care and the communities in which they are located. To take another example, the local authority personal social services should accept the responsibility of concerning themselves with offenders and the families of offenders, co-operating for this purpose with the probation and aftercare service, the prison welfare service, and other statutory and voluntary organisations.

The present structure of the personal social services ignores the nature of much social distress. Since social need is complex it can rarely be divided so that each part is satisfactorily dealt with by a separate service. In the previous chapter we rejected a number of proposals for reform because they allocated the responsibilities of departments according to age or 'types' of problems. This, we believe, reflects an artificial and rigid view of human need. An integrated social service department will impose fewer boundaries and require less arbitrary classification of problems. Of course, important administrative boundaries will remain. Responsibilities for medical care, education and housing will continue to be separate, although the problems they deal with also have an obvious social component.

Because problems are complicated and interdependent, co-ordination in the work of social services of all kinds is crucial. In many cases effective help will continue to depend upon the assistance of more than one organisation. But an integrated social service department will ease problems of collaboration as the number of separate units involved is reduced, and above all as issues of responsibility are clarified.

paras. 141–3

It has been suggested in evidence that a unified social service department would be monolithic. As a result, 'difficult' people who needed its help might be neglected and it could prove unresponsive to the need for change. Though it would provide 'a door on which anyone could knock' it would be the only door and anyone who was turned away would have nowhere else to go; the present untidy pattern, it is argued, allows the public some measure of choice.

In fact, alternative public services hardly exist outside a few authorities; the 'shopping around' between departments within the present structure is accidental and wasteful and the advantages seem to us nebulous. We attach greater weight to the tendency of separate services to concentrate exclusively on the needs of particular groups, and to the temptation to steer 'difficult' people from one department to another. A service with a clear and comprehensive responsibility for meeting social need would provide a more secure base for helping those who are not the concern of any of the present departments; the responsibility for assisting any particular family would be clear and there would be less risk of people falling between departmental stools.

Any organisation which combines professional power with public authority is bound to involve dangers, particularly where poor, vulnerable, inarticulate and sometimes difficult people are concerned. However, placing responsibility for social care on one committee and department would provide a clear and evident system of accountability. The need for safeguards against neglect and the abuse of power, and for the periodic critical review of the services provided, lie behind some of our recommendations in chapter XIX on the *Organisation of the Social Service Department*.

With a unified social service department, elected members and the press would still be able to take up grievances; indeed its comprehensive nature should make this easier. Moreover, if the social service department comes to be used by a broader cross section of the population, that in itself will discourage inconsiderate treatment. Finally, risks such as these can be reduced by effective management within the department, including decentralisation, and by the further development of professional responsibility among the staff.

The issue of size

It has been argued that a unified social service department would be too big for humanity or efficiency and lose the 'personal touch'. We do not believe there is any ground for fear on this score. Most of the present social service departments are, we consider, too small to be fully effective. Appendix N shows that, assuming the combination of welfare and children's departments with the social work parts of health departments, 7 per cent of local authorities would still have fewer than 10 social workers, 51 per cent would have fewer than 30, and only 8 per cent would have more than 100. Including the staffs of residential and day care establishments, the home helps, administrative and clerical staff, the proposed department would not be large by local authority standards.

In their evidence to the Royal Commission on Local Government in England, the Home Office and the Ministry of Health both urged the need for the average local health, welfare and children's authorities to be bigger. Given the present range of sizes, we see great value in combining departments in the smaller authorities, and no harm in combining those in the largest, provided there is delegation of responsibility, especially through area offices. ... As we have noted, the small department is at serious risk of disruption because of absence through illness and leave; it is liable to serious difficulties when senior staff move; it is at a serious disadvantage in arranging in-service training and in seconding staff for full-time courses, and it is hard for it to contribute fieldwork placements for training students. It faces difficulties in maintaining a full range of specialist services and ensuring adequate administrative and clerical support.

paras. 155–60

The new department we have in mind will have responsibilities extending well beyond those of existing local authority departments. Nevertheless, we think it right at this point to specify the main changes in departmental responsibilities which we recommend. They are listed briefly and without argument in this part of the report. The existing services to be included in the new social service department are:

(a) the present services provided by children's departments,
(b) the welfare services provided under the National Assistance Act 1948,
(c) education welfare services and child guidance services,
(d) the home help service, mental health social work services, adult training centres, other social work services and day nurseries, provided by local health departments.
(e) certain social welfare work currently undertaken by some housing departments.

para. 168

THE AREA OFFICE

It was a recurrent complaint in the evidence we received that the way in which the personal social services are housed and located is often a deterrent to those who need them. In county boroughs, the only way to approach the welfare and children's departments is generally to visit one or other of a group of buildings in the centre of the town. For those without their own transport, for mothers with young children, and for the elderly, the journey itself may be a major undertaking, and the difficulties are intensified if the person needing help has to visit more than one department, or goes first to the wrong building. In administrative counties, even though there are usually area or divisional offices, the difficulties are often greater, partly because of the greater distances, but on occasion because the local offices of different departments are in different towns.

para. 583

Despite the advantages of accommodating all staff with related functions under one roof, the size of headquarters buildings and the multiplicity of staff may deter those in need and thus reduce 'effectiveness'. In the larger administrative counties it is usual to have area offices, and progress has already been made in some of them towards bringing the area offices of the personal social service departments together within the same buildings. Besides being generally more acceptable to those in need and convenient for other statutory services, this fosters economy by enabling the area teams from different departments to share clerical services.

In small county boroughs the advantages of decentralising field services are less obvious. People are used to coming to the '*Town Hall*' when they need help, and the administrative centre is often close to the geographical and communications centre of the town. However, in larger towns, and in some of the London boroughs, travel by public transport is so difficult and traffic congestion so bad that both on the scores of accessibility and acceptability there are great advantages to the public and the staff in doing most of the work from area offices, and several authorities are moving in this direction.

paras. 586–7

Experiments in associating area offices with other locally based services should be encouraged: health centres, primary schools, libraries, children's playgrounds, day nurseries or even coffee shops run under Civic Restaurant powers are all possibilities. Multi-purpose development of this kind is difficult at present because of the variety of statutory powers and government departments involved. Simplification of the procedures for obtaining loan sanction for multi-purpose development is, we think, right in itself and likely to be helpful to what we have in mind.

In towns, an area office might be needed for a population of about 50,000–100,000. It would be served by a team of at least 10–12 social workers. In the present state of the services, we do not think a team of less than 10–12 could be fully effective, because of the need to provide adequate supervision, and to cover absences due to sickness, leave or in-service training. The figure of 50,000–100,000 population could, we consider be served by teams of this size assuming the present numbers of health and welfare social workers, child care officers, and education welfare officers, taking account of the fact that some of them will be occupied with duties at headquarters. The figure also looks reasonable from the point of view of accessibility. Each area team would also have to include one or more home help organisers, who on the basis of national figures, would be responsible for the full-time equivalent of 63 home helps. On the basis of national averages, each area team would have contacts with between 40 and 50 general practitioners, 12 health visitors, and 18 home nurses. The numbers of schools in the area would vary considerably according to local circumstances, but would embrace a substantial number of primary schools, a minimum of say four six-form entry secondary schools and often a few nursery and special schools.

paras. 589–90

We attach great importance to the comprehensive area team approach in the search for an effective family social service and, as a concomitant, the delegation of the maximum authority for decisions to the area officers. The effectiveness of the service to the person or family seeking help is in the provision of prompt and skilled assistance. For this reason, we suggest that ideally each area office should be controlled by a senior professionally trained social worker with a grasp of administrative issues and wide powers of decision.

We must also stress that the figures in paragraph 590 are based on the *present situation* and are not optima. If the supply of social workers could be substantially increased, the areas covered by each unit could be reduced. Indeed, with the present numbers of social workers it will not be possible to provide area offices on this scale in sufficient numbers to be readily available to the whole population, so that in addition to the provision of advice and information at the area offices, the social service department may well need to establish (either itself or in conjunction with other agencies including voluntary agencies) more widely distributed advice and information centres in specific sub-areas, neighbourhoods and communities. These advice and information centres too should be located in acceptable and attractively furnished premises, readily accessible to the public generally in the neighbourhood and could also be used by teachers, doctors or nurses as points of referral. Varying local conditions must determine how and where such centres are provided as already indicated by the different forms of family advice centres developed by some children's departments following the increased emphasis placed on preventive work by the Children and Young Persons Act 1963.

The important points are that the social service department can only work effectively through area teams, drawing support from the communities they serve, with a substantial measure of delegated authority to take decisions, and able to call on the more specialised resources, advice and support of the departmental headquarters when the need arises. The effective exercise of delegated authority necessarily implies that the headquarters should produce clear statements of guidance on general policy.

paras. 592–4

THE DIRECTOR OF SOCIAL SERVICES

The principal officer of the new department will have to be an effective administrator, the leader of a group of people with widely differing backgrounds, able to take a broad and informed view of the needs the services ought to be meeting, and capable of looking outwards, well beyond the limits of his own department and authority, and well into the future. He will face problems different from those facing the heads of existing established departments. From the very beginning he will have to win the confidence of members of local authorities, officers of the new department and related departments, and services outside local government. He will have to survey the needs of the area and plan the deployment of workers to meet them, while at the same time taking care not to become remote from the problems of workers in the field and those whom the department is trying to help. If our proposals ... for a new approach to the task of providing services are accepted, he will have the major task of re-training and re-deploying the workers in the new department and persuading many of them to adopt new methods of working within a much larger structure. He will have to weld groups of workers differing widely in training, professional outlook and tradition into a team with common objectives. He must be able to command the confidence of members, to persuade them to provide more resources for the services, to maintain a reasonable balance between the demands made on behalf of different groups in the population, and at the same time to stand up for the department where necessary under pressure to lower professional standards. The work of organising the department will have to be done within a narrow time-span, and under the pressure of having to maintain the existing services at reasonable levels.

It should not be assumed either that the hardest part of the work of the head of a new social service department will be in the early stages of the department. Once the birth pangs of the department have been surmounted, there will be a danger of falling back on routine and failing to see the need to develop in new ways. The head of the social service department, and the committee he serves, must be alert to this danger, and must be prepared to make the effort to consider further adaptation and the introduction of new methods to meet developing needs in a society which is undergoing rapid economic and social change.

What has been said already will have made clear that we see very heavy responsibilities falling on the head of the new department. We think it would be wise to consider the widest possible field of recruitment for the new posts. No single profession in local government at present combines the ideal range of skills which will be required of the head of the department. The objective should be to secure that most of the heads of the social service departments are people professionally qualified in social work (including those qualified in residential care) who have received training in management and administration at appropriate points in their careers, or administrators with qualifications in social work.

paras. 618–20

In paragraphs 618–619 we have tried to describe the qualities required of the principal officer of the new department and the vital importance of the initial appointment to the development of the new service. We are all agreed that local authorities should seek the best advice available in selecting the heads of their new departments and that they should be required to consult the responsible Minister about the composition of the short list and to take account of any observations he may make before making the appointment. The majority of us do however go further and recommend that a minimum requirement should be for ministerial approval for the first appointment and for any further appointment during the first 12 months; some members of the majority wish to see this principle extended indefineitly or until the new organisation is firmly established, which could be some years ahead.

para. 636

10.8 Children and Young Persons Act, 1969

The Children and Young Persons Act, 1969, implemented the main recommendations of the 1968 White Paper, *Children in Trouble*, and sought to transfer a great deal of the responsibility for the care and treatment of delinquent children from the courts to the child care authorities. It brought the care of delinquent children closer to that of other deprived children, in the belief that delinquency more often than not had its roots in deprivation—not of course necessarily of a material kind, but including emotional and social deprivation. The Act was to come into effect in stages, and at the time of writing is not yet fully in operation. Certain provisions came into operation on 1 December 1969, and others on 1 January 1971.

When the Act is fully in operation it will no longer be necessary to bring a child in need of care or control before a court if adequate arrangements can otherwise be made for his supervision by either statutory or voluntary agencies. If a child is brought to court the court will be empowered to place the child under the supervision of a probation officer or of a local authority and this supervision may involve what the White Paper described as 'new forms of treatment, intermediate between supervision in home and committal to care'. The form which this treatment might take, e.g. attendance at a youth club, or participation in an adventure camp, is left to the discretion of the supervisor, as indeed is the question of whether any particular requirement shall be imposed on the child at all. Generally it was intended that facilities used for purposes of intermediate treatment should be of a kind not restricted to offenders, but the Act also provided for the setting up of children's regional planning committees to draw up regional plans for the provision of accommodation and facilities for the care of children, and one of the responsibilities of these committees is to make arrangements with voluntary or statutory bodies to provide facilities for intermediate treatment, and to submit these arrangements for the approval of the Secretary of State. A booklet *Intermediate Treatment* was produced by the Department of Health and Social Security at the beginning of 1972 to help the committees produce schemes of intermediate treatment.

10.9 Local Authority Social Services Act, 1970

The Local Authority Social Services Act, 1970, implemented the main recommendations of the Seebohm Report and required each major local authority to set up a social services committee, appoint a director of social services and establish a social services department. Schedule 1 of the Act specified the functions under previous legislation which were to stand referred to the social services committee but in the body of the Act certain duties under the various Health Acts were carefully specified as not to stand referred to the social services committee. Thus the boundary between health and social services was carefully delineated and resentful medical officers of health were given some protection against further violations of what territory remained to them.

S.4 of the Act permitted two or more local authorities to set up a joint social services committee, and S.6 permitted the joint appointment of a director of social services, but S.10 forbade the delegation of social service functions to district authorities and ordered county authorities to revoke any such delegation of social service functions which was already in effect. S.6 was concerned with the appointment of the director of social services and included a requirement that the Secretary of State should be consulted on the constitution of short lists for such appointments. S.7 laid down that local authorities should act in the exercise of their social services functions, 'under the general guidance of the Secretary of State', while S.11 renamed the existing Council for the Training of Health Visitors and Council for Training in Social Work as the Council for the Education and Training of Health Visitors and the Central Council for Education and Training in Social Work respectively. Many of the professions at this time had grown rather ashamed to use the term 'training', thinking that it put their members on a level with performing seals and semi-skilled operatives in industry. The remaining sections of the Act were concerned with such matters as accounting procedures, the Secretary of State's powers to make orders and regulations under the Act, and protection of the interests of existing local authority staff.

1 April 1971 was set as the date for the creation of the new social service departments and for the directors to take up their appointments. In fact not all local authorities had made their appointments by this date. Although Leicester and Coventry announced the names of their directors-designate in May 1970, and they thus had nearly a year to prepare for the appointed day, some authorities did not appoint their directors until the autumn of 1971. In some cases there were protracted negotiations with the Secretary of State over the authority's wish to appoint as director a person whom he did not regard as suitably qualified. Authorities had been told that in general directors would be expected to be qualified social workers with training in management, or administrators with substantial experience in the social services. Some authorities, however, persisted either in trying to appoint a doctor as director of social services or in attempts to combine health and social service departments under a medical head. The City of London was the only authority eventually allowed to make such a joint appointment, but a handful of other authorities were allowed to appoint as directors of social services doctors who had previously been deputy or assistant medical officers of health, provided that they gave up their health responsibilities. Some appointments went to local authority administrators without social service experience, but the great majority of appointments went to former heads of children's or welfare departments. Not only the appointments made, but the salaries attached to them, marked a significant advance for social work as a profession, and the salaries indeed were a source of envy to, for example, health service non-medical administrators. At the time the post of director of social services for Lancashire was advertised, it attracted a salary of £9,840, considerably more than that of the secretary of Manchester Regional Hospital Board, which covered a rather wider area.

The first task facing the new social service committees and their directors was to merge the former children's and welfare departments, together with those services, such as mental welfare, which were to be transferred from the health department, and to set up a new department capable of providing the 'community-based and family-oriented' services envisaged by Seebohm. They had to do this at a time when new social service responsibilities were being thrust on local authorities as a result of the Health Services and Public Health Act, 1968, and the Chronically Sick and Disabled Persons Act, 1970. Along with the task of reorganization went a responsibility to equip staff to undertake generic social work and to act as a family's point of reference for the full range of local authority social services. Many of the staff involved had worked in highly specialized fields of social work, for example in mental welfare, for many years, and it was not easy for them to adopt a more wide-ranging role. Nor were their colleagues necessarily at ease in dealing with problems that had previously been left to the specialist, with all the legislation at his fingertips.

Some directors claimed that the service to the public necessarily suffered in the early months of the new departments, although the disruption was justified by the long-term benefits it was hoped it would bring.

Select Bibliography

The student will find the following books helpful if he wishes to study in more detail the background to the documents cited in these pages.

General

Bruce, M., *The Coming of the Welfare State* (London, Batsford, 1961).

Cooper, M. H., *Social Policy. A survey of recent developments* (Oxford, Blackwell, 1973).

Family Welfare Association, *Guide to the Social Services* (London, Macdonald and Evans, 1973).

Forder, A. (ed.), *Penelope Hall's Social Services of England and Wales* (London, Routledge and Kegan Paul, 1969).

Fraser, D., *The Evolution of the British Welfare State* (London, Macmillan, 1973).

Griffith, J. A. G., *Central Departments and Local Authorities* (London, Allen and Unwin, 1966).

Sleeman, J. F., *The Welfare State. Its aims, benefits and costs* (London, Allen and Unwin, 1973).

Smith, N. J., *A Brief Guide to Social Legislation* (London, Methuen, 1972).

Part 1 The new poor law

Finer, S. E., *The Life and Times of Sir Edwin Chadwick* (London, Methuen, 1952).

Hodgkinson, Ruth G., *The Origins of the National Health Service: The Medical Services of the New Poor Law 1834–1871* (London, Wellcome Institute, 1967).

Institute of Economic Affairs, *The Long Debate on Poverty* (London, IEA, 1972).

Lewis, R. A., *Edwin Chadwick and the Public Health Movement* (London, Longman, 1952).

Roberts, D., *Victorian Origins of the British Welfare State* (New Haven, Yale, 1960).

Rose, M. E., *The English Poor Law 1780–1930* (Newton Abbot, David and Charles, 1971).

Part 2. Public health and community health services

Brockington, C. F., *Public Health in the Nineteenth Century* (London, Churchill, 1965).

Brockington, C. F., *A Short History of Public Health* (London, Churchill, 1966).

Clark, G. Kitson, *The Making of Victorian England* (London, Methuen, 1970).
Essex-Cater, A. J., *A Synopsis of Public Health and Social Medicine* (Bristol, Wright, 1967).
Finer, S. E., *The Life and Times of Sir Edwin Chadwick* (London, Methuen, 1952).
Frazer, W. M., *A History of English Public Health* (London, Baillière, Tindall and Cox, 1950).
Hodgkinson, Ruth G., *The Origins of the National Health Service: The Medical Services of the New Poor Law 1834–1871* (London, Wellcome Institute, 1967).
Lambert, R., *Sir John Simon 1816–1904* (London, MacGibbon and Kee, 1963).
Lewis, R. A., *Edwin Chadwick and the Public Health Movement* (London, Longman, 1952).
Roberts, D., *Victorian Origins of the British Welfare State* (New Haven, Yale, 1960).

Part 3 Social security

Braithwaite, W. J., *Lloyd George's Ambulance Wagon* (London, Methuen, 1957).
George, V., *Social Security: Beveridge and After* (London, Routledge and Kegan Paul, 1968).
Gilbert, B. B., *The Evolution of National Insurance in Great Britain* (London, Michael Joseph, 1966).
Gilbert, B. B., *British Social Policy 1914–1939* (London, Batsford, 1970).

Part 4 Provision and organization of health services

Abel-Smith, B., *The Hospitals 1800–1948* (London, Heinemann, 1964).
Brown, R. G. S., *The Changing National Health Service* (London, Routledge and Kegan Paul, 1973).
Eckstein, H., *The English Health Service: Its Origins, Structure and Achievements* (Cambridge, Mass., Harvard University Press, 1959).
Jewkes, J., and Jewkes, Sylvia, *The Genesis of the British National Health Service* (Oxford, Blackwell, 1961).
Lindsey, A., *Socialized Medicine in England and Wales* (University of North Carolina Press, 1962).
Willcocks, A. J., *The Creation of the National Health Service* (London, Routledge and Kegan Paul, 1967).

Part 5 Internal administration of hospitals under the National Health Service

Clegg, H. A., and Chester, T. E., *Wage Policy and the Health Service* (Oxford, Blackwell, 1957).
Haywood, S. C., *Managing the Health Service* (London, Allen and Unwin, 1974).
Lindsey, A., *Socialized Medicine in England and Wales* (University of North Carolina Press, 1962).
Milne, J. F., and Chaplin, N. W., *Modern Hospital Management* (London, Institute of Hospital Administrators, 1969).

Part 6 The medical and dental professions

Butler, J. R., in collaboration with J. M. Bevan and R. C. Taylor, *Family Doctors and Public Policy: A study of manpower distribution* (London, Routledge and Kegan Paul, 1973).

Dopson, L., *The Changing Scene in General Practice* (London, Johnson, 1971).

Forsyth, G., *Doctors and State Medicine* (London, Pitman Medical, 1966).

Klein, R., *Complaints Against Doctors. A study in professional accountability* (London, Charles Knight, 1973).

Little, E. M., *History of the British Medical Association 1832–1932* (London, British Medical Association, 1932).

Office of Health Economics, *The Dental Service* (London, OHE, 1969).

Stevens, Rosemary, *Medical Practice in Modern England* (New Haven, Yale, 1966).

Vaughan, P., *Doctors' Commons: A Short History of the British Medical Association* (London, Heinemann, 1959).

Part 7 The nursing and midwifery professions

Abel-Smith, B., *A History of the Nursing Profession* (London, Heinemann, 1961).

Bendall, Eve R. D., and Raybould, Elizabeth, *A History of the General Nursing Council for England and Wales 1919–1969* (London, Lewis, 1969).

Brown, R. G. S., and Stones, R. W. H., *The Male Nurse* (London, Bell, 1974).

Woodham-Smith, Cecil, *Florence Nightingale 1820–1910* (London, Constable, 1950).

Part 8 The paramedical professions

Martin, Margaret, *Colleagues or Competitors* (London, Bell, 1969).

Part 9 Mental disorder

Jones, Kathleen, *A History of the Mental Health Services* (London, Routledge and Kegan Paul, 1972).

Scheff, T. J., *Being Mentally Ill: A Sociological Theory* (London, Weidenfeld and Nicolson, 1966).

Part 10 Social work and family welfare

Halmos, P., *The Faith of the Counsellors* (London, Constable, 1965).

Heywood, Jean S., *Children in Care* (2nd ed. London, Routledge and Kegan Paul, 1965).

Rooff, Madeline, *A Hundred Years of Family Welfare* (London, Michael Joseph, 1972).

Stroud, J., *An Introduction to the Child Care Service* (London, Longman, 1965).

Wootton, Barbara, *Social Science and Social Pathology* (London, Allen and Unwin, 1959).

Index

The main topics covered in each section are listed in the Contents. Names of persons have not been indexed if they appear only in the lists of members of working parties, committees, etc.